ESSENTIALS OF
FORENSIC MEDICINE

Dr. Greeshma Sharma

ALLIED
HEALTH
PRESS

Essentials of Forensic Medicine

Author: **Dr. Greeshma Sharma**

Allied Health Press
4164 Lakeshore Road
Burlington ON L7L 1A4
Canada
www.alliedhealthpress.com
Email: orders@arclereducation.com

ISBN: 978-1-77956-218-0

ABOUT THE AUTHOR

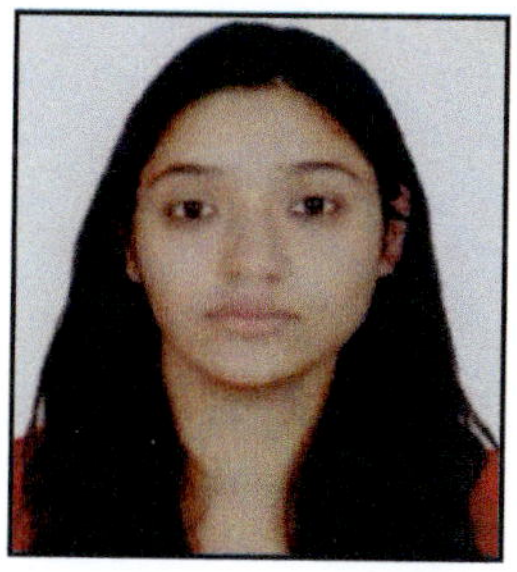

Dr. Greeshma Sharma, a post doctoral Project Scientist, in one of the most reputed research institutes of India. She holds a Ph.D in the field of Maternal and Child health care, with specialization in Neonatalogy, and Molecular Biology. UGC qualified in Forensic Science, with an expertise in Forensic Biotechnology. She has received an international scholarship (Harold Gunson fellowship, International Society of Blood Transfusion) and holds 9+ years of Research experience, which includes reviewing articles, writing research articles as well as proposal for extramural funding. Serving in the field of freelance writing ad research since 2020.

Word Roots, Prefixes, and Suffixes by Chapter

Chapter 1 Basics of Forensic Medicine and Pathology

Forens: pertaining to the law or courts
Path: disease
Necr: dead, death
Tox: poison
Hemo: blood
Cardio: heart
Osteo: bone
Psycho: mind

Chapter 2 The Role of Pharmacogenetics in Forensic Science

pharmaco-: drug, medicine
geno-: gene, genetic
poly-: many
allo-: other, different
anti-: against
auto-: self
bio-: life, living
cyto-: cell

Chapter 3 Forensic Psychiatry

Psycho- (mind, mental)
Neuro- (nerve, nervous system)
Forens- (pertaining to courts or legal)
Patho- (disease)
An- / A- (without, lack of)
Sub- (under, below)

Chapter 4 Forensic Histopathology

Path- (disease)
Necro- (death)
Cyto- (cell)
Micro- (small)
Auto- (self)
Bio- (life)

Chapter 5 Care of Detainees

Anti- (against)
-care (protection, attention)
-pathy (disease, suffering)
-ist (one who specializes)
-ic (pertaining to)
-al (pertaining to)

Chapter 6 Forensic Autopsy

Neo-: new (as in neoplasm)
-opsy: view or examine
Necro-: dead, death
Morto-: death
Histo-: tissue
-logy: study of
-scopy: visual examination
-tomy: cutting, incision

Chapter 7 Virtual Autopsy

ops (view, sight)
auto (self)
Prefixes:
auto- (self)
Suffixes:
-psy (to see, to examine)

Chapter 8 Sexual Assault: Forensic Examination

Non- (as in non-consensual)
Un- (as in unwanted)
-ation (as in violation)
-ment (as in harassment)

Chapter 9 Infectious Diseases: The Role of the Forensic Physician

-itis (inflammation)
-osis (condition)
-emia (blood condition)
-pathy (disease)
-logy (study of)

Table of Contents

LIST OF FIGURES

LIST OF TABLES

PREFACE

Forensic medicine, also known as legal medicine, is the application of medical knowledge to legal issues. This specialized field bridges the gap between the medical and legal worlds, addressing a wide range of problems that require both legal and medical expertise. The origins of both law and medicine are ancient, shrouded in the early history of human civilization, dating back to the beginnings of family and tribal life. Human history, as recorded, extends back approximately 6,000 years, and throughout this time, various civilizations have contributed to the development of forensic medicine.

In the ancient civilizations of Sumeria, Babylon, and Egypt, early forms of forensic medicine began to take shape. Imhotep, an Egyptian polymath, is often regarded as the first true medicolegal expert. His contributions laid the foundation for the integration of medical knowledge with legal principles. In ancient Greece, Hippocrates, often referred to as the "Father of Medicine," made significant contributions to the field, emphasizing the importance of systematic observation and documentation. Similarly, Galen, a prominent Roman physician, advanced medical knowledge and practices that would later influence forensic medicine.

The progress of forensic medicine stalled during the Dark Ages, a period spanning approximately a 1,000 years, during which there was little advancement in science and medicine. However, the Renaissance era, beginning in the late 15th century, marked a resurgence of interest and innovation in many fields, including medicine. During the 17th, 18th, and 19th centuries, forensic medicine experienced significant growth and development, driven by the broader advancements in medical science and the increasing complexity of legal systems.

In the twentieth century, forensic medicine became a recognized and vital field worldwide. The scope of forensic medicine expanded to include various professionals, each contributing their expertise to the investigation of crimes and legal issues. Physicians, coroners, pathologists, medical specialists, and forensic laboratory technicians collaborate to investigate crimes against individuals, determine causes of death, and solve complex issues such as identification, untoward deaths, and apparent drownings. This collaborative approach ensures that forensic medicine continues to play a crucial role in the intersection of law and medicine, providing essential insights and solutions to legal problems.

The purpose of this book, titled "*Essentials of Forensic Medicine*," extends beyond exploring the traditional fields of forensic science, which support the application of criminal law. These traditional areas include forensic pathology, forensic anthropology, forensic hemogenetics, forensic toxicology, and forensic entomology, all of which are examined in their most significant and contemporary scientific contexts. In addition to these established fields, the book aims to cover the most recent and emerging areas of medico-legal disciplines. This involves evaluating injuries and determining compensation in legal disputes. Another critical area is the evaluation of medical liability, where forensic medicine provides insights into cases of alleged medical malpractice. The book also covers clinical forensic medicine, which involves using forensic expertise to support clinical practices, ensuring the accuracy and reliability of medical evaluations in legal contexts.

Moreover, the book addresses the analysis and evaluation of healthcare safety, a vital aspect of forensic medicine aimed at improving patient care and preventing medical errors. Environmental protection is another significant area, where forensic medicine contributes to identifying and mitigating health risks associated with environmental hazards.

The book also explores the broader role of forensic medicine in public health, particularly in protecting individual rights and providing social assistance in states of need. This includes collaboration with various sectors to ensure the well-being and safety of communities, emphasizing the multifaceted nature of forensic medicine in contemporary society. Through these comprehensive studies, the book aims to provide a thorough understanding of both the traditional and modern applications of forensic medicine, highlighting its evolving role in supporting justice and public health.

Chapter 1

BASICS OF FORENSIC MEDICINE AND PATHOLOGY

Contents

Introduction

The aim of this chapter is to explain what legal medicine is (from its background to the present), and forensic pathology in particular—what its objectives are, what forensic doctors do, and when, why, how, and for whom.

Orientation and Directional Terms

Term	Definition	Illustration
Forensic Medicine	A branch of medicine that applies medical knowledge to legal questions and issues, often involving the investigation of injuries and deaths.	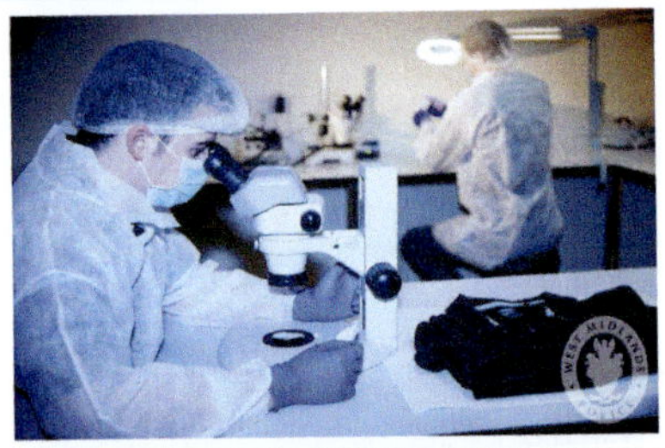
Forensic Pathology	A specialized area within forensic medicine focused on determining the cause of death by examining deceased bodies and analyzing autopsy results.	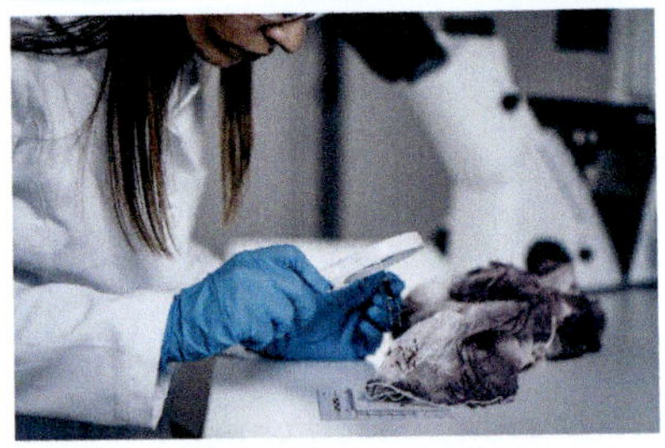
Forensic Anthropology	The study of human skeletal remains to determine the identity, age, sex, ancestry, and other characteristics of deceased individuals in a legal context.	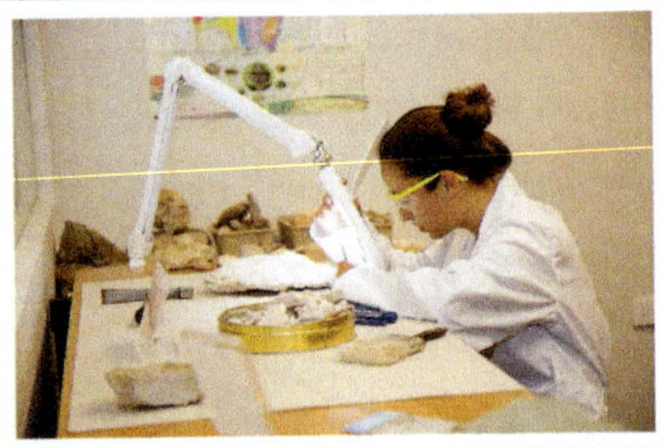
Toxicology	The science of studying the effects, detection, and treatment of poisons and toxins, often used to understand poisoning cases or substance-related harm.	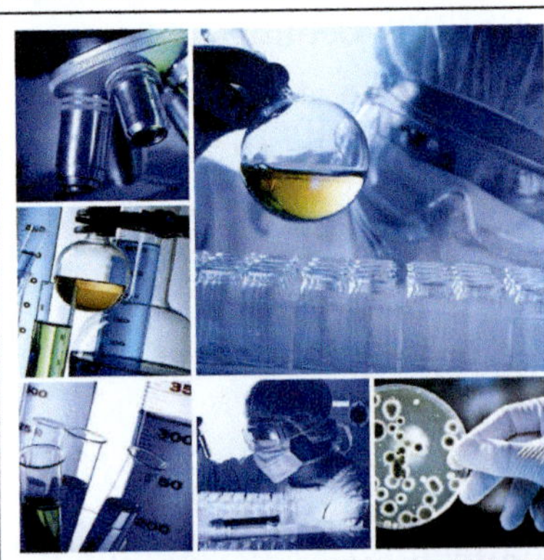
Histology	The study of the microscopic structure of tissues and organs, crucial for diagnosing diseases and understanding pathological changes at a cellular level.	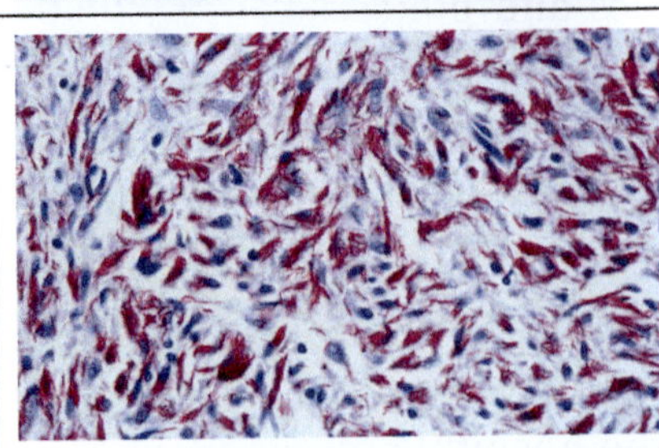

1.1. Forensic Medicine

In today's world, forensic medicine is a vast medical field that encompasses a multitude of subspecialties. On the other hand, when people talk about it or think about it, they immediately think of death, autopsies, and other issues that are associated with it. However, this is only a portion of legal medicine, as new methods and subspecialties are evolving because of developments in medical sciences and changes in sociopolitical conditions all over the world. It is possible that the most prominent examples of these "new sciences" are the fields of forensic anthropology and clinical forensic healthcare.

An introductory section to both forensic pathology and forensic anthropology seems to be an essential component of a book that is intended to serve as a bridge between two sciences that are complementary to one another (forensic pathology and forensic anthropology) for anthropologists, medical doctors, and other professions affiliated with the field. Can you explain what forensic medicine is, beginning with its history and continuing up to the present day, and what exactly is forensic pathology? What are the goals that it serves? What exactly do forensic physicians do? Who, when, why, and how, and for what purpose? In what ways are the challenges present, and what are the anticipated outcomes for the future? This chapter tries to provide answers to all these questions, which are questions that a person who is a medical professional might ask.

The origin of forensic medicine is still unknown, but it is believed to have originated in the distant past when the principles of law and justice collided with those of the medical sciences. Perhaps the Code of Hammurabi (1792–1750 BCE), which imposed punishments for mistakes made in medical and surgical procedures, was the first document to do so. Persia was also subject to the same kind of cruel and unusual punishment. In later times, the Visigoths enacted laws that punished homicide, infanticide, and poisoning as well as other violent crimes.

One way to think of forensic medicine is as a medical trunk that serves the administration of justice. There are many subspecialties within this field. It is likely that forensic pathology is the most representative of all of them. In many Latin American countries, forensic pathology is referred to as tanathology, which is derived from the Greek word Thanatos, which means "death's god." Definitions of forensic pathology are frequently so broad that they would be more appropriate in the field of forensic medicine rather than in this subfield. As far as Di Maio is concerned, it is "a branch of medicine that applies the principles and knowledge of the medical sciences in the field of law." An even larger conception of forensic pathology considers it the study of diseases and injuries of the community, because it involves the knowledge of diagnosis and treatment in every medical specialty, but also requires information in many nonmedical areas, such as chemistry, physics, criminalistics and police sciences, motor vehicle and highway conception, politics, sociology, and even the way of life of a society. According to Williams et al., forensic pathology is a specialized branch of pathology (pathology is the study of disease and tissue injury through scientific methods) that relates within a legal framework to the effects of trauma, poisoning, occupational hazards, and natural disease. This definition brings forensic pathology closer to its objectives and limits.

Forensic dissections of bodies were initiated in the 13th century at the University of Bologna in Italy by Saliceto, a surgeon and anatomy teacher. Interestingly, these forensic dissections preceded the hospital autopsies that began in the late 19th century with Rokitansky, Virchow, and the emergence of the understanding of disease pathogenesis and cellular pathology. However, certain authors attribute the title of the father of legal medicine to the French surgeon Ambrosio Paré, who initiated a genuine scientific era in France in 1575.

Zacchia, the physician of the Pope, is credited with the authorship of the first medicolegal textbook, which was written in 1,601 and taught in Italy. The development of forensic sciences was significantly influenced by this event, as well as by the European codes of the 16th century, such as the Bamberg Code in 1,507 and the Caroline Code in 1,532. These codes mandated that courts must consult specialized doctors to provide expert clarification on forensic matters.

However, the 19th century served as a significant period for the establishment of modern legal medicine, which was formally recognized in multiple countries around the same time. Specifically, it was established in Austria in 1855, Hungary in 1872, Brazil in 1886, Great Britain in 1887, and Portugal in 1889 (when legal medicine was first acknowledged as being legally organized). The 21st century witnessed a remarkable era of advancement in forensic medicine, characterized by rapid yet well-founded growth, particularly in France, Italy, and Germany. In addition, it is worth noting that forensic matters have always been handled with great care in German countries. This is evident from the fact that forensic medicine was taught in some universities as early as 1,720. The advancement of forensic pathology in different countries was influenced by their respective legal systems and sociopolitical conditions.

In the late 19th century, additional scientific fields like toxicology and histology were combined with forensic pathology, leading to the establishment of legal medicine institutes resembling the modern-day medico-legal units. These institutes encompass various areas of expertise related to the administration of justice.

Subsequently, during the latter half of the 20th century, a novel issue about the intersection of medicine and law emerged in Europe and any other regions where roads and automobiles were present. The occurrence of traffic accidents and the subsequent need for legal actions regarding the injuries sustained by the victims has given rise to a specialized field known as clinical forensic medicine, which focuses on the medical examination and assessment of living individuals. The origins of the event can be traced back to Belgium and France, specifically involving individuals named Derobert, Roche, Muller, and Rousseau. Following Deliberation 75 of the Committee of Ministers of the Council of Europe, an "expertise-type" was established to conduct a comprehensive assessment of the consequences arising from bodily injuries caused by accidents to an individual. This process was essential for insurance companies to provide financial compensation for injuries. The ideas, introduced in Portugal by Oliveira Sá, a passionate advocate of this emerging field, were further disseminated to Spain through his strong connections with forensic physicians in the neighboring country. This led to significant advancements, although the practice remained predominantly within private medical settings rather than being centralized in medicolegal institutions. The rapid rise in popularity of this emerging forensic field can be attributed to the escalating global incidence of traffic accidents. After the Iberian Peninsula was successfully conquered, its influence expanded to encompass South and Latin America. The English-speaking nations were the most recent to cultivate this emerging field; only in the past few years has the prevalence of clinical forensic medicine skyrocketed in the United States and the United Kingdom. This field has provided forensic practitioners with the opportunity to achieve economic autonomy, although pathologists have not experienced the same. Adjacent to the field of victimology, this emerging domain encompasses all forms of harm inflicted upon a person, including acts of aggression, sexual assault, determination of age, and, naturally, traffic accidents. According to E. Baccino, forensic doctors should be referred to as "violence medicine doctors" because violence, regardless of its lethality, is the shared element between perpetrators and victims. Violence typically arises from complex interactions between the perpetrator and the victim, and the assessment of injuries is comparable in both living and deceased individuals.

Considering these facts, certain experts (E. Baccino, personal communication) erroneously concluded, contrary to the authors' viewpoint, that forensic medicine is increasingly leaning towards clinical aspects rather than pathological ones.

1.2. Autopsies

1.2.1. Types of Autopsy: Clinical and Forensic

There are two main types of autopsies: clinical or academic autopsies conducted in hospitals, and forensic autopsies performed in medico-legal settings. The primary objective of a clinical autopsy is to ascertain, elucidate, or validate diagnoses that were previously unidentified or insufficiently comprehensible during a patient's hospitalization or stay in a healthcare facility. The forensic autopsy is conducted under the oversight of a legal authority, such as a prosecutor, procurator fiscal, magistrate, judge, coroner, medical examiner, or police. The forensic or medicolegal autopsy primarily investigates deaths resulting from violence, such as accidents, suicides, and homicides. However, it also includes a significant percentage (35–40% based on Portuguese experience) of natural deaths that would typically be examined through a clinical autopsy. Forensic autopsies are necessary to investigate deaths that are suspicious, sudden, unattended by medical professionals, or connected to surgical or anesthetic procedures, to obtain clarification (Figure 1.1).

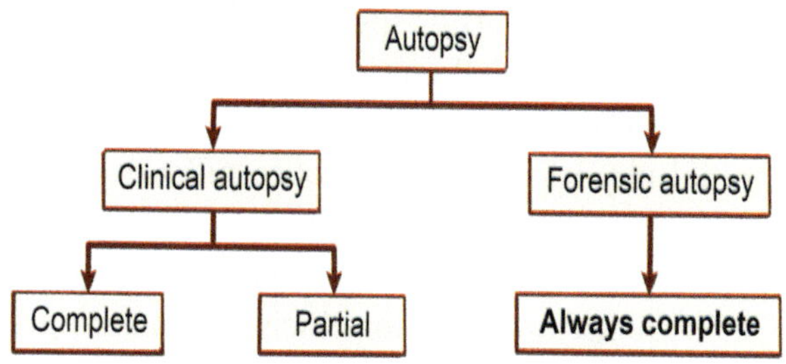

Figure 1.1. *Categorization of autopsy.*

Typically, in most jurisdictions, it is not required to obtain the consent of relatives to conduct an autopsy. Subsequent obstruction of justice is thus prevented. Forensic autopsies in certain areas are classified into two categories: criminal deaths, which include suspicious deaths, murders, homicidal suffocation or smothering, and infanticide; and noncriminal deaths, which encompass suicides, natural deaths, accidents, and so on.

1.2.2. Objectives of a Forensic Autopsy

In recent decades, the primary objective of a forensic autopsy has been to determine the cause and manner of death. While not a new development, another significant objective has recently arisen from ethnic conflicts and genocide: the identification of the victim(s). Hence, the primary goals of a medico-legal autopsy are to determine the cause of death and establish the identity of the deceased. When conducting a standard forensic necropsy on a recognized cadaver, a classification of objectives can be established. Firstly, it is essential to diagnose the cause of death and differentiate it as either natural or violent. This can often be accomplished during the autopsy by relying solely on macroscopic examination. If the case involves a death caused by violence, there are three potential scenarios: traumatic injuries, asphyxia, or intoxication. Subsequently, it is necessary to categorize traumatic wounds based on the specific instrument or weapon that caused them, namely blunt, incised and perforating, or a combination of both. One of the initial inquiries made by police officers at the start of a crime investigation is to ascertain the specific weapon employed, which aids in strategizing the subsequent investigation. Incised wounds are caused by sharp tools while perforating injuries can be caused by a variety of weapons, ranging from pointed, sharp tools to firearms. It is important to acknowledge that the naming of these wounds may not be accurate in every country or language, which often leads to further challenges in understanding an autopsy report.

The conclusive phase of a postmortem examination involving a violent death entails determining the manner of death: homicide, suicide, accident, or undetermined. Several cases, such as intoxications and natural deaths, are not determined during the necropsy procedure and require additional investigation, including supplementary examinations.

In addition to its primary purpose, an autopsy serves several supplementary objectives, including the following:

- To document (diagnose, describe, and measure both external and internal injuries.
- To detect external and internal abnormalities, malformations, and diseases.
- To attribute the death to a particular event—the nexus of causality, a paramount issue in legal medicine.
- To determine other causes that might have contributed to death.
- To collect samples for histological, toxicological, microbiological, orotherancil-laryanalysis.
- To determine the time of death, when necessary and possible.
- To keep relevant organs, tissues, or samples as evidence.
- To provide a full written report of the necropsy findings, giving a serious and competent medicolegal interpretation of the findings.
- To return the body to the family as well presented as possible.

During specific autopsy distinct objectives of a particular expertise can be identified. When a firearm is employed, it is crucial to assess the shot's range, and the trajectory of the bullet, and discern whether the wound is an entry or exit point. Additionally, it is important to ascertain the relative positions of the assailant and the victim.

When investigating delayed deaths, it is important to establish the causal relationship between the initial traumatic event (and resulting injuries) and the presumed "natural cause" of death that is determined. One common error is when general physicians incorrectly attribute "pulmonary embolism" as the natural cause of death for traffic accident victims who suffered traumatic injuries and died in the hospital. This complication is clearly connected to the initial traumatic wounds.

1.2.3. Cause, Manner, and Mechanism of Death

A significant number of individuals, including certain experts in the field, encounter challenges when it comes to differentiating between the cause, manner, and mechanism of death. Cause of death refers to any injury or disease that produces a pathological change in the body resulting in the person's demise. Examples include esophageal carcinoma, myocardial infarction, blunt head trauma, or a thoracic gunshot wound.

The mechanism of death refers to the pathological changes that occur as a result of the cause of death, such as bleeding, infection, or a fatal irregular heartbeat. A potential scenario is that various causes of death may share a common mechanism of demise. For instance, a hemorrhage could occur as a consequence of blunt trauma, stabbing, or lung carcinoma. Conversely, the cause of death can also lead to various mechanisms of death. For instance, a gunshot wound can result in hemorrhage, but if the victim had survived, an infectious complication would be the mechanism.

The term "manner of death," also referred to as "medicolegal etiology" in Latin countries, is used to differentiate between accident, suicide, homicide, or an undetermined cause in cases of violent deaths. It is considered an additional objective of the autopsy. Based on the aforementioned line of thinking, a manner of death can arise from various causes and mechanisms. An illustrative instance is that of a gunshot injury, which can be categorized into four manners of death: homicide (where the victim was shot by someone else), suicide (where the victim shot themselves), accident (where the victim unintentionally shot themselves), and undetermined (where there are no witnesses to the events and the autopsy does not provide clarity on the manner of death). The cause of death may have been hypovolemic shock resulting from hemorrhage. Alternatively, if the person survived, they may have experienced a thromboembolic or infectious complication, such as bronchopneumonia or peritonitis.

Typically, this involves laboratory analysis and relies on information about the circumstances of death, which can be obtained from the police's scene report or the forensic pathologist who recovered the body. However, it can be challenging to reconcile the pathologist's statement with the crime scene report or the police account of the case. In addition, families rarely acknowledge suicide as the cause of death. Hence, it is imperative for the pathologist to meticulously examine each case, possess comprehensive knowledge about the circumstances surrounding the victim, and meticulously record the investigation to arrive at a conclusive judgment.

In cadavers that are not fresh, specifically in various stages of decomposition (more closely related to the subject of this book), the pathologist and forensic anthropologist may occasionally be unable to determine the manner of death, particularly in bodies that have become skeletonized. These are the unresolved cases.

At times, a death can be classified without establishing the specific cause of death. A nurse committed suicide by injecting herself with an anesthetic product, and laboratory analysis did not detect the presence of the toxin. The macroscopic and histological findings were also non-specific. Nevertheless, the situation was undeniably clear – the presence of a syringe in the arm, an empty bottle in the wastebasket, and a farewell letter – leading to the conclusion that it was a case of suicide.

Within the framework of this book, a young pregnant girl was killed by her boyfriend, who confessed to the crime. She was buried and later dug up 2.5 months later. The autopsy was conducted by a team of experts from different fields, but due to the advanced decomposition of the body, it was not possible to determine the cause of death. The organs in the chest were completely decayed, and the larynx apparatus and hyoid bone were not found. However, considering the circumstances and the extensive data collected by the police, it strongly suggests that the death was most likely a result of intentional homicide.

1.3 DNA Profiling

DNA profiling, also known as DNA fingerprinting or genetic fingerprinting, has revolutionized forensic science since its inception in the mid-1980s. This technique involves the analysis of the unique genetic makeup of individuals to identify them. Given the polymorphic nature of DNA, where no two individuals (except identical twins) have the same genetic sequence, DNA profiling has become an indispensable tool in criminal investigations, paternity testing, and identifying disaster victims.

At the core of DNA profiling is the understanding that the human genome is highly variable. While the vast majority of human DNA is identical from one person to the next, certain regions, known as variable number tandem repeats (VNTRs) and short tandem repeats (STRs), exhibit significant variability. VNTRs are longer sequences that repeat a variable number of times, whereas STRs are shorter sequences that repeat. These regions are highly polymorphic, making them ideal for distinguishing between individuals. DNA profiling exploits these variations by comparing specific loci within the genome. Forensic scientists typically analyze 13-20 STR loci, as the probability of two individuals having the same STR profile across these loci is astronomically low. This statistical improbability is what makes DNA profiling a powerful tool in forensic science.

1.3.1 Methodologies of DNA Profiling

The process of DNA profiling involves several key steps: sample collection, DNA extraction, DNA quantitation, PCR amplification, and analysis.

1.3.1.1 Sample Collection

The first step in DNA profiling is collecting a biological sample that contains DNA. This can be anything from blood, saliva, and hair, to skin cells and semen. Proper collection and preservation of samples are crucial to avoid contamination and degradation, which can compromise the integrity of the DNA evidence.

1.3.1.2 DNA Extraction

Once a sample is collected, DNA must be extracted. This involves breaking open the cells to release DNA and then purifying it from other cellular components. Several methods exist for DNA extraction, including organic extraction, Chelex extraction, and silica-based methods. The choice of method often depends on the type of sample and the quality of DNA required.

1.3.1.3 DNA Quantitation

After extraction, the amount of DNA is quantified to ensure there is sufficient material for analysis. This step is critical because too little DNA may not yield a usable profile, while too much can lead to amplification artifacts. Quantitation is usually performed using techniques such as spectrophotometry, fluorometry, or more commonly, quantitative PCR (qPCR).

1.3.1.4 PCR Amplification

The next step is amplifying the DNA regions of interest using polymerase chain reaction (PCR). PCR is a technique that allows for the selective amplification of specific DNA sequences, enabling the creation of millions of copies from a small initial amount. This step focuses on amplifying STR loci, as they are the most informative for forensic analysis. The amplified products are then labeled with fluorescent tags to facilitate detection and analysis.

1.3.1.5 Analysis

The final step in DNA profiling is analyzing the amplified DNA. This is typically done using capillary electrophoresis, which separates DNA fragments based on size and charge. The fluorescent tags attached during PCR allow for the visualization of these fragments, producing a DNA profile. This profile is then compared to profiles from known individuals or entered into DNA databases to search for matches.

1.3.2 Applications of DNA Profiling in Forensic Science

DNA profiling has a wide range of applications in forensic science, including criminal investigations, paternity testing, disaster victim identification, and exoneration of the wrongfully convicted.

1.3.2.1 Criminal Investigations

In criminal investigations, DNA profiling is used to link suspects to crime scenes or exclude individuals from suspicion. Biological evidence left at a crime scene, such as blood or semen, can be analyzed and compared to DNA samples from suspects. A match can provide compelling evidence of a suspect's presence at the crime scene, while a non-match can exonerate them.

1.3.2.2 Paternity Testing

DNA profiling is also widely used in paternity and maternity testing. By comparing the DNA profiles of a child and the alleged parents, scientists can determine with high accuracy whether a biological relationship exists. This application is critical in legal cases involving child support, inheritance disputes, and immigration.

1.3.2.3 Disaster Victim Identification

In mass disaster scenarios, DNA profiling is invaluable for identifying victims. When traditional identification methods such as visual recognition or dental records are not possible, DNA can be used to match remains with DNA samples from personal items or relatives. This was notably used in the aftermath of the 9/11 attacks and the 2004 Indian Ocean tsunami.

1.3.2.4 Exoneration of the Wrongfully Convicted

One of the most profound impacts of DNA profiling has been its role in exonerating individuals wrongfully convicted of crimes. Organizations like the Innocence Project have used DNA evidence to overturn wrongful convictions, highlighting the importance of accurate and reliable forensic analysis.

1.3.3 Ethical Considerations

Despite its many benefits, DNA profiling raises several ethical and legal issues. These include concerns about privacy, the potential for misuse, and the accuracy and reliability of DNA evidence.

1.3.3.1 Privacy Concerns

The collection and storage of DNA profiles raise significant privacy issues. DNA contains sensitive information about an individual's genetic makeup, health, and ancestry. The potential for misuse of this information by law enforcement, employers, or insurers is a significant concern. Ensuring that DNA databases are secure and that access is strictly controlled is essential to protect individuals' privacy rights.

1.3.3.2 Potential for Misuse

There is also the potential for misuse of DNA profiling. For instance, DNA evidence can be planted at a crime scene to falsely implicate someone. Moreover, the expansion of DNA databases to include individuals not convicted of crimes, such as arrestees or even the general population, raises ethical questions about the balance between public safety and individual rights.

1.3.3.3 Accuracy and Reliability

While DNA profiling is highly accurate, it is not infallible. Issues such as contamination, degradation, and human error can affect the reliability of DNA evidence. Furthermore, the interpretation of mixed DNA samples, where biological material from multiple individuals is present, can be complex and contentious. Ensuring that forensic laboratories adhere to stringent standards and that analysts are properly trained is crucial to maintaining the integrity of DNA evidence.

DNA profiling has transformed forensic science, providing a powerful tool for identifying individuals with unprecedented accuracy. Its applications in criminal investigations, paternity testing, disaster victim identification, and exoneration of the wrongfully convicted have had profound societal impacts. However, the use of DNA profiling must be carefully regulated to address ethical concerns and ensure the accuracy and reliability of forensic analysis. As technology advances, the capabilities of DNA profiling will continue to expand, further solidifying its role as a cornerstone of forensic science.

1.4 Forensic Serology and Biology

Forensic serology and biology play pivotal roles in modern criminal investigations, helping to solve crimes through the analysis of biological evidence. These disciplines encompass a range of scientific techniques and methodologies used to identify and analyze bodily fluids, tissues, and other biological materials found at crime scenes. Through the application of serological and biological principles, forensic scientists can provide crucial information about the events that occurred during the commission of a crime and help identify perpetrators.

1.4.1 Historical Background

The use of biological evidence in criminal investigations dates back centuries, but it was not until the late 19th and early 20th centuries that forensic serology began to take shape as a formal scientific discipline. Early pioneers, such as Paul Uhlenhuth and Karl Landsteiner, made significant contributions to the field. Uhlenhuth developed the precipitin test in 1901, which allowed for the differentiation of human and animal blood. Landsteiner's discovery of blood groups in 1900 laid the foundation for modern blood typing, a crucial tool in forensic serology.

The advent of DNA profiling in the 1980s revolutionized forensic biology. British geneticist Alec Jeffreys developed the technique of DNA fingerprinting, which allowed for the unique identification of individuals based on their genetic makeup. This breakthrough marked a significant leap forward in the ability to link biological evidence to specific individuals with a high degree of accuracy.

1.4.2 Forensic Serology

Forensic serology involves the identification and characterization of various bodily fluids, including blood, semen, saliva, and urine. These fluids can provide valuable information about the nature and circumstances of a crime. The following are some key techniques and tests used in forensic serology:

- **Blood Typing**: Blood typing involves determining the ABO and Rh blood groups of a sample. This can help narrow down potential suspects or identify victims. Blood typing is based on the presence of specific antigens on the surface of red blood cells.
- **Presumptive Tests for Blood**: Presumptive tests are used to indicate the possible presence of blood at a crime scene. Common tests include the Kastle-Meyer test, which uses phenolphthalein to detect hemoglobin, and the luminol test, which produces a luminescent reaction in the presence of blood.
- **Confirmatory Tests for Blood**: Confirmatory tests, such as the Takayama and Teichmann tests, are used to definitively confirm the presence of blood. These tests rely on the formation of characteristic crystals when blood is present.
- **Semen Detection**: Semen can be detected using presumptive tests like the acid phosphatase test and confirmatory tests such as the presence of spermatozoa under a microscope. Prostate-specific antigen (PSA) testing is also used to confirm the presence of semen.
- **Saliva Detection**: Saliva can be identified through the presence of amylase, an enzyme found in high concentrations in saliva. The Phadebas test and starch-iodine test are commonly used for this purpose.
- **Urine Detection**: Urine can be identified through the presence of urea and creatinine. Tests like the DMAC (p-dimethylaminocinnamaldehyde) test are used to detect these compounds.

1.4.3 Forensic Biology

Forensic biology encompasses a broader range of biological analyses, including DNA profiling, hair and fiber analysis, and the examination of other biological materials. DNA profiling, in particular, has become the cornerstone of modern forensic biology due to its ability to provide highly specific and reliable results.

- **DNA Profiling**: DNA profiling involves the extraction, amplification, and analysis of DNA from biological samples. The process typically includes the following steps:
  - **DNA Extraction**: DNA is extracted from cells using various methods, such as organic extraction, Chelex extraction, or silica-based extraction.
  - **DNA Amplification**: Polymerase chain reaction (PCR) is used to amplify specific regions of the DNA, making it possible to generate a profile from even small or degraded samples.
  - **DNA Analysis**: Short tandem repeats (STRs) are the most commonly analyzed regions of DNA in forensic biology. STRs are highly variable regions that differ between individuals, making them ideal for identification purposes.

Capillary electrophoresis is used to separate and analyze the amplified STRs, generating a DNA profile.

- **Mitochondrial DNA Analysis**: Mitochondrial DNA (mtDNA) analysis is used in cases where nuclear DNA is degraded or insufficient. mtDNA is inherited maternally and can be used to trace maternal lineage. It is particularly useful in cases involving old or degraded samples, such as skeletal remains.
- **Y-STR Analysis**: Y-STR analysis focuses on the Y chromosome, which is passed from father to son. This type of analysis is valuable in cases involving male-specific biological evidence or in situations where multiple male contributors are present.
- **Hair and Fiber Analysis**: Hair and fiber analysis can provide valuable information about the individuals involved in a crime. Microscopic examination of hair can reveal characteristics such as color, texture, and the presence of artificial treatments. DNA can also be extracted from the root of a hair. Fiber analysis involves the examination of textile fibers to determine their type, origin, and possible sources.
- **Touch DNA**: Touch DNA refers to DNA obtained from skin cells left behind when a person touches an object. This type of evidence can be challenging to analyze due to the small quantity of DNA present, but advancements in DNA extraction and amplification techniques have made it increasingly valuable in forensic investigations.

1.4.4 The Role of Forensic Serology and Biology in Criminal Investigations

Forensic serology and biology are integral to the investigative process, providing critical evidence that can link suspects to crime scenes, victims, or weapons. The following are key roles that these disciplines play in criminal investigations:

- **Identification of Suspects**: Biological evidence can be used to identify suspects through DNA profiling. The comparison of DNA profiles obtained from crime scene evidence with those of known individuals or databases can lead to the identification of perpetrators.
- **Linking Evidence to Crime Scenes**: Blood, semen, saliva, and other bodily fluids found at crime scenes can be linked to suspects or victims. This can help establish the presence of an individual at a specific location and provide insights into the sequence of events.
- **Corroborating Witness Testimony**: Biological evidence can corroborate or refute witness testimony. For example, the presence of a suspect's DNA on a weapon can support a witness's statement that the suspect was armed.
- **Cold Case Resolution**: Advances in DNA technology have led to the resolution of many cold cases. Biological evidence collected years or decades ago can now be re-analyzed using modern techniques, leading to new leads and the identification of suspects.

- **Exoneration of the Innocent**: Forensic serology and biology have also played a crucial role in exonerating individuals wrongfully convicted of crimes. DNA testing has led to the release of numerous innocent individuals who were previously imprisoned based on flawed or insufficient evidence.

1.4.5 Challenges and Future Directions

While forensic serology and biology have revolutionized criminal investigations, they are not without challenges. Contamination, degradation of biological samples, and the interpretation of complex DNA mixtures are ongoing issues. Additionally, the increasing sensitivity of DNA analysis techniques raises concerns about the potential for detecting low-level, incidental DNA that may not be relevant to the crime.

Future directions in forensic serology and biology include the development of more advanced techniques for analyzing degraded and low-quantity samples, as well as the integration of new technologies such as next-generation sequencing (NGS).

NGS allows for the simultaneous analysis of multiple genetic markers and has the potential to provide even more detailed and informative DNA profiles.

Furthermore, the continued advancement of forensic databases and the use of probabilistic genotyping software will enhance the accuracy and reliability of DNA analysis. The combination of forensic serology, biology, and emerging technologies will continue to improve the ability to solve crimes, bring justice to victims, and ensure the integrity of the criminal justice system.

1.5 Sexual Offences

Sexual offences are a grave violation of an individual's bodily autonomy and integrity. These offences encompass a wide range of actions, all of which are rooted in non-consensual sexual behavior. Sexual offences not only inflict severe physical and psychological harm on the victim but also have a profound impact on society, fostering an environment of fear and mistrust. The types of sexual offences are diverse, and understanding them is crucial for addressing and preventing such crimes.

1.5.1 Definition and Legal Framework

Sexual offences are criminal acts that involve unwanted sexual activity, ranging from sexual harassment to rape. The legal definitions of these offences vary across jurisdictions, but they commonly include any act of a sexual nature that is carried out without the consent of the victim. Consent is a fundamental element in distinguishing between lawful sexual activity and a sexual offence. It must be given freely and voluntarily, without any form of coercion or manipulation.

The legal framework for sexual offences is designed to protect individuals from sexual violence and to ensure that perpetrators are held accountable. Laws against sexual offences are enforced through various mechanisms, including criminal prosecutions, civil remedies, and protective orders. These laws also provide for victim support services, such as counseling and medical care, to help victims recover from the trauma of sexual violence.

1.5.2 Types of Sexual Offences

1. Rape

Rape is one of the most severe forms of sexual offence. It involves non-consensual penetration, whether vaginal, anal, or oral, using any part of the body or an object. The defining characteristic of rape is the absence of consent, which can be overridden by force, threats, or incapacitation. Rape is a deeply traumatic experience for the victim, often resulting in long-term psychological effects such as post-traumatic stress disorder (PTSD), depression, and anxiety.

2. Sexual Assault

Sexual assault is a broader category that includes any non-consensual sexual contact. This can range from unwanted touching or groping to more severe forms of sexual violence. Sexual assault is often committed by someone known to the victim, such as a friend, family member, or intimate partner. The impact of sexual assault can be profound, affecting the victim's sense of safety and trust in others.

3. Sexual Harassment

Sexual harassment involves unwanted and inappropriate sexual advances, requests for sexual favors, or other verbal or physical conduct of a sexual nature. It can occur in various settings, including the workplace, educational institutions, and public spaces. Sexual harassment creates a hostile and intimidating environment for the victim, undermining their dignity and well-being. It is often characterized by a power imbalance, where the perpetrator uses their position of authority to exploit the victim.

4. Child Sexual Abuse

Child sexual abuse is a heinous crime that involves engaging in sexual activities with a minor. This can include anything from touching or fondling to more severe forms of sexual exploitation. Children are particularly vulnerable to sexual abuse because they lack the capacity to give informed consent and may not fully understand the nature of the abuse. The psychological and emotional impact of child sexual abuse is profound, often leading to long-term mental health issues and difficulties in forming healthy relationships.

5. Incest

Incest is a specific form of sexual abuse that occurs within a family. It involves sexual activities between close relatives, such as parents and children, siblings, or other family members. Incest is particularly damaging because it violates the trust and safety that are fundamental to family relationships. Victims of incest often experience severe psychological trauma, including feelings of shame, guilt, and betrayal.

6. Human Trafficking and Sexual Exploitation

Human trafficking for sexual exploitation involves the recruitment, transportation, transfer, harboring, or receipt of individuals through force, fraud, or coercion for the purpose of sexual exploitation. Victims of trafficking are often subjected to extreme forms of violence and abuse, and they may be forced into prostitution or other forms of sexual slavery. Human trafficking is a global problem that affects millions of people, particularly women and children.

7. Indecent Exposure

Indecent exposure involves deliberately exposing one's genitals in public or to someone who does not wish to see them. This act is intended to cause shock, alarm, or distress to the victim. While indecent exposure may seem less severe compared to other sexual offences, it can still have a significant psychological impact on the victim, contributing to feelings of violation and fear.

8. Voyeurism

Voyeurism, also known as "peeping," involves secretly observing someone who is undressing, naked, or engaged in sexual activities without their consent. Voyeurism is a violation of the victim's privacy and can cause significant distress and anxiety. With the advent of technology, voyeurism has expanded to include activities such as secretly recording or photographing individuals without their knowledge.

1.5.3 Psychological Impact on Victims

The psychological impact of sexual offences on victims is profound and multifaceted. Victims often experience a range of emotional responses, including shock, fear, anger, and sadness. Many victims develop PTSD, characterized by symptoms such as flashbacks, nightmares, and hypervigilance. Depression and anxiety are also common, as are feelings of guilt, shame, and self-blame.

The long-term effects of sexual violence can include difficulties in forming and maintaining relationships, sexual dysfunction, and problems with trust and intimacy. Victims may also struggle with substance abuse, self-harm, and suicidal thoughts as they attempt to cope with the trauma of their experience.

1.5.4 Societal Implications

Sexual offences have far-reaching implications for society as a whole. They contribute to a culture of fear and mistrust, undermining the social fabric and eroding the sense of safety and security. Sexual violence also has economic costs, including medical expenses, lost productivity, and the cost of criminal justice responses.

Addressing sexual offences requires a comprehensive approach that includes prevention, support for victims, and accountability for perpetrators. Public awareness campaigns, education programs, and legal reforms are essential components of a strategy to prevent sexual violence and support survivors. Additionally, providing access to mental health services and other forms of support can help victims heal and rebuild their lives.

Sexual offences are a serious violation of an individual's autonomy and dignity, with profound psychological and societal implications. Understanding the different types of sexual offences is crucial for developing effective strategies to prevent and address sexual violence. By promoting awareness, supporting victims, and holding perpetrators accountable, society can work towards a future where everyone is free from the threat of sexual violence.

1.6 Forensic Toxicology

Forensic toxicology is a critical field within forensic science that focuses on the study and analysis of drugs, alcohol, poisons, and other toxic substances within biological specimens to determine their influence on a person's death or behavior. A key component of forensic toxicology is the examination of viscera, which refers to the internal organs, particularly those within the abdominal cavity. This examination can provide crucial evidence in criminal investigations, particularly in cases of suspected poisoning or overdose.

1.6.1 Methodologies in Forensic Toxicology: Examination of Viscera

The examination of viscera involves a series of meticulous steps, starting from the collection of samples during an autopsy to the sophisticated analytical techniques used to detect and quantify toxic substances. The primary organs examined include the liver, stomach, intestines, kidneys, and sometimes the heart and lungs. Here's a detailed overview of the process:

1.6.1.1 Sample Collection

The collection of visceral samples is performed during an autopsy, typically by a forensic pathologist. The liver is often the primary organ of interest because it metabolizes many substances and can contain high concentrations of toxins. The stomach contents are also examined to identify recently ingested substances, while the intestines can provide information on substances absorbed over a longer period. The kidneys are analyzed for their role in excreting toxins, and sometimes the heart and lungs are examined for specific toxicants, such as volatile substances.

1.6.1.2 Preservation and Transportation

Once collected, the samples must be preserved properly to prevent degradation of the toxic substances. This usually involves storing the viscera in airtight containers and keeping them at low temperatures. The use of preservatives like sodium fluoride can inhibit bacterial growth and enzyme activity, which might otherwise degrade the toxins. Proper labeling and chain-of-custody documentation are critical to maintain the integrity of the samples.

1.6.2 Analytical Techniques

The analysis of visceral samples involves several sophisticated techniques to detect and quantify toxic substances. The choice of technique depends on the type of substance suspected and the matrix being analyzed. Common analytical methods include:

- **Gas Chromatography-Mass Spectrometry (GC-MS):** This technique is highly sensitive and specific, making it ideal for detecting volatile and semi-volatile substances, including drugs and poisons.
- **Liquid Chromatography-Mass Spectrometry (LC-MS):** LC-MS is used for non-volatile and polar compounds. It is particularly useful for analyzing biological samples for a wide range of toxicants.
- **High-Performance Liquid Chromatography (HPLC):** HPLC is employed for separating and quantifying compounds that may be present in the viscera, including drugs and their metabolites.
- **Immunoassays:** These are used for preliminary screening of biological samples for specific drugs or toxins. They are relatively quick and can indicate the presence of certain substances before more detailed analysis.
- **Atomic Absorption Spectroscopy (AAS) and Inductively Coupled Plasma Mass Spectrometry (ICP-MS):** These techniques are used for detecting and quantifying metals and other elements that may be toxic.

1.6.3 Importance of Viscera Examination in Forensic Toxicology

The examination of viscera in forensic toxicology is crucial for several reasons:

1.6.3.1 Determining Cause of Death

In cases of suspected poisoning or overdose, the analysis of viscera can provide definitive evidence of the presence of toxic substances that contributed to the individual's death. By identifying and quantifying these substances, forensic toxicologists can establish a causal link between the toxicant and the fatal outcome.

1.6.3.2 Supporting Legal Proceedings

Forensic toxicology findings are often pivotal in criminal investigations and legal proceedings. The detection of poisons or drugs in the viscera can support charges of homicide, manslaughter, or negligence. In cases where the cause of death is disputed, toxicological evidence can provide objective data that aids in delivering justice.

1.6.3.3 Understanding Substance Abuse Patterns

The examination of viscera can also reveal patterns of substance abuse, which can be important in both criminal and public health contexts. Identifying trends in drug use or the prevalence of certain poisons can inform preventive measures and policy decisions.

1.6.4 Challenges in Viscera Examination

Despite its importance, the examination of viscera in forensic toxicology presents several challenges:

1.6.4.1 Decomposition and Degradation

Biological tissues begin to decompose soon after death, which can degrade toxic substances and complicate their detection and quantification. The use of preservatives and proper storage conditions can mitigate this, but degradation remains a significant challenge, especially in cases where the body is discovered long after death.

1.6.4.2 Interference from Endogenous Compounds

Visceral samples contain a complex mixture of endogenous compounds that can interfere with the detection of toxic substances. Analytical techniques must be highly specific and sensitive to distinguish between the toxicants and the background biological matrix.

1.6.4.3 Variability in Metabolism

The metabolism of toxic substances can vary significantly between individuals due to genetic, environmental, and health factors. This variability can affect the concentration and form of the substance detected in the viscera, complicating the interpretation of toxicological findings.

1.6.4.4 Limited Sample Volume

In some cases, the volume of viscera available for analysis may be limited, especially if the body has undergone significant decomposition or trauma. This limitation necessitates the use of highly sensitive analytical techniques that can detect and quantify substances in very small amounts.

1.6.5 Advances and Future Directions

The field of forensic toxicology is continually evolving, with advancements in analytical techniques and technologies improving the detection and quantification of toxic substances in viscera. Some of the promising developments include:

1.6.5.1 Enhanced Sensitivity and Specificity

Advancements in mass spectrometry and chromatography are enhancing the sensitivity and specificity of toxicological analyses. These improvements allow for the detection of even trace amounts of toxicants in complex biological matrices.

1.6.5.2 Rapid Screening Techniques

The development of rapid screening techniques, such as portable mass spectrometers and advanced immunoassays, is enabling quicker preliminary analysis of viscera. These tools can provide immediate information that guides further detailed analyses.

1.6.5.3 Integration of Omics Technologies

The integration of omics technologies, such as proteomics and metabolomics, is providing a more comprehensive understanding of the biochemical changes associated with toxic exposure. These approaches can reveal new biomarkers of poisoning and improve the accuracy of toxicological assessments.

The examination of viscera in forensic toxicology is a vital process that provides crucial evidence in the investigation of deaths involving toxic substances. Through meticulous sample collection, preservation, and sophisticated analytical techniques, forensic toxicologists can determine the presence and impact of drugs, poisons, and other toxicants. Despite challenges such as decomposition, endogenous interference, and metabolic variability, ongoing advancements in technology and methodology continue to enhance the field's capabilities. As forensic toxicology evolves, the examination of viscera will remain a cornerstone in the pursuit of justice and the understanding of toxic substance effects on the human body.

1.7. Medicolegal Organizations

Which type of death are examined through a medicolegal autopsy? The classification of deaths varies depending on the legislation of each country. It may include categories such as violent deaths, deaths under suspicious circumstances or of unknown cause, sudden deaths, deaths that occur without medical assistance, deaths that occur in institutions or while in custody, and deaths that are related to surgical or anesthetic procedures. In addition to the violent deaths, a significant number of other deaths can be classified as natural deaths, which constitute most cases handled by most medicolegal institutions. A significant number of pathologists express dissatisfaction with it. However, becoming a proficient forensic pathologist and acquiring the ability to identify a death caused by violence can only be achieved through extensive experience conducting numerous autopsies on deaths resulting from natural causes.

The purpose of this chapter is not to provide a comprehensive review of medicolegal systems worldwide, but rather to offer specific examples that demonstrate the limitations of these frameworks. It aims to highlight the advantages and disadvantages, variations and similarities, as well as the actualities and expectations associated with medicolegal systems.

1.7.1. United States

Medicolegal systems vary across different countries. The situation within states in the United States can differ from one county to another. Nonetheless, there exist two distinct primary systems, namely the coroner system and the medical examiner system.

The coroner system, derived from the English feudal system, operates on the principle of electing an individual to serve as a coroner. The coroner is responsible for ascertaining the manner of death, regardless of whether there is a physician's opinion, following or without reliance on the autopsy report. In previous times, being a physician was not obligatory, however, in numerous regions nowadays, it is mandatory, regardless of whether the physician is not a pathologist. The training for coroners ranges from no training at all to a duration of 1 to 2 weeks. The variation in the coroner's system is due to the historical introduction of the system in different regions of the British Empire in its original "English" form. The rules and subsequent amendments of the Coroner's Act in Great Britain have not been adopted in the United States in recent years.

The implementation of the medical examiner system began in 1877 in Massachusetts and underwent further advancements until 1918 when the first medical examiner was established in New York City. The medical examiner must be a proficient physician specialized in pathology. The contemporary concept observed in the United States today has its origins in the New York system, albeit with some modifications. In contemporary systems, the primary medical examiner must possess expertise in forensic pathology.

In certain states, the medical examiner operates within the framework set by state government agencies or the public health department. However, this arrangement can create complications as it is crucial for the medical examiner to have both technical and economic autonomy to carry out their duties effectively. However, it is important to note that individuals who are not physicians are not authorized to make medical determinations, regardless of their level of training. Being a politically elected official, the coroner may face significant pressure to decide, while a physician is bound by strict ethical guidelines. Although the coroner may depend on a capable physician, they can still be replaced in the upcoming election due to political motives, with a more convenient candidate. Regardless of the specific title given to the system—whether it be medical examiner, coroner, or medical examiner-coroner—the primary concern revolves around the responsibility and methods that these authorities must undertake to ensure scientific and professional excellence.

These systems lack the presence of a scene of crime investigation during every scene examination due to an insufficient number of forensic pathologists available. In the United States, the responsibility of determining whether a death falls under the jurisdiction of the medical examiner's office is assigned to civilian investigators who are employed by the office. If it is not possible to obtain a death certificate, the office will accept the case. Subsequently, these experts generate a report. If the case is not accepted, a physician is required to review the report. In the event of a disagreement between the two parties (which is unlikely to occur), the case will be deemed acceptable. The medical examiner determines whether to conduct solely an external examination, a complete autopsy, or additional laboratory tests.

1.7.2. Northern Europe

The medicolegal external examination system is also utilized in northern European nations, including Finland and Denmark. In the latter scenario, a medical officer of health conducts an examination, either in the presence of or at the request of the police, to determine the need for an autopsy. The presumed cause and manner of death are typically determined following the external examination, although there may be occasional errors in this determination.

1.7.3. Turkey

In Turkey, a comparable system is utilized: the prosecutor directs medicolegal deaths to forensic departments, where a medical doctor conducts an external examination and, if necessary, collaborates with the prosecutor to sign the death certificate, unless an autopsy is deemed necessary.

1.7.4. Great Britain

The evolution of forensic medicine in Great Britain is closely intertwined with the coroner system, which was subsequently adopted in the United States. The process started in the 12th century with the election of county coroners and continued gradually over the following centuries. Forensic medicine originated in the 17th century with the recording of the first autopsy, but it was not until the early 19th century that the first book on the subject was published. The Coroner's Act of 1887, which governs the British medicolegal system, was implemented after the specialty had already been established in Continental Europe.

The Coroner's Amendment Act of 1926 and subsequent regulations revised the original Act. Consequently, the coroners are now responsible for handling a significant number of deaths caused by natural causes. In certain jurisdictions, coroners are affiliated with university departments, while in other areas, Home Office pathologists may be summoned to investigate cases of homicide and suspicious deaths. However, most cases handled by coroners, which include both natural and noncriminal unnatural deaths, are managed by consultant pathologists employed by the National Health Service in general hospitals in Britain.

1.7.5. France

In France, the external examination is consistently mandated by the police or a prosecutor. Nevertheless, a medicolegal autopsy can only be requested by a prosecutor, who has the sole authority to make this decision. French law does not provide any criteria for determining whether to order or refuse a forensic necropsy. The certifying general physician typically does not indicate any "medicolegal impediment" on the death certificate. The forensic doctor, whose opinion is subsequently provided, typically verifies this assertion. There is no postmortem examination in this instance. Consequently, the judicial inquiry into a death often focuses on determining whether it was due to natural causes, suicide, or an accident, without the need for an autopsy. Therefore, in France, suicides are infrequent, which undoubtedly presents challenges in training. For instance, one cannot effectively conduct an autopsy on strangulation without prior experience in examining numerous cases of suicidal hangings.

The situation becomes more dire when a fatal accident occurs at work, as autopsy is often not carried out. Lenoir pertains to investigations where autopsies were conducted, and in 32% of the instances, the examinations took place between 3 and 6 months after death, making them essentially exhumations. These exhumations have significantly restricted diagnostic value when compared to a more recent autopsy. The percentage of recent autopsies conducted on job accidents or professional diseases was below 9%. The evident bias of relatives when it comes to legal disputes involving insurance companies is apparent.

1.7.6. Spain

In Spain, the term "forense" refers to a specialized medicolegal examiner who operates within a specific geographical region of the country. The forensic expert must possess the ability to proficiently handle a wide range of medico-legal examinations, including autopsies and psychiatric evaluations of prisoners. To acquire the necessary credentials, medical practitioners must complete a six-month postgraduate training program encompassing all pertinent fields of forensic science, including pathology, toxicology, genetics, and law. One advantageous feature of this system is its extensive national coverage. However, forensic experts possess significant authority as they are the ones responsible for determining whether an autopsy should be conducted, and only a limited number of autopsies are performed as a result. Furthermore, the limited education in such a vast scientific field is inadequate and unsuitable.

1.7.7. Portugal

According to personal communication from D.N. Viera, Portugal is recognized for having one of the most exceptional medicolegal systems in Europe. Consequently, numerous countries desire to adopt and incorporate this system.

This is why it is important to provide a thorough presentation and acknowledge Duarte Nuno Vieira, the architect of this system and the current president of the National Institute of Legal Medicine (NILM).

The NILM, a self-governing administrative division under the jurisdiction of the Justice Ministry, is situated in the small central town of Coimbra rather than the capital, Lisbon (an exemplary instance of institutional political decentralization). The NILM consists of three primary delegations, which were formerly independent legal medicine institutes. These delegations are in Coimbra, Lisbon, and Oporto. These three delegations are comprehensive "institutes," indicating that they are capable of performing almost all forms of medicolegal expertise at each location. The delegation is organized into various departments, namely forensic pathology (including histopathology), forensic toxicology, forensic genetics, and clinical forensic medicine (which encompasses the areas of sexual abuse and psychiatry). In addition, there are protocols established with other institutions, such as the Anthropology Department of the Sciences and Technology Faculty, for conducting anthropological examinations. Furthermore, hospitals are involved in carrying out more specialized examinations that may be required during medicolegal activities. When a forensic pathologist encounters a non-fresh body during their routine work, they may seek the assistance of forensic anthropologists for examination purposes.

On certain occasions, when the remains consist of desiccated skeletal structures, the anthropologist can conduct the necessary analysis. Nevertheless, in cases where a death certificate is required or when the cause of death can be ascertained, the pathologist is summoned to take part. This assistance encompasses almost the entire country, with only a few exceptions of cases handled by local practitioners who have no communication with the NILM.

Forensic pathology and clinical forensic medicine departments employ full-time medical doctors who have undergone a 5-year training period to specialize in forensic medicine, which is the standard duration for any medical specialty in the country. A proficient pathologist in the histopathology department thoroughly analyzes all the microscopic sections obtained from autopsies conducted within the delegation, as well as those from the regional forensic units mentioned in the subsequent paragraphs. Biologists, biochemists, pharmacists, and chemists possess the necessary qualifications to work in laboratories specializing in toxicology and genetics. They receive comprehensive training to fulfill their responsibilities. A psychiatrist, an orthopedist, and a neurologist are part-time specialists who provide assistance and scientific expertise in medical examinations, particularly in clinical forensic medicine departments. 24/7 X-ray facilities staffed by dedicated radiology technicians are accessible in all medical departments, while the presence of a radiologist, or a specialized medical professional, is typically limited to part-time hours. The entire institution is overseen by an administrative staff equipped with the necessary logistical resources to function effectively.

Medicolegal offices, known as regional forensic units, have been established in smaller towns across the country to centralize and coordinate medicolegal activities in the respective localities. They possess the essential prerequisites to carry out all medicolegal duties, including autopsies, clinical examinations for legal disputes, and investigations related to sexual or drug abuse. However, they do not have any laboratory facilities. When necessary, samples are sent to one of the three primary delegations mentioned earlier. Within these GMLs, there exist medical doctors from various specialties, predominantly general practitioners, who have completed a postgraduate program of 90 hours, which includes practical training in conducting autopsies. It is somewhat adequate, but not enough. Therefore, the NILM must focus on enhancing the training of "regional" specialists to address the current disparity in the quality of medicolegal services between the main delegations (which meet international standards) and the GML.

One notable advantage of the Portuguese system is the legal requirement for a mandatory autopsy in cases of violent deaths or deaths with unknown causes. The decision hinges upon the prosecutor, who considers the police report regarding the circumstances of death and any relevant hospital records (if the deceased was hospitalized). The prosecutor typically conducts interviews with the relatives to gather information regarding the medical history or any other pertinent details related to Law 45/2004, Article 18. Moreover, this legislation mandates that autopsies be conducted in cases of immediate fatalities resulting from traffic or occupational accidents, regardless of the necessity for a necropsy. This system effectively addresses the persistent issue faced by Europe and the United States: the decrease in the number of autopsies being performed. It conducts a substantial number of postmortem dissections in the present era, approximately 6,000 per year for a country with a population of 12 million. In 2002, the percentage of deaths that underwent forensic autopsy was 4.8%, while in 2003 this percentage increased to 5.1%.

One of the services provided by the NILM is always the availability of a forensic doctor in the three main delegations and in many GML. This doctor is responsible for conducting scene examinations in cases of violent deaths, examining victims of assaults (particularly those with minor injuries), and observing victims of sexual assault to ensure that biological evidence is preserved. This community service is of great significance, yielding highly favorable outcomes in aiding subsequent criminal investigations.

There is a strong correlation between the three primary delegations and the leading medicine faculties across the country, where the instruction of legal medicine at the undergraduate level takes place. Forensic medicine professors typically hold joint appointments with their respective faculties and the National Institute of Legal Medicine (NILM). Medical and law students in Portuguese universities are required to complete a legal medicine course for a semester or one year. As part of this course, they must participate in a minimum of two autopsies. This scientific support is also extended to magistrates, prosecutors, and judges, even during their academic education. The NILM and their professionals collaborate with various forensic training programs, ranging from criminal police to mortuary technicians.

The medicolegal council, consisting of university professors specializing in various medical fields and law, representatives from the Portuguese Medical Council, and the directors of the three NILM delegations, serves as a technical scientific advisory body. It provides support to the courts in dealing with complex medical issues that go beyond routine forensic cases and require in-depth and specialized studies or discussions, such as medical responsibility. In addition to the permanent members, other specialists may be summoned to provide their expert opinion in a specific field. The Minister of Justice, the General Prosecutor, the Supreme Council of Justice, and the President of the NILM have the authority to request this council.

1.8. Quality Control and Forensic Pathologist Qualifications

The matter of quality control in autopsies is not a recent concern. In fact, as early as the 19th century, the Austrian decree of 1855 established comprehensive guidelines for conducting medicolegal autopsies. Simultaneously, it transpired in other nations. In Portugal, a questionnaire and detailed instructions were provided through the renowned Decree of February 8, 1900, which remained in effect until the 1980s. Subsequently, the law was updated, and a new medicolegal organization was established, characterized by enhanced expertise and standards.

In contemporary times, it has become imperative to establish uniformity in procedures, particularly within communities like the European Economic Community. In 1991, the United Nations endorsed its model protocol for autopsy, known as the UN Minnesota Protocol. Subsequently, Interpol established its standardized protocol for Disaster Victim Identification. The European Council of Legal Medicine advocated for the standardization of the procedures for medicolegal autopsies. This initiative, known as the "Harmonization of the Performance of the Medicolegal Autopsy," was endorsed in 1995 and served as the foundation for the Recommendation No. R (99) 3 on the "Harmonization of Medico-Legal Autopsy Rules and Its Explanatory Memorandum." The Economic European Community Committee of Ministers adopted this recommendation in 1999. European countries are legally required to integrate these rules into their national legislation. However, as far as is known, this is not the situation in most of them. Harmonizing procedures presents a challenge, while harmonizing systems and qualifications do not.

The professional credentials of individuals conducting medicolegal autopsies differ depending on the location and the specific system in place. Occasionally, such as in the United States, there are regional and intraregional discrepancies. Qualifications for forensic professionals vary widely, ranging from highly trained clinical or anatomic pathologists with postgraduate training in forensics in the United States and United Kingdom, to forensic physicians with specialized training in legal medicine in Portugal. In Spain, the minimum requirement is a half-year training in forensics, although some individuals may have no formal training at all.

The United States mandates that the chief medical examiner must possess board certification as a forensic pathologist. The chief medical examiner is a physician who has successfully completed a series of advanced medical programs and examinations, including those administered by the Residence Review Committee, the Accreditation Council for Graduate Medical Education, and the American Board of Pathology. This training program concludes with a comprehensive year of forensic pathology.

Forensic medicine is recognized as a medical specialty in approximately 20–25 member countries of the European Union, each with its own distinct training programs.

In Yugoslavia and Portugal, physicians can specialize in forensic medicine after completing their medical studies and 2 years of general practice. In Yugoslavia, the specialization lasts for 3 years, while in Portugal it lasts for 5 years. Spanish university hospitals offer a 4-year medical specialization in forensic medicine, which is similar to other programs. Only a select few candidates opt for this path, as it requires a couple of years to attain the same level as those who undergo a 4-year postgraduate course in forensics after completing their undergraduate studies. An admirable characteristic of the Hungarian system is the mandatory periodic training course for each specialist every 5 years, which serves as an excellent model that should be emulated by other countries.

Legal medicine in Belgium is a formally recognized medical specialty since 2002, which necessitates an additional 5 years of study. Regrettably, in numerous locations, individuals lacking adequate skills and experience are conducting crucial criminal necropsies, excluding the programs and qualifications. This phenomenon is not limited to impoverished, underdeveloped nations; it also occurs in Europe and even in the United States. Furthermore, this question holds significant importance as it directly impacts the effectiveness of the justice system and has the potential to result in substantial and occasionally irreversible errors in the administration of justice. An unfavorable opinion is frequently more detrimental than having no opinion at all, as in the latter scenario, a magistrate is acutely aware of the absence of endorsement for their decision. When inexperienced pathologists make unequivocal statements, a judge may accept seemingly indisputable arguments without any scientific basis.

Ultimately, the future success of forensic pathology hinges on its ability to triumph in the crucial arenas of education and training.

1.9. The State of the Art

The medicolegal systems have undergone significant changes in recent decades. In the 1980s, legal amendments in the United States granted families the ability to prevent autopsies in cases that did not appear to be homicides, thereby authorizing only autopsies in clear-cut homicide cases.

Experienced pathologists are aware that the challenge lies not in identifying homicides, but in detecting cases that are disguised as suicides, accidents, or natural diseases. Quatrehomme stated that Brinkmann approximated that in Germany in 1997, 1,200 homicides per year were concealed as natural deaths, and 11,000 deaths that were not natural were mistakenly categorized as natural deaths. The autopsy revealed that the death of an elderly man, who was discovered at his residence three weeks after he had gone missing, was not due to a natural disease as initially believed. Instead, it was determined that he was murdered by a blunt force trauma to the head. Identifying a homicide may not always be feasible until an autopsy is conducted. There are numerous instances of this phenomenon, including child abuse syndrome, asphyxiation, and traffic accidents that were caused by heart attacks.

The implementation of new national legislation had far-reaching ramifications in countries such as the United States, Finland, Denmark, and France. The frequency of autopsies has drastically decreased in numerous regions across the globe. Various reasons have been presented to explain this significant decrease, including the expensive nature of necropsies, limited availability of facilities, challenges in attracting individuals to the field, advancements in modern diagnostic techniques, communication issues between pathologists and clinicians resulting in delays in obtaining necropsy results, the use of technical language by pathologists, and resistance from families due to concerns about mutilation, religious objections, economic interests, or other preferences for funeral directors. Referring to these unfavorable methods that led to the elimination of the minimum autopsy rate mandate by the American Joint Commission on Accreditation of Hospitals, Clark asserts that certain authors perceive hospital autopsies as ineffective, costly, irrelevant, and superfluous. Another significant reason, as mentioned by Tedeschi, is the lack of motivation among clinic pathologists to conduct postmortem examinations. This task is time-consuming and is carried out under unfavorable ergonomic conditions, such as standing up for long periods, exposure to unpleasant odors, and working in an unclean environment with a relative risk of contagious diseases. Furthermore, this work is not socially recognized. They prefer obtaining "clean" biopsies from surgical specimens or engaging in other more intriguing research endeavors. However, the issue at hand is not solely the lack of motivation, but also the inability to provide an answer to the question "Why did he die?" due to the ineffective methodology employed by hospital pathologists in elucidating the cause and manner of death. Considering the recent advancements in clinical pathology worldwide, it is foreseeable that clinical pathologists will no longer be capable of conducting autopsies soon.

It is important to consider the accuracy of mortality statistics when autopsies are conducted in specific populations. This is necessary for health authorities to implement appropriate disease prevention and control measures. However, this is not always the situation. This has a detrimental impact on society: the mass media inundate the public with official statistics immediately following the occurrence of a specific medical condition (such as sudden cardiac death), disregarding the fact that these statistics are often unreliable. For instance, Ambach et al. conducted a study on a substantial group of 1,595 patients. They found that a clinical diagnosis of myocardial infarction, which relied on contemporary techniques such as typical symptoms, electrocardiographic abnormalities, and enzymology, was incorrect in 28% of the cases when compared to autopsy results. Myocardial infarction is excessively diagnosed in clinics, leading to mortality statistics that are 15% higher than the actual number of deaths. Surprisingly, the series included cases of murder by strangulation, which emphasizes the importance of autopsies for clinicians to verify their diagnostic accuracy. Clark demonstrated the effectiveness and utility of hospital autopsies through a study of 1,076 consecutive, unselected cases. The results showed that 90% of cases where the cause of death was determined as "dead on arrival" and 9% of cases with important findings were only identified through autopsies, not through other testing methods. Furthermore, he disproved the notion that clinicians should be afraid of being involved in civil litigation due to potential malpractice, as only a few cases were discovered during the autopsy and none of them were presented as evidence. However, families find solace in the 90% confirmation rate of clinic information and express high satisfaction with the 9% of cases that are initially clinically ambiguous but are ultimately clarified through autopsies. This reduces the number of malpractice claims. Based on the College of American Pathologists units, Clark determines that the actual cost of the procedure is comparable to what previous authors have found. It is important to note that this procedure is not cheap, as conducting 200 autopsies (which is the typical workload for a single pathologist) could potentially prevent 10 instances of malpractice. Malpractice insurance providers for hospitals and physicians should recognize the autopsy as a worthwhile investment and should jointly bear the associated expenses.

Nevertheless, it would be chauvinistic to confine forensic pathology to the narrow confines of "little" Europe or North America, a position that the author strongly disagrees with. The decline of autopsies in the Old World can be attributed to the improvement of citizenship rights and a growing awareness of human rights among the population, particularly in developed countries. In Central and South America, the number of autopsies has not decreased and remains consistently high due to the prevalent violence in those countries. Each day, one of the five local forensic institutes in São Paolo, Brazil, conducts an average of 40–50 necropsies for various types of violent deaths. In Bogotá, Colombia, the institute remains open on weekends to avoid the build-up of corpses on Mondays. In this region, the issue of expertise quality arises. Nevertheless, there are notable exceptions. The Medicolegal Institute of Bogotá (Colombia) has achieved a level of quality that is highly desirable for many departments in the United States and Europe. The primary task for the esteemed forensic community is to disseminate their expertise to these nations as part of a worldwide endeavor to educate their workforce. The initiative has already commenced in Brazil with Portuguese scientists, as well as in Argentina and other Latin American countries with Spanish specialists. However, its scope is restricted to congresses or scientific meetings, which is insufficient. This endeavor requires more than just someone who travels and presents various pieces of "academic" science at conferences. Efficient collaboration is required from professionals in the field who regularly conduct autopsies and possess relevant expertise and uncertainties. These individuals should engage in cooperative efforts and work on-site, undertaking short or medium-term assignments with local physicians to provide ongoing training. Regrettably, this goal is still far from being achieved. Simultaneously, it could also serve as an exceptional opportunity to train professionals in countries such as Portugal, where occurrences of violent deaths are fortunately infrequent. One month of study in a South American institute is comparable to four or five years of training in the local area.

1.10. The Future: A Challenge for All

Education, specifically quality and training, is one of the three fundamental pillars that forensic pathology must focus on in the future. The other two objectives are effective legislation and efficient organization. Renowned specialists have emphasized the challenge at a scientific and quality level. Truth, work, and experience are essential for overcoming the well-known problem, as highlighted by Saukko and Knight, that in many countries, individuals who teach forensic pathology in universities have not had practical experience in the field for many years, sometimes even decades. To be a credible and persuasive teacher, it is essential to have ongoing practical experience in the subject matter. According to Arsenio Nunes, a respected professor of legal medicine in Lisbon during the 1950s, it is important to only teach subjects that one has practical experience in.

To further develop the other platforms (legislation and organization), it is essential to demonstrate the utility and benefits of legal medicine to communities, governments, politics, and influential individuals, such as the mass media.

Firstly, it is important to highlight the direct benefits that arise from the objectives of a forensic necropsy. This procedure serves as a valuable tool in enhancing the administration of justice, aiding law enforcement, prosecutors, and courts, and ultimately benefiting the entire community. Several authors report a margin of error of 4.5% in the determination of the manner of death in a series of clinical autopsies. However, in the context of medicolegal autopsies, the percentage rises to 23.4% when compared to the information provided by the medical external examination and the police. The rate of error in this context has more severe ramifications than clinical errors, as it leads to legal and insurance implications. The majority of the 23.4% incorrect determinations of death were attributed to an unidentified cause of death. Excluding those cases, there were 7.6% of women and 6.9% of men whose autopsies showed incorrect determinations. Among presumed accidental deaths, 6.5% were actually natural deaths. Additionally, 7.5% of natural deaths were accidental, 4% were suicides, and there was one case of homicide (refer to Heading 5 for a similar case where a homicide was initially mislabeled as a natural death). During a consecutive series of 600 forensic necropsies, it was discovered that there was a 10% margin of error in determining the mode of death and a 29.5% margin of error in determining the cause of death.

Forensic pathologists, often referred to as "detectives in white coats," are highly specialized professionals who must possess knowledge in various non-medical disciplines. These include criminology, criminalistics, engineering, highway design, police science, political science, chemistry, atmospheric physics, electricity, toxicology, and genetics, among others. Furthermore, the forensic pathologist must possess a thorough understanding of the distinct characteristics of the community in which they are operating, including aspects such as religion, government, society, and politics. There is no other field of medicine that encounters such an invigorating and demanding task. The relevance of forensic pathology to the community lies in its ability to directly determine the cause and manner of death, thereby preventing injury or disease within the entire community. In Great Britain, following numerous cases of individuals suffocating inside refrigerators, it became mandatory for the appliance to have an internal opening. It was required that rural tractors have a protective roof to prevent potential asphyxiation caused by compression of the chest and abdomen if the vehicle were to overturn on the driver. The immunizations and prophylactic therapies were based on the findings obtained from autopsies of individuals who had infectious diseases. Forensic pathology plays a crucial role in determining the cause of death and providing evidence for legal cases involving financial matters, traffic accidents, and individual rights in relation to law enforcement or political authority. The forensic pathologist is required to provide legal defense of their report in court, analyze the reports of other professionals, possess knowledge about the impacts of cardiopulmonary resuscitation or specific treatments, study the mechanics of motor vehicles, and offer emotional support to grieving mothers who have tragically lost their child to sudden infant death syndrome.

If the department demonstrates exemplary practices and is renowned as a highly proficient center, it will offer long-term exposure to qualified pathologists and exceptional training prospects for aspiring medical doctors.

A Closer Look

Legal Medicine

Legal medicine, also known as forensic medicine, is a specialized field at the intersection of medicine and law. It encompasses the application of medical knowledge and principles to legal questions and issues, playing a crucial role in the administration of justice. This field involves a variety of tasks, including the examination of living individuals and deceased persons to provide evidence in criminal and civil cases. Forensic medicine professionals, such as forensic pathologists, forensic odontologists, and forensic psychiatrists, use their expertise to assist in legal proceedings, offering insights that can influence the outcomes of cases. One of the core functions of legal medicine is conducting autopsies. Forensic pathologists perform post-mortem examinations to determine the cause of death and establish whether it was due to natural causes, accident, suicide, or homicide. The findings from these examinations are crucial for legal investigations and can help clarify whether a death was a result of foul play. In addition to determining cause of death, forensic pathologists also assess injuries and other pathological conditions that might be relevant in legal contexts.

Forensic odontologists specialize in analyzing dental records and bite marks. They are often called upon to identify deceased individuals through dental records, particularly in cases where other identifying features are not available. They also play a role in evaluating bite mark injuries in assault cases, providing critical evidence that can support or refute allegations of criminal behavior.

Forensic psychiatry is another important branch of legal medicine. Forensic psychiatrists assess individuals' mental states in legal contexts, such as determining criminal responsibility or competency to stand trial. They evaluate whether an individual was suffering from a mental disorder at the time of an alleged crime and whether this condition affects their ability to understand or participate in legal proceedings. Their evaluations can influence sentencing, legal outcomes, and treatment recommendations.

Legal medicine also includes the assessment of injuries and the documentation of medical evidence in cases of personal injury, malpractice, and abuse. Forensic experts provide detailed reports and testimony that can impact legal decisions in civil cases, helping to establish the extent of harm and its implications for compensation or liability.

Additionally, legal medicine contributes to public health and safety by identifying trends and patterns in forensic data. Forensic evidence can reveal important information about emerging threats, such as drug overdoses or patterns of violence, thereby informing preventive measures and public health policies. The integration of legal medicine with modern technologies has further enhanced its efficacy. Techniques such as DNA profiling, digital forensics, and advanced imaging technologies have revolutionized the field, enabling more precise and comprehensive analyses. Forensic professionals often work closely with law enforcement, legal professionals, and other experts to provide robust evidence that upholds the principles of justice and supports the legal system in resolving complex cases.

Summary

- "Forensic pathology is the last stronghold of the autopsy," Wright and Tate wrote in their respective works. The deaths of people will continue to occur regardless of what man does or where he lives, and they will frequently be the result of acts of violence or mistakes. There is an expectation that forensic pathology will provide an explanation for these deaths and will suggest measures that could have prevented diseases that were not necessary. Considering forensic pathology in this manner, it is possible to refer to it as "community and public safety pathology."
- To meet the challenge of forensic pathology in the days that lie ahead, education, legislation, and organization will be the magic triangle that will write the future. This is because these three things are more important than financial support. To meet the diverse multidisciplinary missions for which they are employed, day after day, in many parts of this ever-changing world, the bridge between forensic pathology and forensic anthropology will become more solid the stronger and more powerful forensic pathology is.

References

1. Cameriere, R., Scendoni, R., Ferrante, L., Mirtella, D., Oncini, L., & Cingolani, M. (2023). An effective model for estimating age in unaccompanied minors under the Italian legal system. *Healthcare (Basel), 11*(2), 224. https://doi.org/10.3390/healthcare11020224.
2. Cingolani, M., Scendoni, R., Fedeli, P., & Cembrani, F. (2023). Artificial intelligence and digital medicine for integrated home care services in Italy: Opportunities and limits. *Frontiers in Public Health, 10*, 1095001. https://doi.org/10.3389/fpubh.2022.1095001.
3. De Micco, F., Angelakopoulos, N., Martino, F., Corbi, G., Cameriere, C., & Campobasso, C. P. (2022). Skeletal age estimation in a contemporary South African population using two radiological methods (Bo/Ca and TW2). *Australian Journal of Forensic Sciences, 54*(6), 767–784.
4. De Micco, F., Fineschi, V., Banfi, G., Frati, P., Oliva, A., Travaini, G. V., et al. (2022). From COVID-19 pandemic to patient safety: A new "Spring" for Telemedicine or a Boomerang effect? *Frontiers in Medicine (Lausanne), 15*(9), 901788. https://doi.org/10.3389/fmed.2022.901788.
5. Fedeli, P., Scendoni, R., Cingolani, M., Corrales Compagnucci, M., Cirocchi, R., & Cannovo, N. (2022). Informed consent and protection of personal data in genetic research on COVID-19. *Healthcare (Basel), 10*(2), 349. https://doi.org/10.3390/healthcare10020349.
6. McCord, B. R., Gauthier, Q., Cho, S., Roig, M. N., Gibson-Daw, G. C., Young, B., et al. (2019). Forensic DNA analysis. *Analytical Chemistry, 91*(1), 673–688.
7. Monteith, S., Bauer, M., Alda, M., Geddes, J., Whybrow, P. C., & Glenn, T. (2021). Increasing cybercrime since the pandemic: Concerns for psychiatry. *Current Psychiatry Reports, 23*(4), 18.
8. Pennisi, M., Kavasidis, I., Spampinato, C., et al. (2021). An explainable AI system for automated COVID-19 assessment and lesion categorization from CT-scans. *Artificial Intelligence in Medicine, 118*, 102114. https://doi.org/10.1016/j.artmed.2021.102114.
9. Prince, D. A., & Ubelaker, D. H. (2002). Application of Lamendin's adult dental aging technique to a diverse skeletal sample. *Journal of Forensic Sciences, 47*(1), 107–116.

10. Scendoni, R., Fedeli, P., Cannovo, N., & Cingolani, M. (2021). The "magnificent seven errors" in forensic autopsy practice: The Italian context. *Academic Forensic Pathology, 11*(4), 208–214.

11. Travaini, G. V., Pacchioni, F., Bellumore, S., Bosia, M., & De Micco, F. (2022). Machine learning and criminal justice: A systematic review of advanced methodology for recidivism risk prediction. *International Journal of Environmental Research and Public Health, 19*(17), 10594. https://doi.org/10.3390/ijerph191710594.

12. Wankhade, T. D., Ingale, S. W., Mohite, P. M., & Bankar, N. J. (2022). Artificial intelligence in forensic medicine and toxicology: The future of forensic medicine. *Cureus, 14*(8), e28376.

Chapter

THE ROLE OF PHARMACOGENETICS IN FORENSIC SCIENCE

2

Contents

Introduction

Pharmacogenetics refers to the study of how genes affect an individual's response to drugs; it plays a significant role in forensic sciences. This field intersects with forensics primarily in the investigation of drug-related deaths, toxicology, and legal medicine.

In forensic toxicology, pharmacogenetics helps to understand the variability in drug metabolism among individuals. This understanding is crucial when investigating death due to drug overdoses or poisonings.

Certain genetic variants can lead to slower or faster metabolism of drugs, affecting their toxicity. For example, variations in the CYP450 enzyme family can influence how different individuals metabolize common drugs like opioids, benzodiazepines, or antidepressants. Identifying these genetic differences post-mortem can provide insights into whether a drug level found in the body was within a therapeutic range, a lethal dose, or indicative of an overdose.

The variability in the human genome plays a pivotal role in pharmacogenetic studies. Each individual's unique genetic makeup can significantly influence how they respond to various drugs. Pharmacogenetic variability in drug response can explain why some individuals experience severe side effects, while others do not, despite taking the same medication at the same dose. By identifying genetic factors that affect drug response, forensic scientists can better predict and understand adverse drug reactions, therapeutic failures, and cases of drug toxicity.

Genetic approaches to understanding individual differences in susceptibility to drugs and xenobiotics responses are crucial in forensic pharmacogenetics. These approaches involve identifying specific genetic polymorphisms that influence drug metabolism and response. For instance, polymorphisms in genes encoding for drug-metabolizing enzymes, drug transporters, and drug targets can all affect an individual's reaction to a drug. Understanding these genetic differences can help forensic scientists make more accurate determinations about drug-related deaths and adverse reactions.

Ethical issues relating to the collection of genetic data are also a critical aspect of forensic pharmacogenetics. The collection, storage, and use of genetic information must be handled with care to protect individuals' privacy and rights. Ethical considerations include obtaining informed consent for genetic testing, ensuring confidentiality of genetic data, and addressing potential discrimination based on genetic information. These issues must be carefully navigated to balance the benefits of pharmacogenetic insights with the need to protect individual rights.

This chapter will focus on:

1. adverse drug reactions;
2. drug addiction;
3. variability in the human genome;
4. pharmacogenetic variability in drug response;
5. genetic approaches to understand the individual differences in susceptibility to drugs/ xenobiotics responses; and
6. ethical issues relating to the collection of genetic data.

Through these focal points, the chapter will examine the significant role pharmacogenetics plays in enhancing forensic investigations, improving the accuracy of toxicological analyzes, and contributing to the broader understanding of drug-related fatalities. This integration ultimately aids in the delivery of justice by providing more precise and individualized insights into drug metabolism and its forensic implications.

Orientation and Directional Terms

Term	Definition	Illustration
Forensic Toxicology	The branch of toxicology that focuses on the application of toxicological principles to legal issues, often involving the investigation of poisons, drugs, and other substances in criminal cases.	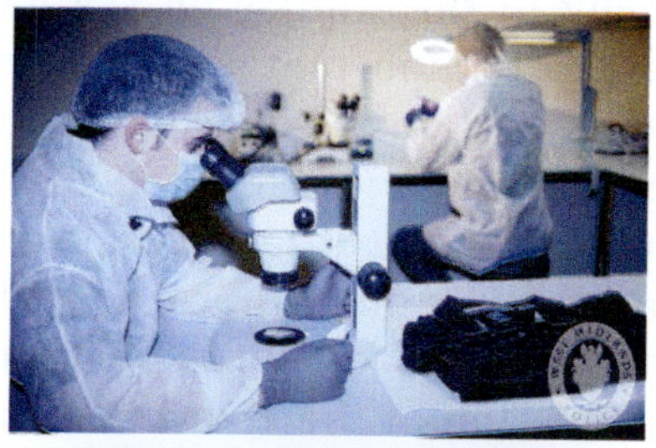
Genetic Variants	Alterations in the DNA sequence that make up a gene, which can result in different traits or susceptibility to diseases. Variants can be inherited or acquired.	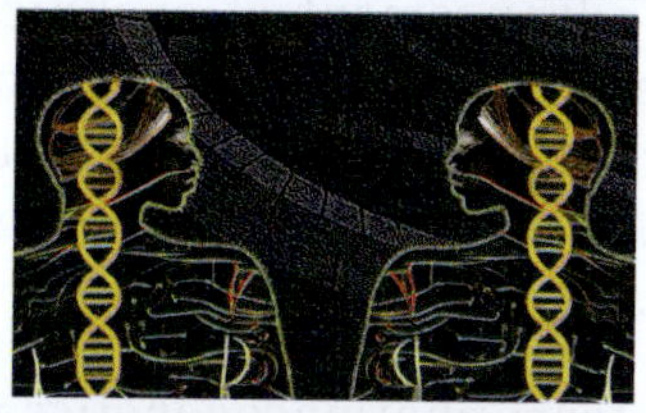
Opioids	A class of drugs that include both prescription pain relievers (like morphine and oxycodone) and illegal substances (like heroin). They work by binding to opioid receptors in the brain and can be highly addictive.	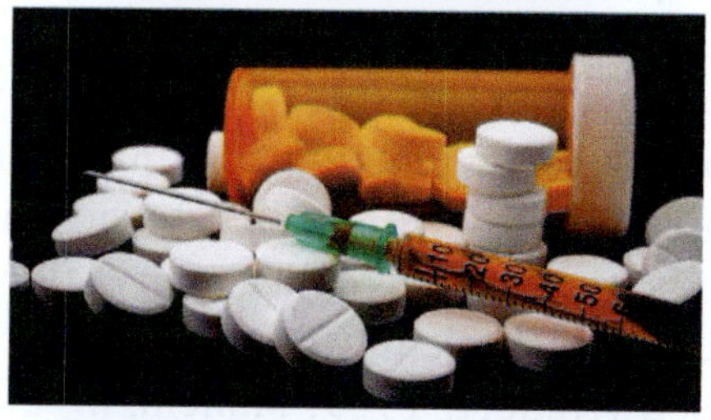
Benzodiazepines	A group of medications commonly prescribed for anxiety, insomnia, and other conditions. They work by enhancing the effect of a neurotransmitter called GABA in the brain.	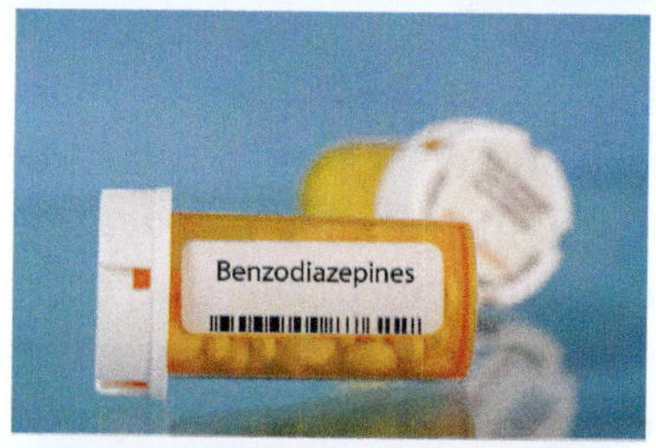
Human Genome	The complete set of genetic information in humans, contained within DNA, including all of the genes and non-coding sequences. The Human Genome Project mapped this entire set of genes.	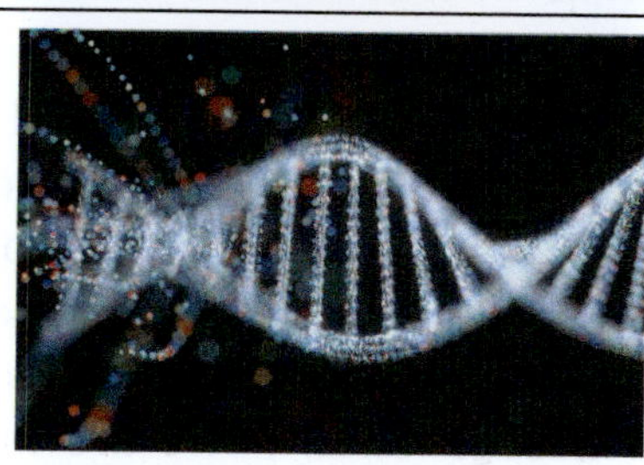

2.1. Concept of Pharmacogenetics

Especially in the studies on the genetic basis of the most important inherited arrhythmia syndromes responsible for sudden cardiac death, which is a major cause of death worldwide, and of individual differences in response to potential toxicants, where a new emerging area of interest is known as pharmacogenetics, the completion of the Human Genome Project and the advancement of analytical technology with the large-scale identification of genome polymorphisms have contributed to the field of forensic science (also known as forensic science).

The term pharmacogenetics was first used in the late 1950s (Clayman, 1952) and can be defined as the study of variability in drug responses as a function of genetic differences among individuals; applied to nontherapeutic foreign substances, collectively referred to as xenobiotics, the equivalent term toxicogenetics is used (Nebert, 1999; Mancinelli, 2000; Wolf, 2000; Park & Pirmohamed, 2001; Roses, 2002). The term "pharmacogenomics," which was more recently coined, typically refers to alterations in gene expression that occur because of exposure to drugs. On the other hand, we frequently use the terms pharmacogenetics and pharmacogenomics interchangeably.

The identification of the molecular genetic bases for interindividual variations in susceptibility to the anticipated effects of a drug or of xenobiotics is one of the goals of pharmacogenetics (Pirmohamed & Park, 1999). This is one of the goals of the field of pharmacogenetics. If we are interested in providing a contemporary interpretation of the well-known assertion made by Paracelsus (1493–1541), it is true that "the dose makes the poison," but the degree to which this is true varies from person to person, depending on the genetic characteristics of the individual.

Despite extensive and well-regulated registration processes for proving drug efficacy and drug safety, adverse drug reactions (ADRs) are a common cause of morbidity and mortality. Furthermore, they are associated with substantial costs of medical care (Lazarou, 1998; Pirmohamed, 1999). There is no doubt that ADRs are a common cause of morbidity and mortality.

The origins of addictions, which are a diverse set of common and complex diseases that are, to some extent, linked together by shared genetic and environmental etiological factors (Kendler, 2003; Goldman, 2005), could also be clarified through genetic studies. From the level of the individual to that of the family, community, and society, the use and abuse of substances, whether they are legal or illegal, is a global public health priority that includes repercussions that extend beyond the individual.

2.2. Adverse Drug Reactions

According to Edwards (2000), when a substance can produce a therapeutic effect, it also has the potential to produce unwanted or adverse effects. The risk of such effects can range from almost nonexistent to exceptionally high. According to the World Health Organization's definition, an adverse drug reaction (ADR) is "a response to a drug that is noxious, unintended, and undesired effect of a drug, which occurs at doses used in man for prophylaxis, diagnosis, or therapy of disease, or for modification of physiological function." This definition pertains to the adverse effects that a drug may have on a person. This definition does not include therapeutic failures, intentional and accidental poisoning (also known as overdose), or drug abuse. Furthermore, this does not include adverse events that are the result of errors in drug administration or non-compliance (taking more or less of a drug than the prescribed amount). Furthermore, by using this narrow definition, it is possible to avoid overestimating the incidence of adverse drug reactions (Lazarou, 1998). The terms "adverse reaction" and "adverse effect" are interchangeable; however, it is important to keep in mind that the "drug" is the one that is experiencing an adverse effect, while the "patient" is the one who is experiencing an adverse reaction during treatment. However, it is important to differentiate between these two terms and the term "adverse event," which refers to a negative outcome that takes place while a patient is taking a medication but is not necessarily attributable to the medication itself (Edwards, 2000).

The thalidomide tragedy that occurred in the 1960s sparked an interest in adverse drug reactions (ADRs), and over the course of the past few years, ADRs have garnered attention all over the world. The Food and Drug Administration (FDA) has planned a system of pharmacovigilance that will be followed by regulatory agencies, pharmaceutical companies, and individual health care providers (U.S. Department of Health and Human Services Food and Drug Administration, 2005).

There is a correlation between the occurrence of adverse drug reactions (ADRs) and morbidity and mortality, as well as substantial costs associated with medical care. There are a great number of studies that provide a wide variety of epidemiological data concerning adverse drug reactions. In the United States, adverse drug reactions (ADRs) are one of the top 10 causes of death, accounting for more than 100,000 deaths each year. According to Lazarou (1998), adverse drug reactions are responsible for approximately 2–5% of all hospital admissions. As a result of an adverse drug reaction (ADR), 328 patients out of a total of 1937 patients who visited emergency departments in French public hospitals consulted a physician in 1999 (Queneau, 2007). This represents 21% of the patients who visited the emergency departments. In the year 2000, a prospective study was conducted in Italy over the course of two observational periods of 10 days each in 22 emergency departments. The study involved a total of 18 854 patients who were enrolled in the study. Out of these patients, 629 (3.3%) were affected by adverse drug reactions (ADR), and 244 (38.8% of ADR patients) reported experiencing a serious event (Trifirò, 2005). The incidence of lethal adverse drug reactions was estimated to be 0.95 percent in a prospective study conducted in Scandinavia with 13.992 patients who were receiving internal medicine treatment (Ebbesen, 2001).

According to the findings of another prospective study carried out in the United Kingdom, approximately 6.5% of hospital admissions were related to adverse drug reactions in a total of 18.820 patients (Pirmohamed, 2004). Throughout a six-year period (2001–2006), a nationwide study was conducted in Spain, which revealed that the total number of hospitalized patients with an adverse drug reaction (ADR) diagnosis was 350,835. This represents 1.69% of all acute hospital admissions (Carrasco-Garrido, 2010). Similarly, in the Netherlands, in 2001, 12 249 hospitalizations were coded as being related to an adverse drug reaction (1.83% of all acute hospital admissions) (van der Hooft, 2006).

The unfortunate reality is that a significant number of medical professionals continue to view adverse drug reactions as an exception rather than a primary diagnosis. Furthermore, adverse drug reactions have evolved into instances of medical professional liability, leading to a significant rise in the number of lawsuits (Wooten, 2010).

Type A reactions are common, predictable, and therefore potentially preventable, based on the pharmacological action of the drug, whereas type B reactions are more troublesome, uncommon, and unpredictable. The classification of adverse drug reactions (ADRs) distinguished dose-related reactions from non-dose-related reactions, using the names type A and type B, respectively. In more recent times, additional types have been introduced, including chronic (type C) and delayed (type D) effects, as well as withdrawal or end-of-use syndromes (type E) and therapeutic failures (type F) (Edwards, 2000). It is important to note that these types exist.

According to Mancinelli (2000) and Meyer (2004), different subjects with the same diagnosis may have different responses to the same drug when it is administered at the same dose. These responses may include a diminished, absent, or excessive response from the drug, or an interaction with other medications. Patients' age, gender, race, nutritional status, organ function, particularly of the liver and kidneys, co-morbidities, co-medication, as well as certain lifestyle variables (smoking habits, concurrent use of alcohol and drugs), and, of course, genetics are all potential risk factors for adverse drug reactions (ADRs). Previously thought to be unpredictable, some adverse drug reactions (ADRs) caused by genetic variation may now be preventable. According to estimates, genetic factors are responsible for 15–30% of the interindividual differences in drug metabolism and response. However, for certain drugs, this percentage can reach as high as 95%. (2006) Evans (2004) and Weinshilboum (2003)

The implementation of "personalized medicine," which involves the screening of patients for polymorphisms associated with a drug response, typically carried out before the beginning of therapy, has the potential to reduce adverse drug reactions (ADRs). There are several gaps that limit the application of pharmacogenetics due to the complex nature of the drug response itself (Gervasini, 2010). Despite the significant progress that has been made in this field, only a small number of drugs, including cetuximab, dasatinib, maraviroc, and trastuzumab, are required to undergo a pharmacogenetic test before being prescribed.

In the field of genetics, in particular, this kind of policy anticipates the introduction of new and more advanced tests, such as DNA microarrays or DNA chips respectively.

2.3. Drug Addiction

Compulsive drug-seeking and drug-taking behavior persist despite serious negative consequences; continued use induces adaptive changes in the central nervous system that lead to tolerance, physical dependence, sensitization, craving, and relapse (Goodman, 2008). Drug addiction is a chronic disorder that relapses, and it is characterized by the presence of relapses. Since it is linked to a significant amount of morbidity and mortality, as well as violence and legal issues, this mental health disorder places a significant burden on those who are directly affected by it, as well as on health care systems and society in general.

The World Health Organization (WHO) estimates that approximately 2 billion people around the world consume alcoholic beverages, 1.3 billion people consume nicotine, and 185 million people use illegal drugs across the globe. The use of alcohol, nicotine, and illegal substances accounts for 10%, 12%, and 2% of the total cost of illness in Europe, respectively. They are responsible for these percentages (WHO, 2002).

The style of consumption that is becoming increasingly prevalent among younger subjects is characterized and defined using polydrug use, which includes the use of both legal and illegal psychoactive substances. There is yet another emerging market all over the world for an increasing number of psychoactive substances. These substances are difficult to recognize, which causes the diagnosis and treatment of patients to be delayed. Additionally, the compositions of these substances are not well known, and the effects of these substances have not yet been recorded by medical professionals.

Furthermore, in recent years, there has been a notable shift in the marketing of both legal and illegal drugs through online pharmacies, eliminating the need for a prescription. This is a phenomenon that has occurred in recent years. The younger generations are especially susceptible to this risk because they are more likely to make use of new technologies than older generations already are.

An additional significant emerging problem on a global scale is the use of prescription or over the counter (OTC) medications for purposes other than medical treatment. The term "over the counter" (OTC) medications refers to pharmaceuticals that are found on the shelves of markets, stores, and pharmacies and do not require a prescription to be purchased.

The several classes of medications that are commonly abused include analgesics opioids, which are most often prescribed to treat severe pain (morphine, oxycodone, hydrocodone, hydromorphone, codeine); central nervous system depressants, commonly prescribed to treat anxiety and sleep disorders (barbiturates and benzodiazepines); stimulants, which are used primarily to treat attention deficit disorder, attention deficit hyperactivity disorder (ADHD) and narcolepsy (dextroamphetamine and methylphenidate). Over-the-counter medications, such as certain cough suppressants (dextromethorphan), sleep aids (doxylamine), antihistamines (diphenhydramine), decongestants can be abused due to the psychoactive effects that they have (Lessenger, 2008).

There were approximately 7 million (M) people in the United States who reported using psychotherapeutic drugs for non-medical purposes in the previous month, according to the figures reported by the National Institute on Drug Abuse (NIDA) in 2009. Abuse of pain relievers (5.3. M), tranquilizers (2.0. M), stimulants (1.3. M), and sedatives (0.4. M) are the medications that are most frequently abused. According to the National Institute on Drug Abuse (2010), among boys aged 12 to 17 years, 8.3% reported abusing Vicodin (hydrocodone), and 5% reported abusing Oxycontin (oxycodone hydrochloride). This indicates that drug abuse is especially problematic, especially among adolescents.

Abuse of any substance has the potential to cause dependence and withdrawal symptoms associated with the substance. It is currently a challenge to transfer the significant increase in knowledge regarding the neurobiology of addiction in patients who are struggling with addiction and to identify specific genes that are responsible for the vulnerability or resistance to addiction. According to Merikangas (2003), there are schools of thought that addiction can be completely avoided through the implementation of appropriate legislative measures and the exercise of individual choice. These schools of thought also assert that genetic research in this area should be considered a low priority. On the other hand, genetic research plays a very significant role because the origins of addiction susceptibility are multifaceted and extensive. It is necessary to identify the underlying genetic factors to solve the mystery of what causes these pervasive and relatively intractable disorders (Goldman, 2005).

According to Bevilacqua (2009), the initiation of the use of addictive agents and the conversion from use to addiction are both influenced by a combination of genetic and environmental factors. The percentage of the risk of developing a substance abuse disorder that is due to genetic factors varies depending on the substance (Nestler, 2000). The evidence that comes from studies involving twins and adoption suggests that the risk is between 40 and 60%. Those who are addicted are suffering from complex disorders that involve the interaction of multiple genes and the environment (G x E). This variation could add to allelic variations that could produce effects on addiction susceptibility phenotypes through other routes.

These other routes could include differences in the pharmacokinetic characteristics of the substance, such as metabolism and biodistribution; differences in the rewarding properties of the drug; differences in the traits manifested by the addict, including personality differences; and differences in the addict's psychiatric comorbidities (Uhl, 2004). Genetic influences are more prominent in the later phases of developmental progression toward substance dependence. This indicates that there are two broad types of genetic predisposition to addiction: genetic profiles that make people more likely to find the acute effect of drugs rewarding, and genetic profiles that make people more or less likely to develop addiction if they use drugs (EMCDDA, 2009). Both types of predispositions are associated with the development of addiction. In conclusion, there is evidence that suggests that there is a genetic predisposition that is shared between the various substance use disorders. According to Young (2006), nearly 25–36% of the genetic influences of alcohol, nicotine, and cannabis problem use are attributable to factors that overlap with one another.

The inheritance of addictions has been investigated in a variety of ways, including research on families and adoptees; however, the patterns of correlations in monozygotic (MZ) and dizygotic (DZ) twins provide the primary reference for our understanding of the phenomenon. It has been demonstrated that the overall genetic influence on substance use disorders is consistent, and it is estimated that the heritabilities for most substance use disorders range from moderate to high (Wong, 2008). The fact that addiction is initially dependent on an individual's choice to use an addictive agent may appear to be a paradox on account of this moderate to high inheritance. Cocaine and opiates, which are among the substances that are the most addictive, are also among the substances that are the most heritable. Hallucinogens, on the other hand, are among the substances that are the least addictive and the least heritable (Bevilacqua, 2009).

There are a great number of genes that are involved in the diagnosis of the condition (Kreek, 2005). There is a lack of clarity regarding the heritability of addiction to drugs of abuse, and the phenotype with which addiction to drugs is associated is not well defined. According to Buckland (2008), knowing the genetic factors that play a role in the etiology and treatment response may make it possible to facilitate the individualization of both prevention and treatment, as well as the identification of new therapeutic targets.

2.4. Pharmacogenetic Approaches

Two different methodological approaches can be utilized in pharmacogenetic research: the candidate gene approach and the genome-wide linkage analysis procedure. To determine whether alleles of marker genes are found more frequently in individuals who have the disease than in healthy subjects, linkage analysis is applied to families that contain multiple affected individuals. Markers that are uniformly distributed on all chromosomes are used to analyze the entire genome. The goal of this analysis is to identify regions of the genome that may contain genes that are involved in the susceptibility to complex disorders. There is only a search for the linkage in more recent ancestors. Linkage analysis is likely to uncover large gene regions that contain hundreds or even thousands of genes. This is because only a small number of recombination events are involved in the situation. There has been a significant amount of use of genetic association studies to identify regions of the genome and candidate genes that contribute to complex disease. These studies evaluate the correlations between genetic variants and differences in traits on a population scale.

A disease-associated single nucleotide polymorphism (SNP) that is located within a gene can provide information on the mechanistic basis for disease. On the other hand, an SNP that is in linkage disequilibrium with a genetic allele that confers disease predisposition can be used to identify individuals who are susceptible to disease. Naturally, this can include genetic variations that influence relative susceptibility or resistance to toxicants (Roses, 2000). In association studies of complex diseases, the most common types of errors that can occur are as follows: a small sample size, subgroup analysis and multiple testing, random error, a poorly matched control group, failure to attempt study replication and failure to detect linkage disequilibrium with adjacent loci, overinterpreting results and positive publication bias, and unwarranted candidate gene declaration after identifying association in an arbitrary genetic region (Cardon, 2001). According to Risch (2000), the power of association analysis to detect genetic contributions to complex diseases can be significantly greater than that of linkage studies. This is even though these limitations are already known.

Family-based association studies, which employ the transmission disequilibrium test, and population-based association studies, which employ case-control testing, are two distinct types of association studies. With case-control studies, researchers compare the genes of two distinct groups of people: healthy and diseased. In an ideal scenario, the two groups should be identical, with subjects matching for characteristics such as age, ethnicity, years of education, and marital status, and the only thing that would differentiate them is the disease that was researched. Allele frequency of gene markers, such as single nucleotide polymorphisms (SNPs), that are located in or close to the genes is analyzed, and frequency differences between the groups are taken into consideration to determine whether or not the gene is a contributor to the disease.

Since association studies are based on historical recombination, disease-associated regions in outbred random mating populations are extremely small and consist of only a single gene or gene fragment. The mutation that causes the disease will be separated from the alleles that make up its original haplotype through the process of recombination as it is passed down from one generation to the next.

Using association studies, it is possible to determine a particular genetic profile, also known as a haplotype, which is the combination of allelic states in a set of polymorphic markers that are located on the same chromosome. This is accomplished by analyzing several markers of a particular chromosome region in a group of affected subjects and in a control group, specifically in a case-control study. A population can contain a variety of haplotypes because of genetic recombination because of mutation. The genetic distance between markers and the characteristics of the locus where they are found (also known as recombination hotspots) are the primary factors that determine the recombination. The phenomenon known as linkage disequilibrium (LD) is characterized by the presence of markers that do not undergo recombination. Due to decreased rates of genetic recombination or the absence of genetic recombination, certain alleles at distinct loci tend to be co-inherited. This tendency can lead to the association of these alleles in a population, which is referred to as LD. At least in certain regions of the genome, recent LD studies that employed the analysis of SNP haplotypes have suggested the existence of a block structure. It is possible to recognize haplotype blocks as regions that are composed of consecutive alleles that are inherited together. Considering the limited haplotype diversity that exists within blocks, several SNPs will be redundant. This will allow for a minimum number of informative markers to be utilized to identify the common haplotypes that are present in each block. These markers are referred to as tag-SNPs. Different block structures can be found in different populations, which has significant implications for association studies. This is because tag-SNPs that are identified in one population will be useless in another population if they are found in different blocks.

2.5. Ethical Issues

It is imperative to contemplate the utilization of information derived from the human genome. The gathering of genetic data has garnered significant public scrutiny due to the potential ethical, moral, and political implications associated with its utilization. Genome-wide association studies, which aim to identify genes that have a minor impact on common diseases, can only be conducted on a global level. Furthermore, it is increasingly evident that genomic information is difficult to conceal. Therefore, the conventional assurance in research that privacy will be safeguarded seems to be less feasible. The decoding of the genetic code may jeopardize the safeguarding of an individual's privacy; certain variations that forecast drug response also serve as indicators for susceptibility to diseases. This could potentially result in medico-legal consequences, specifically regarding the matter of data confidentiality. It raises the question of whether employers and insurance companies should have the authority to access genetic data (Koo, 2006). Having access to genetic information could potentially result in discrimination against individuals who have an unfavorable genetic makeup. For instance, individuals who have a genetic predisposition for a particular condition or who require expensive medications may be subjected to higher insurance premiums (Vijverberg, 2010).

Most European nations have implemented genetic anti-discrimination laws, with Belgium being the pioneer in 1990, subsequently inspiring several other countries to do the same. The Genetic Information Nondiscrimination Act (GINA) was enacted into law on May 21, 2008, following a 13-year struggle in Congress, which was longer than the time it took to map the human genome. Francis Collins, the director of the National Human Genome Research Institute, stated that the enactment of the legislation was crucial for the achievement of personalized medicine.

According to Van Hoyweghen and Horstman, the genetic non-discrimination laws in Europe may not actually offer effective protection. They argue that these laws only create the appearance of safeguarding individuals from discrimination based on predictive medical information, but the level of protection against such risks is still insufficient. Certain insurance companies may continue to utilize genetic test results or genetic information obtained from physician records or insurance questionnaires (Van Hoyweghen, 2008). The prevalence of this practice is primarily attributed to a lack of knowledge, perplexity, and misinterpretation. Additionally, the absence of precise legal definitions for 'genetic data' and 'genetic tests' contributes to this issue (Vijverberg, 2010). A comprehensive analysis was conducted on the definitions of genetic testing employed by 65 different organizations and entities, such as genetics professional organizations, insurance companies, pharmaceutical firms, and legal entities. The study revealed a significant degree of variability in the definitions used, ranging from DNA testing alone to encompassing any reliable source of genetic information, including family history (Sequeiros, 2005).

Roses (2002) suggests that ethical concerns regarding the use of genetic data can be reduced by focusing on selecting single nucleotide polymorphisms (SNPs) that have pharmacogenetic and toxicogenetic significance, and avoiding those that are associated with genetic diseases.

Toxicogenetics can benefit from the knowledge and techniques used in forensic sciences. One such technique, known as "genetic fingerprinting," involves the use of a small number of genetic markers that are highly variable and not linked to any known health implications in individuals (Orphanides & Kimber, 2003).

A Closer Look

Opiods in Forensic Science

Opioids, a class of drugs primarily used for pain relief, have become a significant focus in forensic science due to their complex effects on human health and their role in the ongoing public health crisis of opioid addiction. In forensic science, opioids are studied extensively to understand their impact on individuals, their potential for abuse, and their involvement in deaths and other legal matters.

Opioids include a range of substances, from prescription medications like oxycodone, hydrocodone, and morphine to illicit drugs such as heroin. Their primary mechanism of action involves binding to opioid receptors in the brain and spinal cord, which can provide effective pain relief but also leads to the risk of dependence, addiction, and overdose. In forensic contexts, opioids are scrutinized to determine their presence and role in cases of overdose deaths, drug-related crimes, and various legal investigations.

One of the critical applications of forensic science concerning opioids is the investigation of overdose deaths. Toxicologists and forensic pathologists perform detailed analyses to detect the presence and concentration of opioids in biological samples such as blood, urine, and tissue. These analyses are essential for confirming opioid toxicity and understanding its role in causing death. In cases of suspected overdose, forensic experts assess whether opioids were the primary cause or if there were contributing factors such as poly-drug use or underlying health conditions.

Forensic toxicology involves not only detecting opioids but also identifying their metabolites. Metabolites are the byproducts of drug metabolism, and their presence can provide information about the timing of drug use and the level of exposure. Forensic scientists use sophisticated analytical techniques such as gas chromatography-mass spectrometry (GC-MS) and liquid chromatography-tandem mass spectrometry (LC-MS/MS) to achieve accurate and reliable results. These methods allow for the precise quantification of opioid levels, which can be crucial in legal cases to establish whether an overdose was accidental or intentional.

In addition to their role in overdose investigations, opioids are also examined in the context of drug-related crimes. Forensic scientists may be involved in analyzing drug seizures, identifying counterfeit or adulterated drugs, and tracing the sources of illegal opioid distribution. The presence of opioids in a suspect's possession, or evidence of opioid trafficking, can significantly impact legal proceedings, influencing charges, sentencing, and criminal investigations.

The opioid crisis has led to increased scrutiny of opioid prescribing practices and regulatory compliance. Forensic experts may be called upon to review medical records and prescription histories to determine whether opioids were prescribed appropriately and whether there were signs of misuse or diversion. This aspect of forensic science is essential for addressing the broader implications of opioid addiction and ensuring that medical practices align with legal and ethical standards.

The intersection of opioids and forensic science also includes the development and evaluation of harm reduction strategies. Forensic professionals contribute to public health initiatives by providing data on overdose patterns, evaluating the effectiveness of interventions such as naloxone (an opioid antagonist used to reverse overdoses), and supporting policy changes aimed at mitigating the impact of opioid misuse.

From investigating overdose deaths and drug-related crimes to evaluating prescribing practices and contributing to public health efforts, forensic scientists provide critical insights that help address the complexities of opioid use and its consequences. Their work is essential for understanding and managing the challenges associated with opioids, ultimately contributing to the broader goal of improving public safety and health.

Summary

Pharmacogenetics is currently in its early stages but has the potential to significantly enhance clinical practice as a valuable biomedical tool in the post-genomic era. The objective is to assist physicians in selecting the appropriate medication for an individual, to achieve optimal effectiveness and minimal toxicity. This is done through a genetic test, in accordance with the new approach known as "personalized medicine." The concept involves prescribing the correct drug at the correct dosage to the appropriate patient, considering their specific health requirements and individual traits.

Forensic practice should incorporate advanced diagnostic analyzes, genetic counseling, and an interdisciplinary and multidisciplinary approach that encompasses neurobiological, genetical, toxicological, psychological, and social sciences.

Pharmacogenetics, although a new idea in forensic science, has the potential to aid in understanding drug-related deaths, especially in cases of unintentional drug poisonings where the cause of death is uncertain (Pilgrim, 2010). The 11th recommendation of the report from the National Academy of Sciences (NAS) titled "Strengthening Forensic Science in the United States: A Path Forward" focuses on enhancing medicolegal death investigations. It suggests that best practices should involve the use of advanced technologies, such as laboratory testing to examine the molecular causes of diseases.

However, the forensic science community has not fully implemented this directive, and only a few studies have been able to establish a correlation between genotype and phenotype for a limited number of drugs and link them to death (Levo, 2003; Koski, 2006, 2007; Launiainem, 2010).

The relationship between genotype and phenotype continues to be a constraint in a molecular autopsy and is complex for several reasons. Only individuals who completely lack the activity of the enzyme (PMs) show a strong correlation with the expected phenotype. There is significant similarity in the activity observed both within and between the different phenotypic classes. Even individuals with the same genetic makeup can display varying phenotypic activities, which can be attributed to factors specific to certain populations. These factors include unidentified genetic elements, such as other enzymes and proteins, as well as non-genetic factors like diet. Furthermore, the genetic variation may have specific effects on substrates, such as drugs or their metabolites, as demonstrated by Gaedigk (2008) and Sajantila (2010).

Pharmacogenetics provides new opportunities for forensic scientists to analyze genetic variations associated with the risk of adverse drug reactions (ADRs) or susceptibility to drug addiction. These analyzes are highly valuable in evaluating drug addiction at all stages of its development, from initiation to advanced stages. Gaining a more comprehensive comprehension of the genetic predisposition to addiction could also be valuable for determining the origins and conditions leading to death. Certain genetic variants may indeed make certain individuals more susceptible to the substance, resulting in a higher risk of toxic effects, potentially even leading to death.

References

1. Esposito, M., Montana, A., Liberto, A., Filetti, V., Nunno, N. D., Amico, F., Salerno, M., Loreto, C., & Sessa, F. (2021). Anaphylactic death: A new forensic workflow for diagnosis. *Healthcare, 9*(1), 117. https://doi.org/10.3390/healthcare9010117.
2. Ferrara, M., Sessa, F., Rendine, M., Spagnolo, L., De Simone, S., Riezzo, I., & Maglietta, F. (2019). A multidisciplinary approach is mandatory to solve complex crimes: A case report. *Egyptian Journal of Forensic Sciences, 9*(1), 1–7. https://doi.org/10.1186/s41935-019-0133-2.
3. Filetti, V., Di Mizio, G., Rendine, M., Fortarezza, P., Ricci, P., Pomara, C., & Sessa, F. (2019). Volatile organic compounds: Instrumental and canine detections link an individual to the crime scene. *Egyptian Journal of Forensic Sciences, 9*(1), 1–11. https://doi.org/10.1186/s41935-019-0146-x.
4. Fineschi, V., Neri, M., Di Donato, S., Pomara, C., Riezzo, I., & Turillazzi, E. (2006). An immunohistochemical study in a fatality due to ovarian hyperstimulation syndrome. *International Journal of Legal Medicine, 120*(5), 293–299. https://doi.org/10.1007/s00414-006-0125-1.
5. Kupiec, T. C., Raj, V., & Vu, N. (2006). Pharmacogenomics for the forensic toxicologist. *Journal of Analytical Toxicology, 30*(1), 65–72. https://doi.org/10.1093/jat/30.1.65.
6. Ledda, C., Iavicoli, I., Bracci, M., Avola, R., Senia, P., Santarelli, L., Pomara, C., & Rapisarda, V. (2018). Serum lipid, lipoprotein, and apolipoprotein profiles in workers exposed to low arsenic levels: Lipid profiles and occupational arsenic exposure. *Toxicology Letters, 282*, 49–56. https://doi.org/10.1016/j.toxlet.2017.11.013.
7. Ledda, C., Pomara, C., Bracci, M., Mangano, D., Ricceri, V., Musumeci, A., & Rapisarda, V. (2016). Natural carcinogenic fiber and pleural plaques assessment in a general population: A cross-sectional study. *Environmental Research, 150*, 23–29. https://doi.org/10.1016/j.envres.2016.05.012.
8. Lötsch, J., Skarke, C., Liefhold, J., & Geisslinger, G. (2004). Genetic predictors of the clinical response to opioid analgesics: Clinical utility and future perspectives. *Clinical Pharmacokinetics, 43*(14), 983–1013. https://doi.org/10.2165/00003088-200443140-00001.
9. Maiellaro, A., Perna, A., Giugliano, P., Esposito, M., & Vacchiano, G. (2021). Sudden death from primary cerebral melanoma: Clinical signs and pathological observations. *Healthcare, 9*(2), 341. https://doi.org/10.3390/healthcare9020341.
10. Monda, V., Salerno, M., Sessa, F., Bernardini, R., Valenzano, A., Marsala, G., Zammit, C., Avola, R., Carotenuto, M., Messina, G., et al. (2018). Functional changes of orexinergic reaction to psychoactive substances. *Molecular Neurobiology, 55*(8), 6362–6368. https://doi.org/10.1007/s12035-017-0602-2.
11. Montana, A., Rapisarda, V., Esposito, M., Amico, F., Cocimano, G., Nunno, N. D., Ledda, C., & Salerno, M. (2021). A rare case of suicide by ingestion of phorate: A case report and a review of the literature. *Healthcare, 9*(1), 131. https://doi.org/10.3390/healthcare9010131.
12. Orban, G., Bombardi, C., Marino Gammazza, A., Colangeli, R., Pierucci, M., Pomara, C., Pessia, M., Bucchieri, F., Benigno, A., Smolders, I., et al. (2014). Role(s) of the 5-HT2C receptor in the development of maximal dentate activation in the hippocampus of anesthetized rats. *CNS Neuroscience & Therapeutics, 20*(8), 651–661. https://doi.org/10.1111/cns.12151.

13. Pirmohamed, M. (2011). Pharmacogenetics: Past, present and future. *Drug Discovery Today, 16*(17–18), 852–861. https://doi.org/10.1016/j.drudis.2011.07.002.

14. Pomara, C., Fiore, C., D'Errico, S., Riezzo, I., & Fineschi, V. (2008). Calcium oxalate crystals in acute ethylene glycol poisoning: A confocal laser scanning microscope study in a fatal case. *Clinical Toxicology, 46*(4), 322–324. https://doi.org/10.1080/15563650801975692.

15. Poolsup, N., Li Wan Po, A., & Knight, T. L. (2000). Pharmacogenetics and psychopharmacotherapy. *Journal of Clinical Pharmacy and Therapeutics, 25*(3), 197–220. https://doi.org/10.1046/j.1365-2710.2000.00278.x.

16. Rapisarda, V., Loreto, C., Castorina, S., Romano, G., Garozzo, S. F., Musumeci, A., Migliore, M., Avola, R., Cinà, D., Pomara, C., et al. (2018). Occupational exposure to fluoro-edenite and prevalence of anti-nuclear autoantibodies. *Future Oncology, 14*(1), 59–62. https://doi.org/10.2217/fon-2017-0357.

17. Roses, A. D. (2000). Pharmacogenetics and the practice of medicine. *Nature, 405*(6785), 857–865. https://doi.org/10.1038/35015703.

18. Sessa, F., Franco, S., Picciocchi, E., Geraci, D., Chisari, M. G., Marsala, G., & Salerno, M. (2018). Addictions substance free during lifespan. *Acta Medica Mediterranea, 34*(6), 2081–2087.

19. Sessa, F., Salerno, M., & Pomara, C. (2021). Autopsy tool in unknown diseases: The experience with coronaviruses (SARS-CoV, MERS-CoV, SARS-CoV-2). *Medicina, 57*(3), 309. https://doi.org/10.3390/medicina57030309.

20. Spagnolo, L., Bertozzi, G., Ferrara, M., Fiore, C., & Sessa, F. (2018). From crime scene investigation to the identification of the cause of death: A muscle-popping case report. *Romanian Journal of Legal Medicine, 26*(4), 340–343. https://doi.org/10.4323/rjlm.2018.4.340.

21. Spear, B. B., Heath-Chiozzi, M., & Huff, J. (2001). Clinical application of pharmacogenetics. *Trends in Molecular Medicine, 7*(6), 201–204. https://doi.org/10.1016/S1471-4914(01)02058-1.

22. Tamminga, W. J., Wemer, J., Oosterhuis, B., De Zeeuw, R. A., De Leij, L. F., & Jonkman, J. H. (2001). The prevalence of CYP2D6 and CYP2C19 genotypes in a population of healthy Dutch volunteers. *European Journal of Clinical Pharmacology, 57*(10), 717–722. https://doi.org/10.1007/s002280100344.

23. Wolf, C. R., Smith, G., & Smith, R. L. (2000). Pharmacogenetics. *BMJ, 320*(7238), 987–990. https://doi.org/10.1136/bmj.320.7238.987.

Chapter 3

FORENSIC PSYCHIATRY

Contents

Introduction

Forensic psychiatry is a specialized field of psychiatry that focuses on the intersection between mental health and the legal system. It involves addressing the challenges that arise when dealing with mentally ill individuals who have committed crimes, and understanding how they navigate through various social systems. Modern forensic psychiatry has been positively influenced by four significant advancements: the improved comprehension and recognition of the connection between mental illness and criminal behavior; the refinement of legal criteria for determining legal insanity; the emergence of innovative treatment approaches for mental disorders that offer alternatives to incarceration; and the shifting societal attitudes and perceptions towards mental illness. This chapter examines the present extent of forensic psychiatry and the ethical quandaries that this specialized field is encountering on a global scale.

Forensic psychiatrists, originally a small and lesser-known group of psychiatrists focused on studying mental conditions and treating prisoners, have now become a well-established and respected group of highly specialized professionals. They have gained influence and are significantly impacting the field of psychiatry, as well as making significant contributions to the legal system. There have been doubts and concerns about the fundamental nature of forensic psychiatry, as well as its usefulness and ethical implications, associated with this status.

Modern forensic psychiatry has been positively influenced by four significant advancements: the progression in the medico-legal comprehension and recognition of the connection between mental illness and criminal behavior; the advancement of legal criteria to define legal insanity; the emergence of new treatment methodologies for mental conditions that offer alternatives to confinement; and the shifts in public attitudes and perceptions regarding mental conditions as a whole. The recent growth of forensic psychiatry has extended its focus beyond criminal prosecutions and the treatment of mentally ill offenders to encompass various other areas of law and mental health policy. This expansion can be attributed to four key factors (Dom et al., 2018; Khalil et al., 2022; Unützer, 2022).

Orientation and Directional Terms

Term	Definition	Illustration
Forensic Psychiatry	A branch of psychiatry that intersects with the legal system, focusing on the assessment and treatment of individuals involved in legal cases and their mental health evaluations.	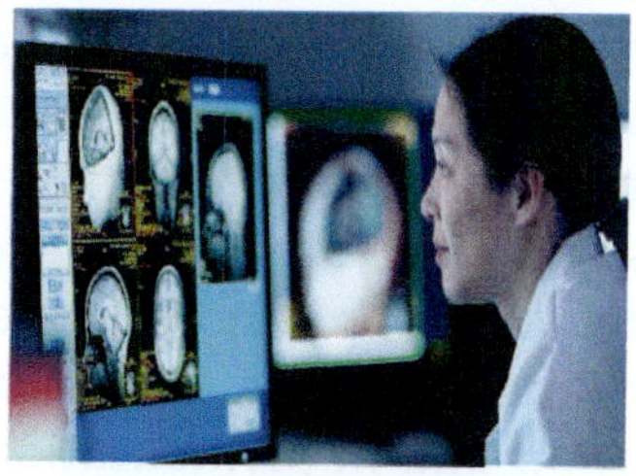
Mental Illness	A broad term encompassing various disorders that affect mood, thinking, and behavior, causing significant distress or impairment in functioning.	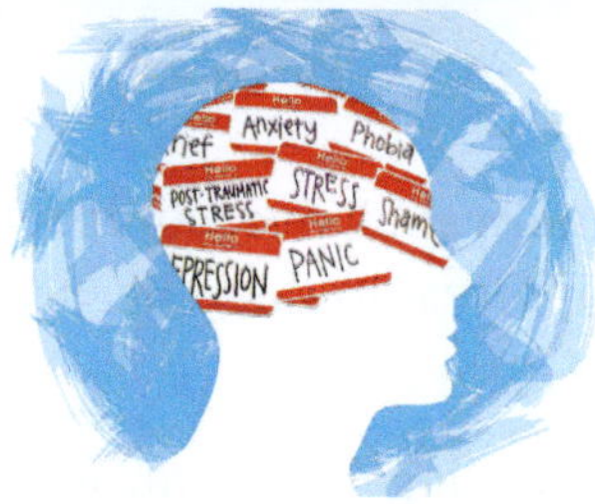
Psychiatrist	A medical doctor specializing in the diagnosis, treatment, and prevention of mental illnesses and emotional disorders, often prescribing medication and providing psychotherapy.	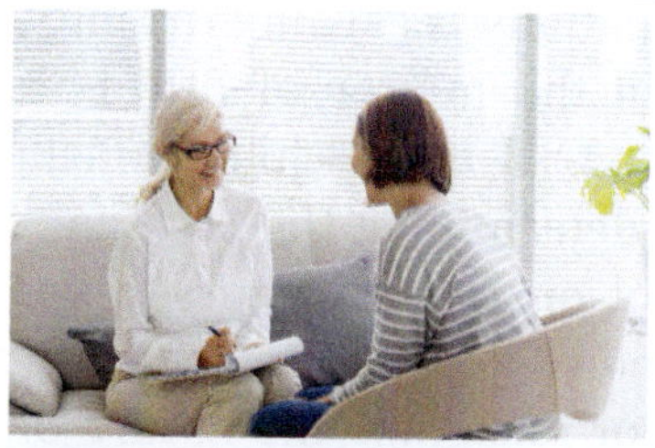
Neurocognitive Disorders	Disorders characterized by a decline in cognitive functioning such as memory, attention, and problem-solving skills, often associated with conditions like dementia.	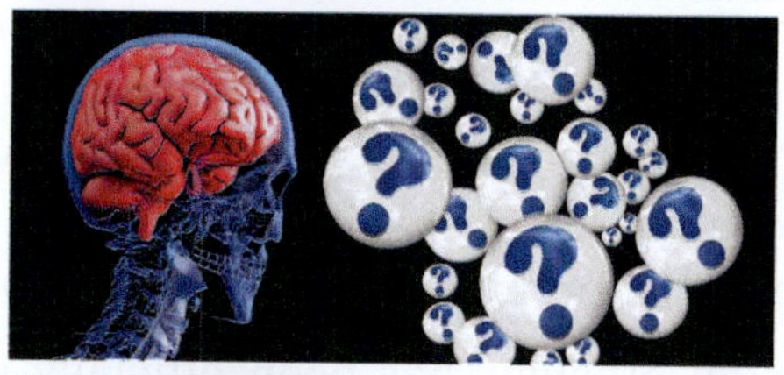
Penal Law	A body of laws that define criminal offenses, establish punishments, and regulate the legal procedures for addressing criminal behavior.	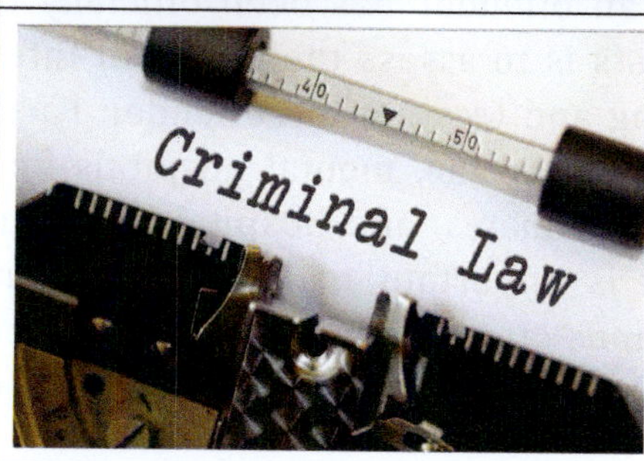

3.1. Scope and Challenges

Forensic psychiatry is a specialized field of psychiatry that focuses on the intersection between psychiatry and the legal system. However, this definition is somewhat limited as a significant portion of the work in forensic psychiatry involves assisting mentally ill individuals who have legal issues in navigating three distinct and incompatible social systems: mental health, justice, and correctional. The definition should be revised to state that forensic psychiatry is the field of psychiatry that addresses matters that arise at the intersection of psychiatry and the legal system, as well as the progression of mentally disordered offenders through various social systems. Forensic psychiatry focuses on matters that intersect with penal or criminal law, as well as evaluations in civil law cases and the creation and implementation of mental health legislation.

3.1.1. Penal Law

Globally, a more comprehensive comprehension of the correlation between mental states and criminal behavior has resulted in an escalated utilization of forensic specialists in various tiers of legal proceedings.

When entering the legal system, it is important to consider three main areas: the ability to stand trial, regulations regarding insanity, and applications related to dangerousness. Significant advancements in the matter of fitness to stand trial involve the decision to send defendants deemed unfit for trial to psychiatric facilities, to restore their ability to be tried. Clinicians face the question of determining the criteria to predict the likelihood of restoring competence, which should be based on a satisfactory response to treatment. Insanity regulations refer to legal criteria employed to determine whether the influence of mental illness on an individual's ability to comprehend or recognize the nature of a crime can be invoked to declare the offender as "not criminally responsible due to a mental condition," "not guilty because of insanity," or any other terminology employed in various countries. Applications to designate an individual as a "dangerous offender" typically require a significant level of proficiency from forensic experts. These experts are responsible for furnishing courts with technical and scientific data regarding the evaluation of risk and the forecasting of future acts of violence.

After an offender has been officially determined guilty, a crucial responsibility for forensic psychiatrists is to assess the extent of interaction between various types of institutions involved in receiving and treating the offender. Facilities catering to the mentally ill, such as hospitals for the criminally insane, mental hospitals for civilly committed patients, penitentiary hospitals for mentally ill inmates, and hospital wings in local jails, are all components of the mental health system. It is important to recognize their interdependence to achieve system integration and allocate funds effectively. The management of mentally ill inmates in prisons is a significant cause for concern. Table 3.1 displays a selection of the presently accessible options.

Table 3.1. Models for the Delivery of Mental Health Care to Mentally Disordered Offenders

Ambulatory treatment within prison
Mental patients remain with other inmates in the regular cells and tiers of the prison and come for visits to the infirmary during psychiatric clinic
Special wing within the prison
Mental patients are transferred to this wing for the duration of the episode or duration of their incarceration
Specialized security hospitals (penitentiary hospitals)
Mental patients or those with special criminal pathology such as sexual offenders are transferred out to these hospitals, usually for the duration of their incarceration
Contractual arrangements with outside psychiatric facilities
Mental patients are transferred out to these hospitals or psychiatric units for the duration of the episode
Forensic community corrections
Every effort is made to prevent that mental patients enter the prison system or, if released from prison, to ensure that they not go back

Source: Watson, R., Stimpson, A., & Hostick, T. (2004).

Upon release from the legal-correctional system, forensic psychiatrists are responsible for offering their specialized expertise in areas including parole eligibility, recidivism predictions, relevant commitment laws for released offenders, and the occurrence of repeated incarcerations and hospitalizations for mentally ill individuals.

3.1.2. Civil Law

Psychiatrists and other mental health professionals frequently need to perform assessments to ascertain the existence of mental or emotional issues in one of the individuals involved. These assessments are necessary in various scenarios, including exams to determine the effects of injuries on a third party in a car accident, assessments of the ability to create a will or engage in contracts, psychological investigations to evaluate mental capacity in cases of suicide or sudden death, and evaluations to determine fitness for work and eligibility for disability insurance benefits. Typically, these situations involve assessing an individual's ability and expertise to carry out a specific task, or evaluating the independent decision-making abilities of individuals with impairments. When someone is deemed incapable and incompetent, it is a way for society to exert control over them and justify imposing certain restrictions on that person. Clinicians are obligated to ensure that their decisions are thoroughly grounded in the most reliable clinical evidence, which entails an elevated ethical responsibility.

Typically, there is an assumption of capability and, therefore, that a specific individual is proficient. An individual is presumed to possess the necessary skills and abilities to make decisions unless evidence is presented to demonstrate otherwise. Merely having a significant mental or physical ailment does not automatically result in a lack of ability, either in general or for particular tasks. Furthermore, even if a person has a condition that could potentially impact their ability, they may still possess the necessary skills to perform certain tasks. This is mainly due to the fact that their capacity may vary over time, and because competence is not a binary concept, but rather depends on the particular decision or function at hand.

Furthermore, a determination of incapacity should be subject to a specific time constraint, necessitating periodic reassessment. For instance, if someone has suffered a stroke, they may be unable to drive a motor vehicle and therefore considered unfit to drive. However, they may still possess the ability and skill to engage in contractual agreements or handle personal financial matters. Over time and through appropriate rehabilitation, the individual may regain the ability and skill to operate a vehicle. Typically, to assess a person's incapacity or gather information from them, their consent is required or a legal order must be obtained to compel their cooperation. It is recommended to utilize a capacity screening test and proceed with a comprehensive assessment only if the individual does not pass the screening test. This will avoid placing a difficult burden on the individual being assessed if they can easily pass the screening test.

3.1.3. Mental Health Legislation and Systems

Forensic psychiatrists have gained a profound understanding of the connections between the mental health system, the justice system, and the correctional system due to the recurring pattern of mentally ill individuals moving back and forth between mental institutions and prisons, known as the double revolving door phenomenon. Due to their participation in legal affairs, forensic psychiatrists have developed a significant interest in the creation and implementation of mental health laws. This is particularly focused on matters such as involuntary commitment, which in many countries is determined by the level of danger posed rather than solely the need for treatment. They also study the management of mentally ill offenders and the legal safeguards for individuals who are deemed incompetent. Forensic psychiatrists, who specialize in evaluating violence and predicting future violent behavior, are often asked to determine the level of risk posed by civilly committed patients with a history of violence.

The relationship between legislation, the establishment of comprehensive mental health systems, and the provision of care, whether in institutional settings or within the community, is highly interconnected. The mental health system in many countries is perceived to be adrift due to a combination of factors. These include mental health legislation that has excessively restrictive commitment clauses, even for short-term commitments. Additionally, the closure of old mental hospitals has led to deinstitutionalization. Furthermore, changes in health care delivery systems have resulted in shorter admissions to general psychiatric units and subsequent treatment in the community. Lastly, a significant number of mental patients are ending up in jails. The expansion of forensic psychiatry can be attributed to legal reforms and a greater willingness to embrace psychiatric interpretations of behavior. However, a more immediate factor is the substantial population of mentally ill individuals residing in forensic facilities, jails, prisons, and penitentiaries. The failures of the overall mental health system may be the underlying cause of the increasing significance of forensic psychiatry.

The primary factor frequently cited to account for the significant increase in mentally ill individuals entering the justice/correctional system is the deinstitutionalization policy that governments have adopted in the last five decades. Deinstitutionalization, in broad terms, refers to the legislative actions taken to shut down large mental hospitals and relocate patients to the community. This involves offering brief stays in general hospital psychiatric units, outpatient treatment choices, psychosocial rehabilitation, alternative housing, and other community services. Occasionally, these decisions were made without any deliberate planning or evaluation of the requirements of the patients who were to be relocated or released from institutional care. There was a lack of clarity regarding the nature of services to be provided and the characteristics of the communities where patients would be relocated. Consequently, the decisions were primarily based on rhetorical and political ideologies rather than sound scientific reasoning.

The concept and strategies of deinstitutionalization have received both acclaim and criticism. For certain individuals, deinstitutionalization is regarded as an enlightened, progressive, and compassionate collection of policies that have prioritized the well-being of mentally ill individuals in numerous communities. Deinstitutionalization has proven to be highly effective in this regard. Deinstitutionalization has been attributed to several positive outcomes. Firstly, it has led to greater patient engagement in their own care and rehabilitation. Secondly, it has prompted critical inquiries that challenge the prevailing therapeutic pessimism of the past. Thirdly, it has enhanced the visibility of mental patients in both the community and mainstream healthcare settings. Fourthly, it has facilitated a more accurate understanding of the disease process, which was previously distorted due to the adverse effects of long-term institutionalization. Additionally, it has stimulated research and learning in the field. Lastly, it has heightened awareness of the human and civil rights of individuals with mental illnesses.

However, deinstitutionalization has also been attributed to a multitude of adverse consequences. From a legal standpoint, deinstitutionalization has been criticized for contributing to an increase in litigation and the excessive legal and regulatory burden on psychiatric practice. On a social level, the mentally ill have been directly affected by a series of harmful consequences. These reports have documented the presence of "revolving door patients" (patients who require frequent and repeated admissions) and the increase in the proportion of chronically mentally ill individuals among the homeless population, which is estimated to be at least 30%. Even when housing is accessible, it is frequently found in dilapidated tenements located in inner cities or psychiatric enclaves within large urban areas. In these places, mentally ill individuals who have been displaced and disoriented wander aimlessly, engaging in self-conversations. Moreover, they are highly vulnerable to incidents of theft, sexual assault, mistreatment, and physical aggression. Some individuals perish due to hypothermia while living on the streets during extremely cold winter nights. Deinstitutionalization has been attributed to the criminalization and migration of mental patients from the mental health system to the justice/correctional system, as well as the manifestation of violent behavior among certain mental patients in the community.

The primary criticisms of deinstitutionalization now focus on the implementation of the idea, rather than the concept of reintegrating patients into their communities. Due to financial limitations or short-sighted management, mental hospitals in numerous communities have been rapidly emptied without the simultaneous development of sufficient community resources and alternatives, as originally intended by the policies.

To address the negative consequences of deinstitutionalization, it is important to recognize that there are alternative treatments to institutional care. These include improved medications that are more effective and widely accessible, as well as psychosocial treatment approaches that have been proven to effectively manage mentally ill individuals in the community. The establishment of mental health courts, diversion programs as alternatives to imprisonment, assertive community treatment, intense case management, and the implementation of community treatment orders, along with improved housing policies, indicate a societal effort to address the disparities resulting from deinstitutionalization and ensure stable housing for individuals with mental illness. Simultaneously, assessments of anti-stigma programs suggest that certain initiatives are effectively altering public perceptions of mental illness and enhancing understanding of the human rights concerns surrounding the treatment and care of individuals with mental health conditions in numerous countries (Dom et al., 2018; Khalil et al., 2022; Unützer, 2022).

3.2. Ethical Controversies

The practice of forensic psychiatry worldwide is filled with ethical dilemmas due to its dual role in medicine and law. A forensic psychiatrist is primarily a clinician who possesses both theoretical and practical expertise in general psychiatry and forensic psychiatry. They also have the necessary experience to make logical decisions based on a well-defined scientific foundation. Forensic psychiatrists are required to possess a comprehensive understanding of the legal definitions, policies, procedures, and precedents that pertain to the specific question or case at hand. Forensic psychiatrists need to be familiar with courtroom proceedings and can effectively and succinctly communicate their findings, even when faced with the challenging circumstances of cross-examination. Forensic psychiatry is a subspecialty that combines expertise in both psychiatry and law, allowing practitioners to apply their knowledge in legal contexts. This unique combination of knowledge forms the ethical basis for the field. The duality of expertise should be evident from the outset in how the forensic psychiatrist initially agrees to participate in an evaluation, how they approach the individual being evaluated, and the necessary precautions that must be taken. At this stage, the primary concern for the forensic psychiatrist is to ensure that the person being evaluated does not mistakenly believe that the psychiatrist will be acting as a regular doctor, with the duty to prioritize the patient's well-being and maintain privacy and confidentiality. In the field of forensic psychiatry, the evaluator is required to maintain a neutral stance and is unable to provide reassurance regarding confidentiality or privacy. This lack of reassurance can potentially harm the person being evaluated, regardless of their health status and the evaluator's medical background. As a result, forensic psychiatrists may also be involved in the process of treating mentally ill individuals as criminals.

Forensic psychiatrists are seen by some commentators as having a distinct social control function that distinguishes them from the ethical principles of medicine and psychiatry. These commentators are uncertain about whether forensic psychiatrists are functioning as physicians in their legal work – a perspective that has sparked significant controversy. The forensic psychiatrists' authority to act, from the beginning to their appearance in court, is derived from their status as a physician and their obligation to uphold medical ethics. However, the ultimate impact of forensic evaluations is typically determined by other parties. Forensic psychiatrists have an ethical duty to carefully examine their own intentions as well as the intentions and potential outcomes of those who employ them for evaluations. This includes assessing the methods used to gather data, the process by which the evaluator forms opinions, the preparation of legal materials such as reports, memos, and expert evidence, and, most importantly, the intended purpose of their findings.

A significant dispute arises from the dual responsibilities of forensic psychiatrists and other psychiatrists, including those in the military, regarding the utilization of psychiatric judicial hospitals in the Soviet Union and China. This controversy also involves psychiatrists' involvement in interrogations of prisoners and detainees, which may give rise to accusations of torture, particularly in the current context of heightened apprehension about terrorist activities. This entails surrendering confidential psychiatric records to interrogators, which could be utilized to identify the prisoner's weaknesses and vulnerabilities. It also involves offering advice on interrogation methods or actively engaging in deceptive tactics to gather intelligence. Forensic psychiatrists and physicians in general should not overlook the underlying motivations of those advocating for evaluations, considering the circumstances at hand. Engaging in any activity that may result in torture would be a significant violation of medical ethics. This serves as a clear reminder to forensic psychiatrists that they must adhere to medical ethical principles, regardless of the demands made by their superiors.

3.2.1. Psychopathology and Criminal Behaviors

Psychopathology is a scientific field that focuses on the study and analysis of psychological disorders. Psychopathology is frequently employed in practical contexts as a synonym for psychological distress, in addition to its primary definition. Psychological discomfort refers to a distinct clinical condition characterized by a significant decline in the cognitive, emotional, and behavioral functioning of an individual. The 5th edition of the Diagnostic and Statistical Manual of Mental Disorders, commonly known as DSM5, is the most extensively utilized reference for classifying and providing detailed explanations of psychological disorders along with their symptoms. This study provides a detailed discussion of various mental disorders outlined in the 5th edition of the Diagnostic and Statistical Manual of Mental Disorders. These include neurodevelopmental disorders, disorders associated with schizophrenia and other psychotic disorders, bipolar and bipolar-related disorders, depression disorders, anxiety disorders, obsessive-compulsive disorders, dissociation disorders, somatic symptom disorders, eating disorders, impulse disorders, sleep-wake disorders, sexual dysfunctions, gender complaints, disruptive disorders, substance use disorders, neurocognitive disorders, personality disorders, sexual deviation disorders, drug-induced movement disorders, side effects of medications, and other conditions that may be of clinical interest.

It is crucial to comprehend the symptoms of mental disorders and categorize them based on their symptoms in order to implement preventative measures for safeguarding mental well-being and providing treatment for declining mental health. Comprehending and categorizing the symptoms of mental disorders is crucial not only for safeguarding, preserving, and enhancing compromised health, but also for establishing, safeguarding, and maintaining social order. When considering social order, one of the initial concepts that arises is the presence of norms, rules, rights, laws, and the justice system. The presence of both the mental health field and the rights-law and justice system in establishing, protecting, and maintaining social order has paved the way for the development of forensic psychology.

Forensic psychology is a specialized field of applied psychology that involves the application of psychological knowledge and expertise in gathering, assessing, and presenting evidence for legal purposes. Throughout history, there has been a longstanding connection between the mental state and the law, which has led to the development of forensic psychology. Plato's "The Republic" delves into the psychological underpinnings of laws from previous periods. During the Middle Ages, there were continuous debates surrounding the issue of "insanity and criminal liability" in legal proceedings. This discussion also required an analysis of the correlation between psychopathology and criminal behavior. This study focused on periodically examining the psychological symptoms of prisoners in the context of their incarceration. Additionally, efforts were made to understand the impact of psychopathology on the development of criminal behavior. This study will focus on the impact of psychopathology on the development of criminal behavior. It will emphasize the significance of comprehending psychopathology in preventing criminal behavior, to avoid the labeling of criminals as "individuals with psychological disorders" and thereby avoid stigmatization (Dom et al., 2018; Khalil et al., 2022; Unützer, 2022).

3.2.2. The Relationship Between Psychopathology and Criminal Behavior

When analyzing the correlation between criminal behavior and psychopathology based on the DSM-5, it is important to initiate the investigation by focusing on neurodevelopmental disorders. Neuro-developmental disorders are defined by developmental disabilities that cause disturbances in individual, social, educational, and occupational abilities. These disabilities typically manifest in early childhood, often before the child begins formal education. Neuro-developmental disorders encompass a range of conditions such as intellectual disability, communication disorders, autism spectrum disorder, attention deficit hyperactivity disorder, specific learning disorder, motor disorders, and tic disorders. Neuroimaging studies provide evidence indicating that social cognition is processed in networks that involve the prefrontal cortex. Deficits in empathy are commonly seen in individuals with damage to the prefrontal cortex. Neurodevelopmental disorders, such as ADHD, autism spectrum disorders (ASD), specific learning disorders (SLD), and intellectual disability, have been found to hinder the development of empathy. The increasing prevalence of violent behavior in our society can be attributed to two key factors: the inability to accurately assess the underlying motivations behind others' emotions and actions, as well as the presence of anger control disorders. Thus, it can be asserted that there exists a direct correlation between a lack of empathy and engagement in criminal activities.

Expanding on the topic of schizophrenia and related psychotic disorders, schizophrenia is a psychiatric condition distinguished by the presence of delusions, hallucinations, disorganized behaviors, negative symptoms, and impaired social functioning. The 10th edition of the International Classification of Diseases (ICD) by the World Health Organization (WHO) categorizes schizophrenia and its related disorders as "Schizophrenia, Schizotypal and Delusional Disorders." Research has demonstrated that the presence of delusions, hallucinations, and confusion in individuals with schizophrenia can lead to engagement in criminal activities.

Regarding bipolar and related disorders as well as depression disorders, there have been studies indicating that individuals with manic disorders, characterized by explosive and exuberant affect, may have an increased propensity for violence. The risk of experiencing manic episodes is consistently higher in individuals who exhibit grandiosity, high self-confidence, and temper tantrums. Sexual harassment, fraud, and theft crimes can occur during the mania process. The motivation for impulsive murders committed by individuals diagnosed with depression can be attributed to factors such as narcissistic injury, perceived humiliation, or feelings of shame. Furthermore, it has been documented that cases of post-homicide suicide are commonly observed in individuals with psychotic disorders or severe depression.

Anxiety disorders involve a sense of uncertainty about present and future events. Anxiety can be described as a state of worry and uneasiness about a subjective situation that is unlikely to occur. The findings of the studies indicate that anxiety disorders are a consequence of criminal behavior rather than a causal factor for criminal behavior. The underlying cause for this phenomenon is believed to be the profound anxiety experienced by individuals who have engaged in criminal activities. This anxiety stems from the impending loss of personal freedom upon arrest, the prospect of cohabitating with unfamiliar individuals during detention, and the subsequent societal labeling as an "ex-convict" which erodes trust in them.

In the context of obsessive-compulsive disorder and related disorders, the psychoanalytic perspective suggests that obsessions stem from suppressed impulses. Obsessive-compulsive personality exhibits anal characteristics and demonstrates fixation on the anal stage of development. Freud posited that individuals who experience conflict arising from unresolved oedipal desires, which in turn causes anxiety, may revert back to the anal stage of psychosexual development as a means of alleviating this anxiety. Regression impacts both the ego and the superego, causing the superego to become more inflexible and primal. Essentially, three defense mechanisms are employed to manage aggressive and sexual impulses. The three psychological mechanisms are isolation, undoing, and opposition formation (also known as reaction formation). The process involves isolating and maintaining the impulse at the level of consciousness, separate from its emotional components, while focusing solely on its cognitive content. Undoing is the act of reversing or nullifying a previously performed or presumed action, by performing the opposite action, to avert negative consequences. The compulsive action can potentially be counteracted by a subsequent action, allowing the individual to alleviate ego-threatening and distressing obsessive thoughts. The opposite reaction refers to the emergence of behavioral patterns that are diametrically opposed to one's primary impulses.

No empirical research examining the relationship between Obsessive–Compulsive Disorder and Criminal Behavior has been identified in the existing body of literature. This is attributed to the notion that the inflexible superego inhibits the individual from surpassing societal norms. Nevertheless, in the presence of a stressful circumstance, an individual may also engage in criminal behavior by either interfering with their usual actions or persisting compulsively in their usual actions. This phenomenon is readily apparent in the criminal activities carried out by individuals in professional or high-status occupations.

Imagine a situation in which a doctor is highly anxious about catching a disease and declines to physically interact with a patient who has minor allergies. Similarly, a nurse who is excessively distrustful may administer additional medication to a patient because of uncertainty regarding their adherence to the prescribed medication schedule. If the patient dies as a result of the doctor's failure to intervene promptly and the nurse's administration of an excessive dose of medication, the nurse would be held accountable for committing a criminal act.

Continuing the discussion on trauma-related disorders and their triggering factors, this particular disorder is classified as a post-traumatic mental disorder that elicits fear, helplessness, or horror reactions in individuals. The condition is distinguished by the recurrence of the traumatic event, the avoidance of stimuli related to the trauma, and symptoms of heightened arousal. Research indicates that individuals who have experienced trauma often display heightened levels of anger and resort to alcohol and drug use as a means of managing the feelings of guilt and hyperarousal that arise from their inability to prevent the recurrence of the traumatic event. This intense manifestation of anger will heighten the inclination to engage in criminal conduct, including perpetrating acts of violence against others and participating in unlawful activities while under the influence of alcohol or drugs.

Dissociative disorders are a type of mental illness characterized by difficulties in memory, identity, emotion, perception, behavior, and sense of self. These symptoms have the potential to impair all aspects of mental functioning. Three prevalent symptoms of this disorder include amnesia, fugue, and multiple personality. Multiple personalities refer to the phenomenon where an individual experiences distinct and separate personalities and identities within themselves. At that moment, the dominant personality takes control of their attitudes and behaviors, as if the other personality is nonexistent. When the patient undergoes a shift to a second identity, they frequently experience a lack of recollection of their true personality. The true essence of one's character remains oblivious to the existence of any other personality. The shift from one personality to another is frequently abrupt. Every individual possesses distinct traits and qualities that define their personality. When exposed to a two-person psychological test, they yield entirely disparate outcomes. During abrupt shifts in personality, individuals may experience difficulty in recognizing and comprehending their surroundings and the individuals they are interacting with. Consequently, there is an elevated likelihood of engaging in criminal behavior.

Somatic symptom disorder refers to the condition in which an individual experiences heightened and disproportionate anxiety in response to physical symptoms. As previously stated, research findings indicate that anxiety disorders are a consequence of criminal behavior rather than a cause of criminal behavior. Anxiety disorders are a psychological state that occurs subsequent to engaging in criminal activities. The root cause of this phenomenon is thought to stem from the deep-seated anxiety felt by individuals involved in criminal behavior. This anxiety stems from the impending loss of personal freedom upon arrest, the prospect of cohabitating with unfamiliar individuals in confinement, and the subsequent societal labeling as an "ex-convict" upon release, which leads to a lack of trust from others.

Eating disorders are psychiatric disorders characterized by deteriorations in eating attitudes and behaviors, as well as the manifestation of weight control behaviors, leading to impairment in psychosocial and physical functions. Given that eating disorders involve behaviors aimed at weight control, their association with criminal behaviors is believed to be primarily confined to the realm of suicide.

Expulsion disorders, specifically excretion disorders, are frequently observed in childhood and have a detrimental impact on both the child and their family. These disorders are characterized by the child's inability to control their bladder or bowel movements following their age and developmental stage. Based on the definition of expulsion disorders, it is believed that there is no direct correlation with criminal behaviors.

In the context of sleep-wake disorders, the International Classification of Sleep Disorders categorizes sleep disorders into two main types: "dyssomnia" and "parasomnia." Dyssomnia refers to difficulties in starting or maintaining sleep, characterized by alterations in the duration, quality, and timing of sleep. Parasomnia, in contrast, refers to alterations and decline in behavioral and physiological aspects that occur during sleep, coinciding with the sleep phase. When analyzing the defenses in criminal cases, numerous instances of sleep disorders, particularly parasomnias, are employed as a defense strategy. Specifically, there were numerous instances in American courts where the occurrence of sleepwalking persuaded the jury of the defendant's innocence. These findings indicate that the occurrence of sleepwalking in parasomnia is associated with criminal behaviors.

Regarding sexual dysfunctions, gender complaints, and sexual perversion disorders, it is important to note that physiological responses to sexual stimuli in humans can be categorized into four distinct stages: arousal, plateau, orgasm, and resolution. Sexual dysfunctions refer to the lack of response or excessive stimulation in any of the stages of sexual activity. Sexual dysfunctions are typically categorized into three main groups: paraphilias, sexual identity disorders, and sexual dysfunctions. Perpetrators with these disorders were observed engaging in acts such as violating sexual autonomy and displaying sexually aggressive behaviors towards children, violating privacy and the inviolability of homes, and desecrating the body of the deceased after their death. Furthermore, the inclusion of the term "perpetrator" implies that the behaviors in question are indeed criminal in nature.

Disruptive disorders refer to a group of conditions that involve difficulties in controlling impulses and conduct. Impulse control disorders are marked by the repetitive inability of an individual to refrain from engaging in actions that are clearly harmful to themselves or others. On the other hand, destructive behavior disorders are characterized by behavioral issues such as aggression and non-compliance with rules. As per the DSM-5, the disorder can manifest in two different forms: one that begins in childhood and another that begins in adolescence. During the early stages of development, children with this disorder commonly exhibit physical aggression and struggle with forming relationships with their peers. The symptoms of the disorder typically manifest before the age of 10. ADHD and ODD are frequently present alongside the clinical presentation of other disorders. In the adolescent-onset subtype, there is no evidence of the disorder before the age of 10, and the disorder's impact on violent behavior and peer relationships is relatively mild. The magnitude of this disorder, characterized by physical aggression and disruption in peer relationships, is strongly correlated with criminal behavior, particularly in regard to violent conduct.

Substance addiction, also known as substance use disorder according to DSM-V, is a neurological condition characterized by a persistent or intermittent craving for substances and accompanying behavioral disturbances. These cravings are driven by the desire to experience the pleasurable effects of the substance or to alleviate the discomfort caused by its absence. Although numerous factors contribute to individuals engaging in criminal behavior, drug addiction can also be a significant catalyst for such actions. An individual's actions and behavior can potentially make them vulnerable to becoming a target of criminal activity. Upon reviewing the literature, one finds mention of the correlation between illicit drug use and criminal activities involving violence, aggression, and theft. In addition to drug-induced violence, aggression, and theft, crimes such as traffic accidents, media couriers, and sexual assault can also occur. Furthermore, individuals who are under the influence of substances may engage in various criminal activities, including but not limited to behavioral disorders, provocation, aggression, fraud, armed and unarmed attacks, blackmail, threats, and murder, all in pursuit of obtaining the substance they are using. Additionally, substance use can lead to traffic accidents, sexual abuse, and behaviors that pose harm to oneself and others. They have the potential to contribute to accidents and engage in criminal activities, such as substance abuse, while incarcerated.

When it comes to personality disorders, defining them can be extremely challenging. Personality disorders are widely recognized as the primary topic of diagnostic debate within the field of psychiatry. It is widely acknowledged that individuals who are not affected by mental disorders and exhibit persistent adjustment disorders are prevalent in all societies. The distinguishing factor between personality disorders and personality structure lies in the intensity or severity of the traits. To diagnose a personality disorder, it is necessary for the individual to exhibit significant disturbances over an extended duration, while still maintaining their capacity to function in society, hold steady employment, and maintain stable relationships. These ingrained behavioral patterns, which are inherent to the individual, persist without displaying adaptability and result in substantial impairment in both societal and professional settings. Numerous subcategories of personality disorders exist. Antisocial personality disorder (APD) is diagnosed in individuals who struggle to conform to social norms and consistently engage in behaviors that are deemed criminal by society. Individuals diagnosed with this condition are characterized by an inability to assume the required responsibilities in both familial and social settings. They frequently exhibit impulsive behavior and often demonstrate aggression.

Borderline personality disorder (BPD) is characterized by intense anger and impulsive behaviors. However, individuals with BPD also experience transient paranoid thoughts or severe dissociative symptoms during times of intense stress. These additional features increase the likelihood of engaging in criminal behavior. Furthermore, it is established that individuals with paranoid, passive-aggressive personality disorders and narcissistic tendencies have a higher likelihood of engaging in violent criminal activities during their adolescence and young adulthood. Individuals with multiple personality disorders may experience sexual dysfunctions, including sadomasochism, pedophilia, zoophilia, exhibitionism, and erotic asphyxia. These manifestations can occur in individuals regardless of their sexual orientation (Dom et al., 2018; Khalil et al., 2022; Unützer, 2022).

A Closer Look

Penal Law

Penal law in forensics is a fundamental aspect of the criminal justice system, guiding the application of legal principles to the investigation, prosecution, and adjudication of criminal cases. This area of law defines what constitutes criminal conduct, prescribes appropriate punishments, and establishes procedural rules for handling evidence and conducting trials. Understanding the interplay between penal law and forensic science is crucial for ensuring justice and maintaining the integrity of legal proceedings. Penal law are the statutes and regulations that delineate criminal offenses. These laws categorize crimes into various classifications, such as felonies, misdemeanors, and infractions, each with distinct legal implications and penalties. Forensic professionals must be adept at interpreting these classifications to align their investigative practices with legal definitions. For instance, the classification of a crime as a violent offense versus a property crime can significantly influence the type of forensic evidence that is relevant and the methods used to collect it.

Forensic science encompasses a wide range of disciplines, including forensic biology, chemistry, toxicology, and digital forensics. Each of these fields must operate within the confines of penal law, which dictates how evidence is to be collected, preserved, and analyzed. One of the key principles in penal law is the chain of custody, which requires meticulous documentation of evidence handling to prevent contamination, loss, or tampering. Forensic experts must follow strict protocols to ensure that evidence remains intact and admissible in court. Any deviation from these protocols can jeopardize the integrity of the evidence and, consequently, the outcome of the case.

Penal law also outlines the procedures for conducting criminal investigations. This includes the rights of suspects, such as the right to remain silent and the right to legal representation. Forensic professionals must be knowledgeable about these rights to ensure that their work respects legal protections and does not infringe upon constitutional guarantees. For example, evidence obtained through unlawful searches or coerced confessions may be deemed inadmissible in court, potentially undermining the prosecution's case.

The presentation of forensic evidence in court is another critical aspect governed by penal law. Forensic experts often serve as expert witnesses, tasked with explaining complex scientific findings to judges and juries in an understandable manner. Their testimony must be based on sound scientific principles and methodologies, as any lapses in accuracy or credibility can impact the verdict. Penal law sets the standards for the admissibility of expert testimony, ensuring that only reliable and relevant evidence is considered during legal proceedings.

The intersection of penal law and forensic science is crucial for maintaining the integrity of the criminal justice system and ensuring that legal proceedings are conducted with rigor and respect for individual rights.

Summary

- It is recognized that numerous mental disorders listed in DSM-5 are linked to criminal conduct, whereas some are associated with criminal behavior despite not directly causing it. Nevertheless, the aforementioned data should be utilized to enhance proactive mental health services, rather than categorizing wrongdoers as "mentally ill." Neurodevelopmental disorders are associated with impaired empathy and a propensity for impulsive behavior, which can contribute to an increased likelihood of engaging in criminal activities. While engaging in therapy with these individuals, the question arises: "What was his statement and what was my comprehension?" It is feasible to deter individuals from engaging in criminal activities by engaging in exercises or practicing impulse control techniques to enhance their capacity for empathy. To mitigate criminal behavior associated with schizophrenia, one can employ techniques such as recording phone calls during therapy sessions to demonstrate that auditory hallucinations are not grounded in reality or using video cameras to capture visual hallucinations. In the context of bipolar disorder, during a manic episode, the risk of engaging in criminal behavior can be mitigated by bolstering social support networks and ensuring close supervision by family or trusted individuals. To mitigate criminal behavior in individuals with sleep-wake disorders, it is advisable to implement basic precautions like securing the bedroom door, particularly for those who sleepwalk.
- Hormonal therapy can be used to treat sexual dysfunctions and prevent deviant behavior. Alternatively, individuals with sexual dysfunction can engage in daily activities to redirect their energy away from sexuality. To mitigate the likelihood of criminal behavior among children with impulse control and conduct disorder, it is crucial to offer early therapeutic intervention and enhance the awareness of their families. To prevent the development of antisocial personality disorder, it is important to apply appropriate treatment methods when childhood conduct disorder is detected in individuals with personality disorders. Furthermore, individuals diagnosed with borderline personality disorder can be deterred from engaging in criminal behavior through the implementation of impulse control investigations as part of their therapy.

References

1. Abi-Dargham, A., Moeller, S. J., Ali, F., DeLorenzo, C., Domschke, K., Horga, G., Jutla, A., Kotov, R., Paulus, M. P., Rubio, J. M., et al. (2023). Candidate biomarkers in psychiatric disorders: State of the field. *World Psychiatry*, *22*(2), 236–262. https://doi.org/10.1002/wps.21037.
2. Borum, R. (2003). Understanding the terrorist mind-set. *FBI Law Enforcement Bulletin*, *72*(1), 7–13.
3. Borum, R., & Fein, R. (2017). The psychology of foreign fighters. *Studies in Conflict & Terrorism*, *40*(4), 248–266. https://doi.org/10.1080/1057610X.2016.1155821.
4. Crouse, J. J., Ho, N., Scott, J., Parker, R., Park, S. H., Couvy-Duchesne, B., Mitchell, B. L., Byrne, E. M., Hermens, D. F., Medland, S. E., et al. (2022). Dynamic networks of psychological symptoms, impairment, substance use, and social support: The evolution of psychopathology among emerging adults. *European Psychiatry*, *65*, e32. https://doi.org/10.1192/j.eurpsy.2022.32.

5. D'Souza, D. C. (2023). Cannabis, cannabinoids and psychosis: A balanced view. *World Psychiatry*, *22*(2), 231–232. https://doi.org/10.1002/wps.21036.

6. Dom, G., Schouler-Ocak, M., Bhui, K., Demunter, H., Kuey, L., Raballo, A., Frydecka, D., Misiak, B., Gorwood, P., & Samochowiec, J. (2018). Mass violence, radicalization and terrorism: A role for psychiatric profession? *European Psychiatry*, *49*, 78–80. https://doi.org/10.1016/j.eurpsy.2017.11.002.

7. Doosje, B., Moghaddam, F. M., Kruglanski, A. W., De Wolf, A., Mann, L., & Feddes, A. R. (2016). Terrorism, radicalization and de-radicalization. *Current Opinion in Psychology*, *11*, 79–84. https://doi.org/10.1016/j.copsyc.2016.06.004.

8. Fusar-Poli, P., Sunkel, C., Larrauri, C. A., Keri, P., McGorry, P. D., Thornicroft, G., & Patel, V. (2023). Violence and schizophrenia: The role of social determinants of health and the need for early intervention. *World Psychiatry*, *22*(2), 230–231. https://doi.org/10.1002/wps.21035.

9. Isayeva, U., Manchia, M., Collu, R., Primavera, D., Deriu, L., Caboni, E., Iaselli, N., Sundas, D., Tusconi, M., Pinna, F., et al. (2022). Exploring the association between brain-derived neurotrophic factor levels and longitudinal psychopathological and cognitive changes in Sardinian psychotic patients. *European Psychiatry*, *65*, e71. https://doi.org/10.1192/j.eurpsy.2022.71.

10. Kestel, D. (2022). Transforming mental health for all: A critical role for specialists. *World Psychiatry*, *21*(3), 333–334. https://doi.org/10.1002/wps.21032.

11. Khalil, J., Horgan, J., & Zeuthen, M. (2022). The Attitudes-Behaviors Corrective (ABC) model of violent extremism. *Terrorism and Political Violence*, *34*(3), 425–450. https://doi.org/10.1080/09546553.2021.1910507.

12. McCauley, C., & Moskalenko, S. (2008). Mechanisms of political radicalization: Pathways toward terrorism. *Terrorism and Political Violence*, *20*(3), 415–433. https://doi.org/10.1080/09546550802073307.

13. McCauley, C., & Moskalenko, S. (2017). Understanding political radicalization: The two-pyramids model. *American Psychologist*, *72*(3), 205–216. https://doi.org/10.1037/a0040366.

14. McGilloway, A., Ghosh, P., & Bhui, K. (2015). A systematic review of pathways to and processes associated with radicalization and extremism amongst Muslims in Western societies. *International Review of Psychiatry*, *27*(1), 39–50. https://doi.org/10.3109/09540261.2014.973081.

15. Meyer-Lindenberg, A. (2023). The non-ergodic nature of mental health and psychiatric disorders: Implications for biomarker and diagnostic research. *World Psychiatry*, *22*(2), 272–274. https://doi.org/10.1002/wps.21042.

16. Misiak, B., Samochowiec, J., Bhui, K., Schouler-Ocak, M., Demunter, H., Kuey, L., Raballo, A., Gorwood, P., Frydecka, D., & Dom, G. (2019). A systematic review on the relationship between mental health, radicalization and mass violence. *European Psychiatry*, *56*, 51–59. https://doi.org/10.1016/j.eurpsy.2018.10.005.

17. Moghaddam, F. M. (2005). The staircase to terrorism: A psychological exploration. *American Psychologist*, *60*(2), 161–169. https://doi.org/10.1037/0003-066X.60.2.161.

18. Rejek, M., & Misiak, B. (2023). Dimensions of psychopathology associated with psychotic-like experiences: Findings from the network analysis in a nonclinical sample. *European Psychiatry*, *66*, e56. https://doi.org/10.1192/j.eurpsy.2023.56.

19. Schmid, A. (2013). Radicalization, de-radicalization, counter-radicalization: A conceptual discussion and literature review. *Terrorism and Counter-Terrorism Studies*, *4*(1), 1–24.

20. Steger, M. F. (2022). Meaning in life is a fundamental protective factor in the context of psychopathology. *World Psychiatry*, *21*(3), 389–390. https://doi.org/10.1002/wps.21040.

21. Tumminelli, G. (2020). Radicalization. In *Migrazioni in Sicilia 2019* (pp. 306–314). Mimesis Edizioni.

22. Unützer, J. (2022). Psychiatry in the 21st century: The glass is half full. *World Psychiatry*, *21*(3), 422–423. https://doi.org/10.1002/wps.21041.

23. Voineskos, A. (2023). The time is now to start evaluating biomarkers in the clinic. *World Psychiatry*, *22*(2), 267–268. https://doi.org/10.1002/wps.21038.

24. Yatham, L. N. (2023). Biomarkers for clinical use in psychiatry: Where are we and will we ever get there? *World Psychiatry*, *22*(2), 263–264. https://doi.org/10.1002/wps.21039.

Chapter 4

FORENSIC HISTOPATHOLOGY

Contents

Introduction

Forensic histopathology involves the use of histological techniques and examination in the field of forensic pathology. It is a distinctive and specialized facet of pathology practice. This chapter emphasizes various disparities in the practice of forensic histopathology in comparison to clinical and surgical histopathology. The different functions of microscopic tissue examination in the field of forensic pathology are classified and analyzed. These purposes include establishing a clear pathological diagnosis, verifying uncertain and hidden pathology, creating a permanent record, and offering valuable material for education and research. Case examples are provided to demonstrate the influence of routine histological examinations, special stain techniques, and immunohistochemistry, when applicable, on relevant pathological diagnoses. These diagnoses may or may not directly contribute to determining the cause of death. Finally, the chapter also seeks to emphasize recent breakthroughs and the obstacles that lie ahead in this area.

Orientation and Directional Terms

Term	Definition	Illustration
Histology	The branch of biology that studies the microscopic structure of tissues and organs. It involves examining tissues at the cellular level to understand their function and structure.	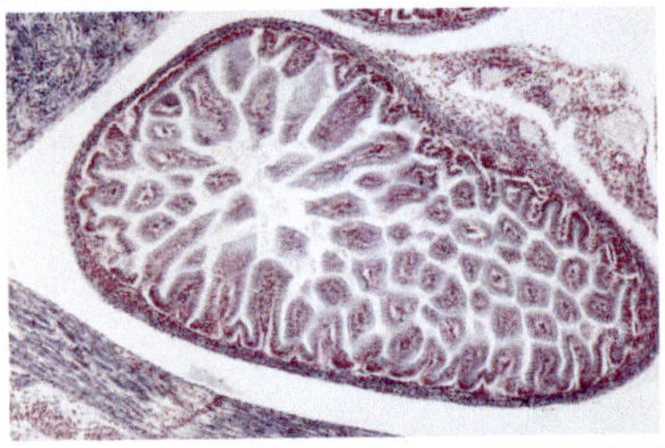
Lung	Pair of respiratory organs located in the chest cavity that facilitate the exchange of oxygen and carbon dioxide between the blood and the environment.	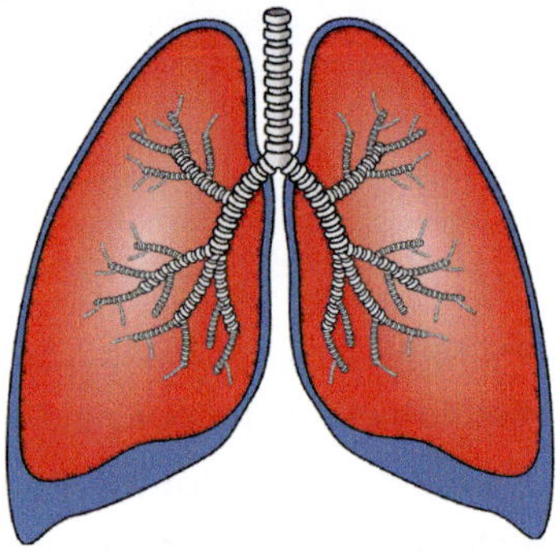
Liver	A large, vital organ located in the upper right abdomen that performs various functions, including detoxifying harmful substances, synthesizing proteins, and producing bile.	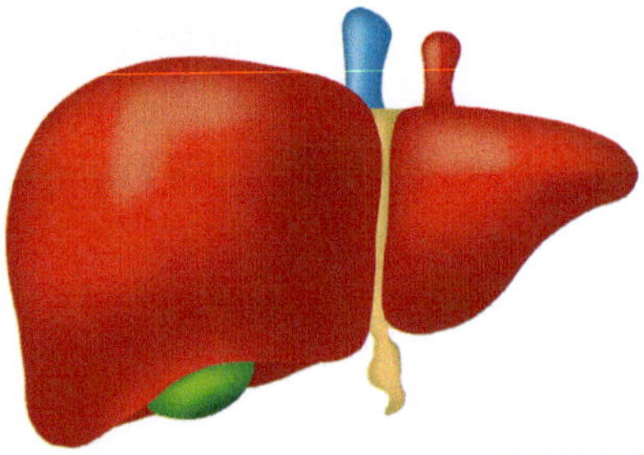
Brain	The central organ of the nervous system located in the skull that controls thought, memory, emotion, touch, vision, breathing, and all other activities that regulate the body.	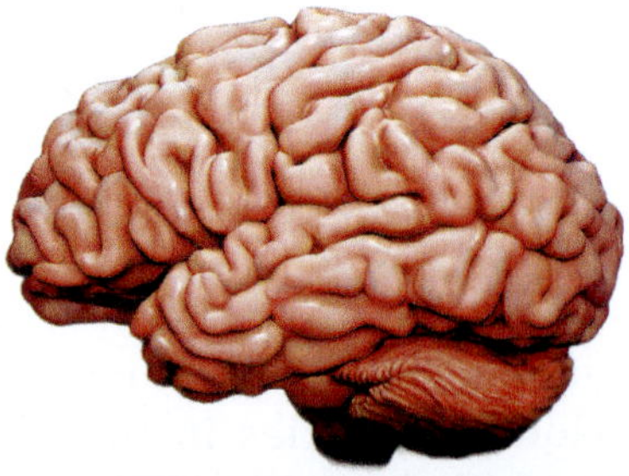
Kidney	Pair of bean-shaped organs located in the lower back that filter blood to remove waste products and excess substances, producing urine as a byproduct.	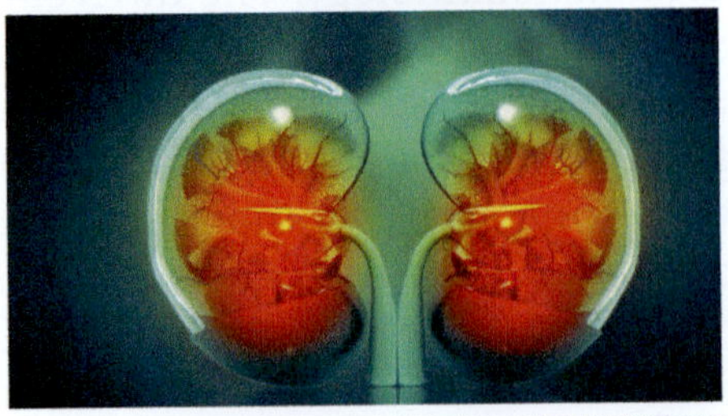

4.1. Histological Techniques in Forensic Pathology Practice

The utilization of histological methodologies and analysis in the field of forensic pathology is a distinct and specialized facet of pathology practice. There are several notable differences between clinical histopathology practice and the application of similar techniques. Specimens in forensic pathology practice and clinical histopathology practice differ significantly in nature. In the field of clinical histopathology, specimens and biopsies typically consist of portions, fragments, or sections of different organs. Diagnoses are made by examining histological sections of tissues that have been obtained through targeted sampling of the specimens, usually after proper fixation. On the other hand, the forensic pathologist regularly examines organs completely and initially in their unfixed condition.

The organs frequently exhibit varying degrees of autolysis and putrefaction. The initial stage of histological sampling and examination diverges from the beginning. Furthermore, there is a divergence in the range of organ and tissue analysis between the field of clinical histopathology and forensic pathology. Small biopsies of the breasts, aerodigestive tract, female genital tract, and other areas are essential components of the workload in histopathology practice. Biopsies of various organs, including the heart, lungs, liver, brain, and kidneys, are commonly analyzed in specialized histopathology practices. However, the forensic pathologist regularly examines complete hearts, lungs, livers, brains, and kidneys, albeit with a slightly different focus and emphasis. Although the breasts, intestines, and lymph nodes are also subject to examination, they receive less emphasis compared to the major organs that are more commonly linked to the cause of death. Being able to recognize visible abnormalities in unprocessed entire organs is a necessary requirement in the field of forensic pathology.

However, the forensic pathologist needs to possess the ability to identify abnormalities in all organs, thoroughly examine them, and provide accurate reports. Furthermore, the primary focus of histological examination of surgical and clinical specimens is to determine the diagnosis and predict the prognosis. The precise measurement of the distance between the edge of surgical specimens and neoplastic lesions is crucial for determining the appropriate course of action for further treatment and management.

The precise grading, meticulous typing, and accurate classification of different neoplasms are crucial for determining the appropriate treatment and predicting the prognosis. Conversely, the primary objective of the forensic postmortem examination is to accurately ascertain the cause of death. Frequently, the reason for death is readily apparent upon macroscopic examination, without the need for histological analysis. In such instances, all additional factors, such as incidental pathologies, can be regarded as having secondary or academic importance.

Thus, in the field of forensic pathology, it is frequently unnecessary to perform extensive tissue sampling of the primary parenchymatous organs for histology to determine the exact cause of death. Nevertheless, histological examination holds considerable influence in various cases (Sacco et al., 2022; Zapico & Adserias-Garriga, 2022).

4.2. The Roles of Histology in Forensic Pathology Practice

The major roles of histology in forensic practice are as follows:

1. As a primary ancillary investigation in cases where macroscopic examinations fail to yield a specific or diagnostic pathology that accounts for death
2. To confirm and refine macroscopic diagnoses including incidental pathologies identified at autopsy
3. To confirm or refute antemortem diagnosis and clinical suspicions
4. To evaluate medical and surgical interventions as a means of medical audit
5. As a form of permanent documentation of pathologies identified at autopsy
6. As an essential source of material for medical undergraduate and postgraduate teaching
7. As a source of research

The authors recommend the practice of routine sampling of major parenchymatous organs such as the heart, lungs, liver, and kidneys for histological examination. At the very least, this could sharpen the forensic pathologist's approach in correlating macroscopic pathology, observed or suspected, with microscopic pathology.

In the following sections, the roles of histological analysis in routine forensic pathology practice are illustrated.

4.2.1. To Establish the Cause of Death

The identification of the exact cause of death may rely on clarifying the microscopic characteristics of hidden or uncertain visible abnormalities. In such instances, the absence of a clear-cut pathology or the existence of borderline pathology necessitates additional confirmation for the diagnosis. Instances of abrupt fatalities caused by viral myocarditis are one such example, where the cellular reaction may exhibit a localized or scattered pattern, rather than being widespread.

Amniotic fluid embolism in cases of maternal deaths is diagnosed by observing the presence of amniotic fluid components in the pulmonary microvasculature, and sometimes in other organs like the kidneys and liver. The identification of epithelial squames, mucin, vernix caseosa (resembling fat), and sometimes lanugo hair can be effectively done using Attwood's stain (for squames and mucin). Alternatively, immunohistochemical epithelial markers, such as AE1/3, Cam 5.2, LP34, CK 7, and CK 20 can be used if needed.

To diagnose disseminated intravascular coagulation, it is crucial to detect microscopic fibrin thrombi in the pulmonary microvasculature and renal glomeruli. This can be done using Martius Scarlet Blue or phosphotungstic acid hematoxylin.

During the recent outbreak of severe acute respiratory distress syndrome (SARS), histological examination played a crucial role in confirming the diagnosis of a severe infectious disease caused by a new strain of coronavirus. The histological analysis of the lungs of individuals affected by SARS revealed widespread damage to the alveoli, with varying levels of organization. There were concurrent cellular changes observed, including abnormal cell morphology of lung cells, fusion of cells to form syncytia, and the formation of large multinucleated cells. These observations were made in deceased patients who had spent an extended duration in intensive care units and had received mechanical ventilation during that time (Figure 4.1).

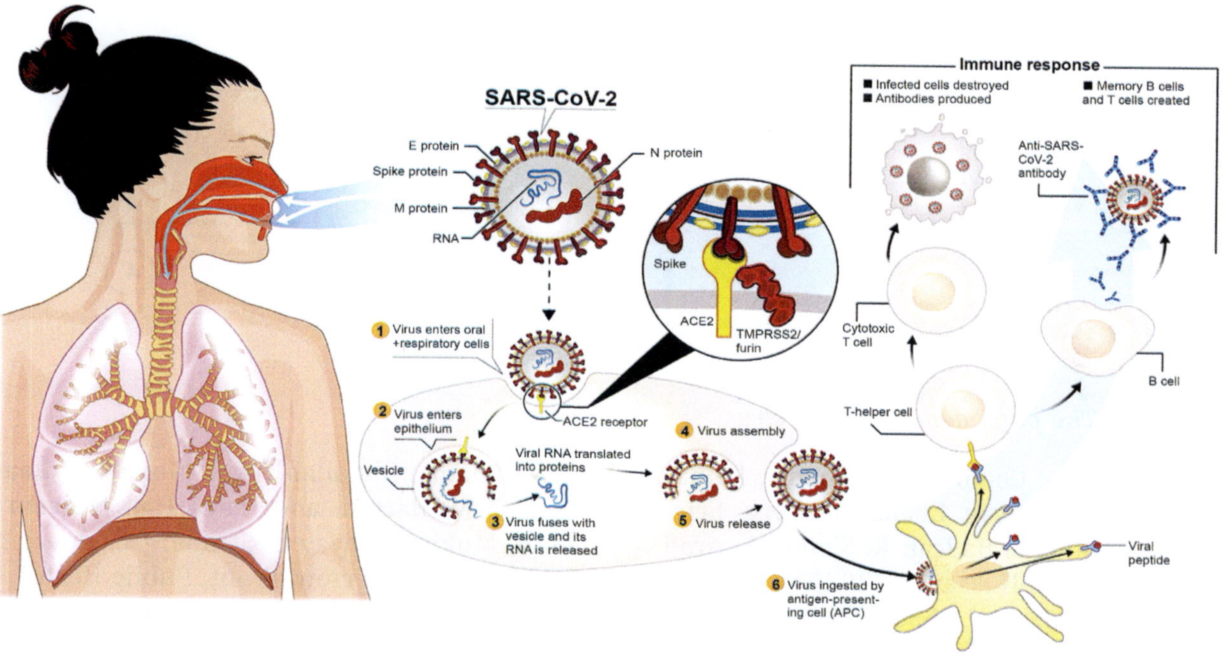

Figure 4.1. *The transmission of SARS.*

Source: By Colin D. Funk, Craig Laferrière, and Ali Ardakani. Graphic by Ian Dennis – http://www.iandennisgraphics.com – Funk CD, Laferrière C y Ardakani A (2020) Una instantánea de la carrera mundial de vacunas dirigidas contra el SARS-CoV-2 y la pandemia COVID-19. Parte delantera. Pharmacol. 11:937. Funk CD, Laferrière C, & Ardakani A. (2020) A snapshot of the global race for vaccines targeting SARS-CoV-2 and the COVID-19 pandemic. Front. Pharmacol. 11:937. https://doi.org/10.3389/fphar.2020.00937, CC BY 4.0, https://commons.wikimedia.org/w/index.php?curid=99473789.

The SARS coronavirus was detected in the cytoplasm of cells that line the alveoli using a technique called in-situ hybridization. This technique involved using a specific probe that targets the nuclear capsid region of the virus (Figure 4.2).

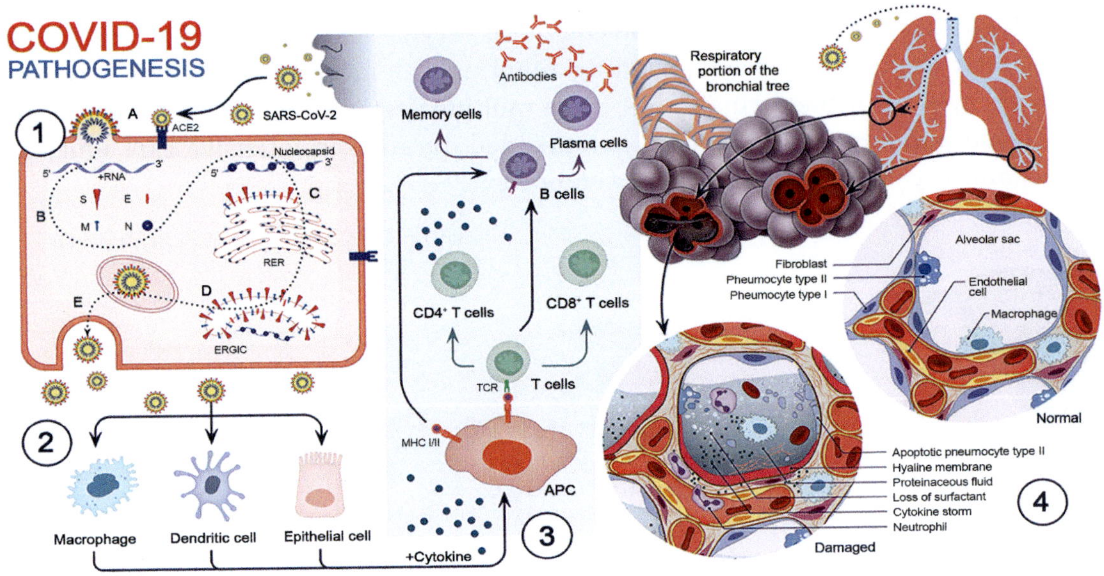

Figure 4.2. *The pathogenesis of the virus.*

Source: By Nour Chams, Sana Chams, Reina Badran, Ali Shams, Abdallah Araji, Mohamad Raad, Sanjay Mukhopadhyay, Edana Stroberg, Eric J. Duval, Lisa M. Barton, and Inaya Hajj Hussein – Chams N, Chams S, Badran R, Shams A, Araji A, Raad M, Mukhopadhyay S, Stroberg E, Duval EJ, Barton LM & Hajj Hussein I. (2020) COVID-19: A multidisciplinary review. Front. Public Health, 8, 383. https://doi.org/10.3389/fpubh.2020.00383, CC BY 4.0, https://commons.wikimedia.org/w/index.php?curid=99750049.

4.2.1.1. Case #1: Unexpected Fatality Resulting from Acute Viral Myocarditis in a Previously Asymptomatic 12-Year-Old Female

A 12-year-old female patient presented at the emergency department in a state of profound physical and mental deterioration. The attempt to revive the individual was not successful. The parents of the deceased provided information that she had been in good health before but had recently experienced symptoms of fever and headache for the past few days.

Upon examination after death, there were no apparent visible abnormalities that could explain the cause of death. The primary discovery was the presence of non-specific acute pulmonary edema. The cause of death remains undetermined, awaiting additional investigations. The histological analysis of the heart showed a concentrated and extensive inflammatory infiltration consisting primarily of lymphocytes within the myocardium. This was linked to the death of the myocardial fibers. The observed characteristics were indicative of acute viral (lymphocytic) myocarditis (Figure 4.3). On a histological level, the heart exhibited a significant and widespread infiltration of lymphocytes in the myocardium, accompanied by myonecrosis.

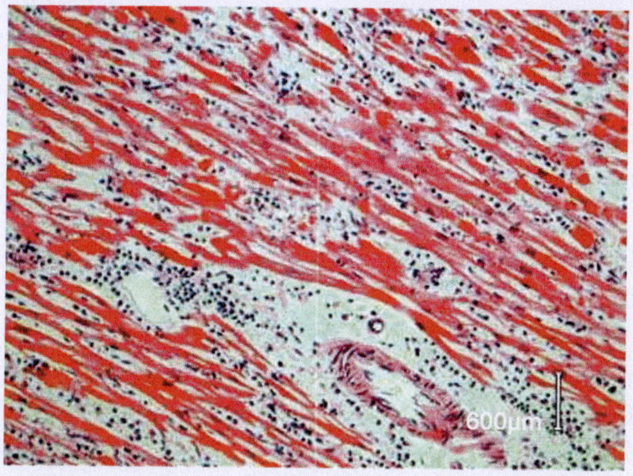

Figure 4.3. *The patient has viral myocarditis, characterized by a significant infiltration of lymphocytes in the myocardium, along with necrosis of the myocardial fibers (H&E ×400).*

Source: Lau G, Lai SH. 2008.

4.2.2. To Confirm and Refine the Diagnosis of Macroscopic Pathological Lesions

4.2.2.1. Confirmation of Macroscopic Pathological Lesions

During an autopsy, pathology can manifest in various ways, not limited to being hidden or concealed as shown in the previously presented cases. Lesions can be categorized as identified, suspected, or incidental. Often, the visible characteristics of lesions such as bronchopneumonia, myocardial infarction, tuberculosis, pneumoconiosis (such as asbestosis, silicosis, berylliosis, siderosis), or malignant tumors (such as mesothelioma, lymphoma) may not clearly indicate their complete nature. Postmortem histopathology can significantly contribute to the evaluation of such cases.

Figures 4.4 and 4.5 depict the macroscopic and microscopic characteristics of an electrical burn that is considered suspicious.

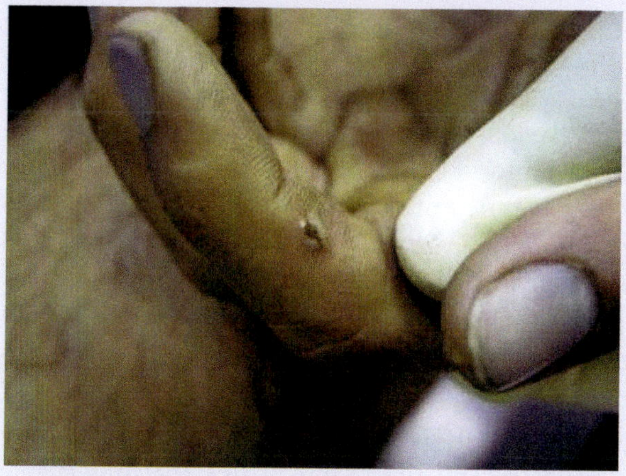

Figure 4.4. *Small, almost innocuous, dry blister on the finger.*

Source: Lau G, Lai SH. 2008, Creative Commons License.

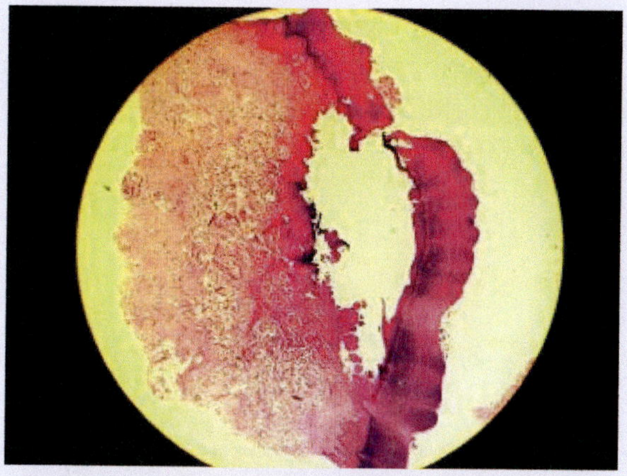

Figure 4.5. *The blister depicted in Figure 4.4 exhibited characteristic attributes of electrothermal damage in its edges and floor (H&E × 40).*

Source: Lau G, Lai SH. 2008, Creative Commons License.

4.2.2.2. Case #2: Sudden Death Due to Acute Pulmonary Embolism by Right Atrial Myxoma

A 27-year-old woman was hospitalized due to a three-week duration of elevated body temperature. The investigations uncovered a high erythrocyte sedimentation rate (ESR) of 93 mm/h. The concentration of C-reactive protein (CRP) was significantly increased to 40.4 mg/L. Nevertheless, there was no abnormal increase in white blood cell count and the proportions of different types of white blood cells were within the expected values. The microbiological and serological investigations conducted to identify a particular microorganism consistently yielded negative results. She was released from the hospital after a few days with a diagnosis of viral fever. Approximately seven days later, she was discovered deceased at her residence.

The autopsy findings showed the presence of numerous gelatinous tumor fragments obstructing the main pulmonary artery, as well as the right and left pulmonary arteries and the lobar pulmonary arterial branches in both lungs. The primary tumor was a polypoid, gelatinous, reddish fleshy mass that was connected to the wall of the right atrium. It had dimensions of 4.0 × 3.5 × 3.0 cm (Figure 4.6).

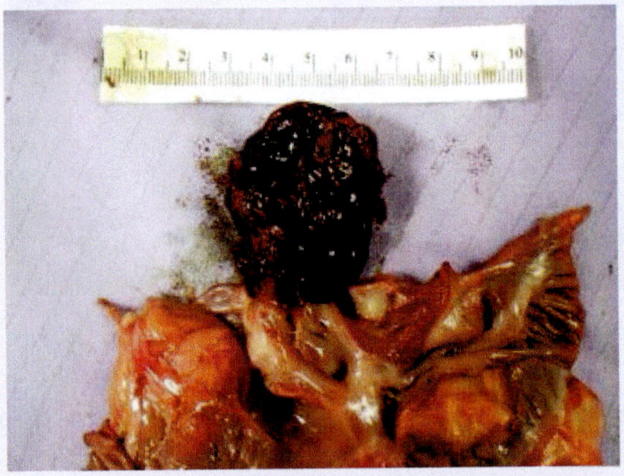

Figure 4.6. *Friable, fleshy and jelly-like polypoid tumor attached to the medial wall of the right atrium.*

Source: Lau G, Lai SH. 2008, Creative Commons License.

The tumor was examined under a microscope and found to have two distinct components. The initial observation consisted of stellate or spindle-shaped myxoma cells that contained a moderate amount of eosinophilic cytoplasm. These cells were occasionally seen forming clusters around blood vessels. The second component consisted of glandular elements that were covered by cuboidal epithelium. The cytoplasm of these elements showed positive staining with mucicarmine, PAS-diastase, and Alcian blue. The epithelial components were encircled by a wide myxoid stroma exhibiting significant regions of bleeding. Figure 4.7 shows the presence of fibrin and hemosiderin deposition in the stroma.

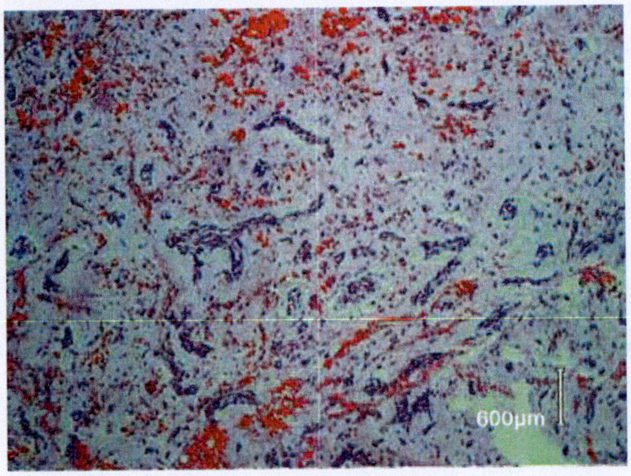

Figure 4.7. *The tumor was examined under a microscope and showed the presence of scattered myxoma cells and glandular elements within a large myxoid stroma. Regions of fibrin and hemosiderin accumulation were observed in certain areas.(H&E ×100).*

Source: Lau G, Lai SH. 2008, Creative Commons License.

The observed characteristics corresponded to a right atrial myxoma that had broken into pieces and traveled through the pulmonary arterial system, resulting in death due to a severe acute embolism of pulmonary tumors.

4.2.2.3. Case #3: Confirmation of Alzheimer's Disease

The deceased was a septuagenarian woman with a medical history of Alzheimer's disease. She was discovered unconscious at her residence in the bathroom and was transported to the emergency department in a state of extreme physical weakness. Efforts to revive the individual were not successful. The autopsy findings indicated that the cause of death was bronchopneumonia. The weight of the brain was 1,210 grams. Under microscopic examination, it was observed that there was a decrease in neurons and an increase in glial cells, which were accompanied by numerous clumps of abnormal protein deposits called neuritic plaques and twisted fibers within the neurons known as intraneuronal fibrillary tangles. The specimens were initially observed using the standard hematoxylin and eosin (H&E) staining method. However, a more effective demonstration of the specimens was achieved by employing the Bielchowski technique, as shown in Figures 4.8 and 4.9. The lesions were detected in multiple regions of the brain, including the hippocampi and cerebral cortices. The histological characteristics confirmed the clinical diagnosis of Alzheimer's disease made before death.

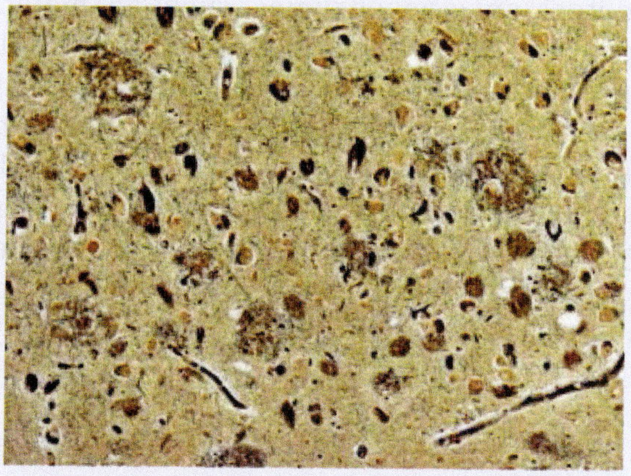

Figure 4.8. *Numerous neuritic plaques are present in the brain (Bielchowski ×200).*

Source: Lau G, Lai SH. 2008, Creative Commons License.

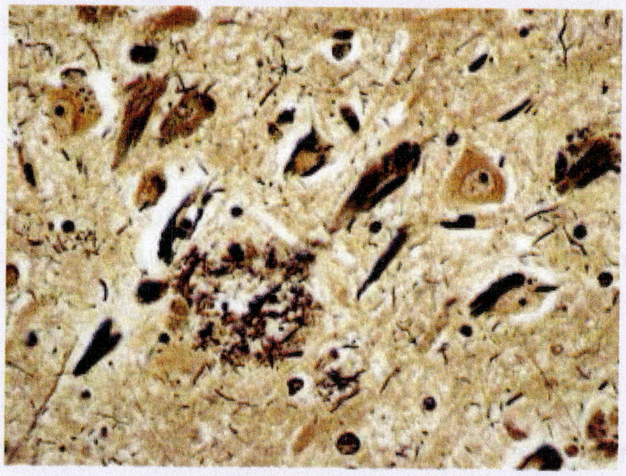

Figure 4.9. *At a higher level of magnification, there is a presence of neuritic plaques and intraneuronal fibrillary tangles.*

Source: Lau G, Lai SH. 2008, Creative Commons License.

4.3. Histological Aging of Lesions

The histological aging of lesions allows the pathologist to determine if a specific lesion or injury is consistent with having been inflicted or sustained within a claimed time period. Typical instances include the following.

4.3.1. Aging of Wounds

Determining the age of wounds, such as incised wounds and lacerations, can be challenging due to the variability in the appearance of inflammatory and histochemical changes that occur during the healing process. Typically, there may be the presence of polymorphonuclear and mononuclear infiltrates after 8 and 16 hours, respectively. Lesions that occur earlier can be aged using enzyme histochemistry on fresh frozen tissue samples stained for histamine and serotonin within the first hour of injury. Subsequently, adenosine triphosphatase and esterase can be used to age lesions that are older than 1 hour. Aminopeptidase can be used to age lesions that are 2 hours old, acid phosphatase for lesions that are 4 hours old, and alkaline phosphatase for lesions that are 8 hours old.

4.3.2. Subdural Hematoma

The age of recent and chronic subdural hemorrhage can be determined using various histological criteria, specifically those established by Munro and Merritt. Similar to the process of aging cerebral contusions, determining the temporal relation between an injury and alleged battery, homicide, or accident is often complex. However, these criteria, while not definitive, can be helpful guidelines in assessing this relationship.

4.3.3. Pulmonary Thromboembolism

The forensic significance of determining the age of pulmonary thromboembolism in relation to lower limb traumatic injury, as well as significant or severe trauma to other body parts (such as in the aftermath of a road accident), is apparent. It is important to examine the residual deep venous thrombi, which are typically found in the deep veins of the lower limbs or the iliac veins, rather than focusing solely on the embolus itself. The evaluation of the thrombo-endothelial junction provides valuable chronological information (Figure 4.10).

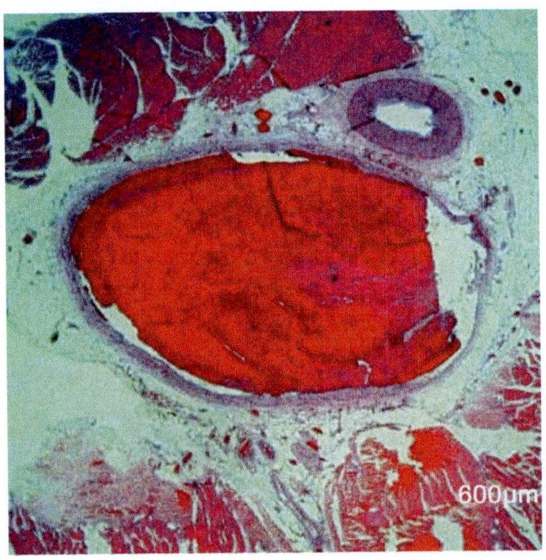

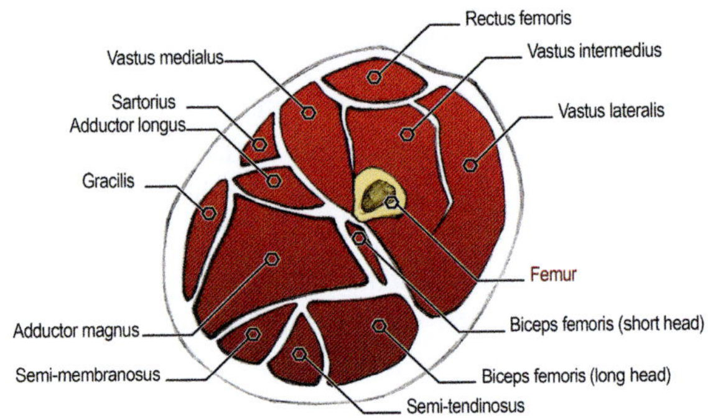

Figure 4.10. *Cross-section of the calf muscles displaying a deep vein thrombosis (H&E ×100).*

Source: Lau G, Lai SH. 2008, Creative Commons License.

4.3.4. Myocardial Infarction

Myocardial infarctions can occur in cases of suspected battery or homicide, or can complicate injuries sustained in an accident. The process of myocardial infarction aging is determined through the application of standard histology techniques using H&E staining, along with the use of specific stains to enhance the visibility of these lesions (such as Masson-Trichrome, acid fuchsin, and PTAH). Infarcts that occur shortly before death can be identified using histochemistry to detect specific enzymes such as malate, succinic, or lactic dehydrogenase. Additionally, the presence of basement membrane components like fibronectin and laminin, cytoskeletal proteins such as actin, desmin, α- and β-tubulin, cell-matrix adhesion molecules like vinculin and Talin, fatty acid binding protein, and other molecules can also be observed (Sacco et al., 2022; Zapico & Adserias-Garriga, 2022).

4.4. Corroborating and Refuting Antemortem Diagnosis and Clinical Suspicions

4.4.1. Histological Evidence of Drug Dependency

Foreign body granuloma, which develops around talc, starch, and other impurities present in recreational and street drugs such as heroin, cocaine, amphetamine derivatives, and their analogs, can be detected at the injection sites or throughout the body, primarily in the lungs and occasionally in the liver and kidneys.

Furthermore, the misuse of cocaine can potentially lead to myocardial contraction band necrosis induced by catecholamines, eosinophilic myocarditis, or infective endocarditis. Heroin abuse can lead to the development of renal amyloidosis and focal segmental glomerulosclerosis. These substances of misuse can also lead to potentially fatal rhabdomyolysis and subsequent kidney failure.

4.4.2. Drug Abuse

An unconscious 27-year-old male was discovered in the kitchen of a relative's residence. He was declared deceased upon arrival at the hospital. According to the police, the deceased had a previous record of drug abuse.

The autopsy findings showed non-specific characteristics of acute pulmonary edema. Under microscopic examination, both lungs exhibited numerous foreign-body granulomas, which were clearly visible when viewed under polarized light. These granulomas were distributed randomly throughout the lung tissue. The granulomas were commonly found in perivascular locations. Additionally, there were sporadic multinucleated giant cells. Excluded were other frequent factors that can cause granulomatous inflammation in the lungs. The observed characteristics were consistent with those commonly found in individuals with a condition known as "junkie's lung," which is often associated with a past history of intravenous drug use (Figure 4.11).

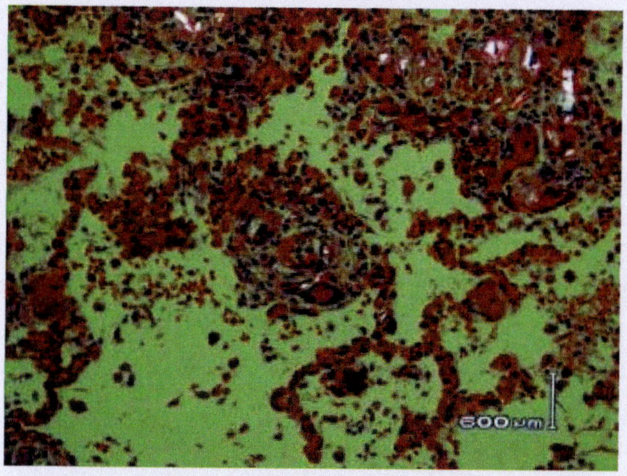

Figure 4.11. *In a case of intravenous drug abuse, there is the presence of birefringent foreign bodies surrounded by granulomatous inflammation in the perivascular space of the lung parenchyma (H&E ×400).*

Source: Lau G, Lai SH. 2008, Creative Commons License.

Postmortem blood samples were subjected to toxicological analyzes, which indicated elevated concentrations of midazolam beyond therapeutic levels. Additionally, therapeutic levels of ephedrine and orphenadrine were detected, along with the presence of several other medications including paracetamol, codeine, and promethazine. Significantly, buprenorphine was also identified in a blood sample taken after death. An analogous profile was acquired from the urine sample collected after death.

There have been numerous reports in the past decade regarding the risks associated with the misuse of buprenorphine and its concurrent misuse with benzodiazepines. After ruling out other potential causes of death, it was determined that the individual died as a result of a mixed drug reaction.

4.4.2.1. Evaluation of Adverse Drug Reactions and Poisoning

Specific histological characteristics can serve as supporting evidence in cases of suspected lethal adverse drug reactions, which can present as mucocutaneous eruptions, hepatotoxicity, nephrotoxicity, cardiotoxicity, and neurotoxicity. Examples of toxic effects include centrilobular fatty change in the liver and hepatocellular necrosis in cases of chloroform poisoning, perivenular, mid-zonal or massive hepatocellular necrosis in cases of paracetamol poisoning, and acute pulmonary hemorrhage followed by massive fibrosis and type II pneumocyte hyperplasia induced by paraquat poisoning. Paraquat poisoning may also lead to toxic myocarditis, as well as hepatic and renal tubular necrosis.

Ethylene glycol poisoning is characterized by chemical meningoencephalitis, renal tubular degeneration, myocardial degeneration with cardiac dilatation, and bronchopneumonia. These conditions are associated with the deposition of calcium oxalate crystals in the respective tissues. Please refer to Figure 4.12 for visual representation.

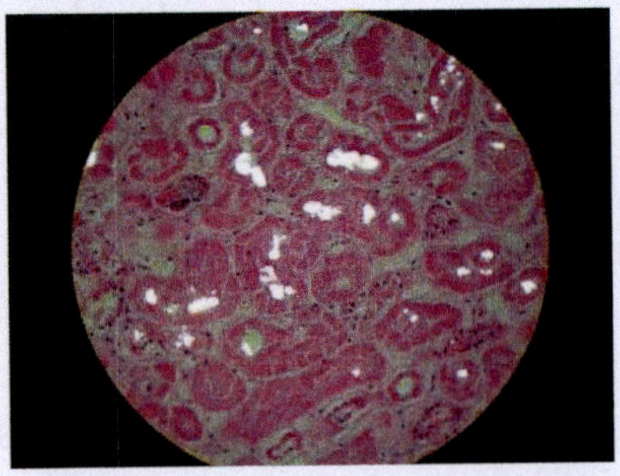

Figure 4.12. *Oxalate crystals within the renal tubules of a victim of ethylene glycol poisoning (H&E ×400).*

Source: Lau G, Lai SH. 2008, Creative Commons License.

4.4.3. Case #5: Massive Hepatocellular Necrosis, Possibly Induced by Orlistat

A 62-year-old man experienced worsening jaundice after taking orlistat at a dose of 120 mg three times a day for 10 days, to lose weight. His drug history involved sporadic consumption of paracetamol, with no more than two to four tablets taken in a single day. Furthermore, he had no prior record of consuming herbal preparations. Furthermore, there was no documented history of any drug allergy or recent international travel. In addition to mild systemic hypertension and occasional alcohol consumption, he had no other noteworthy medical history.

The initial post-admission liver function tests revealed a significant impairment in hepatic functions. Further investigations were conducted to identify markers for various hepatitis viruses, including anti-HAV IgM, anti-HBs, anti-HBc IgM, anti-HBe, HBsAg, anti-HCV, HCV RNA (Chiron), anti-HEV IgM, anti-EBV IgM, anti-CMV IgM, and anti-leptospiral antibodies. Tests for HIV-1 and -2, as well as autoimmune diseases (anti-mitochondrial and anti-nuclear antibodies), were also performed. The results of these investigations were mostly negative, except for the presence of anti-smooth muscle antibodies, which were found at a low level (1:100). Tests for malarial parasites and Clostridium difficile toxin in the stool sample yielded negative results. A clinical drug screen conducted on a blood sample taken on the second day after admission revealed a non-toxic concentration of orlistat at 33 mg/L (μg/mL). Simultaneous clinical investigations ruled out Wilson's disease, Budd-Chiari syndrome, and biliary disease.

The patient was diagnosed with fulminant liver failure, which is believed to be caused by an adverse reaction to orlistat. Despite being deemed eligible for liver transplantation, the patient succumbed to a nosocomial infection and experienced renal failure within a little over three weeks of being admitted to the hospital.

The liver was examined histologically after death, revealing a complete absence of the typical structure of the liver and extensive death of liver cells, along with significant blockage of the bile ducts near the portal and periportal areas (Figure 4.13). Additionally, there was a breakdown of the reticulin framework (Figure 4.14). The liver showed a moderate and persistent inflammation in the portal area, with sporadic preservation of a small number of hepatocytes surrounding the portal veins in certain regions. Perivenular fibrosis was observed, however, veno-occlusive disease and hepatic cirrhosis were not present. The residual hepatocytes did not exhibit any Mallory bodies, giant mitochondria, or steatosis. The toxicological analysis yielded negative results.

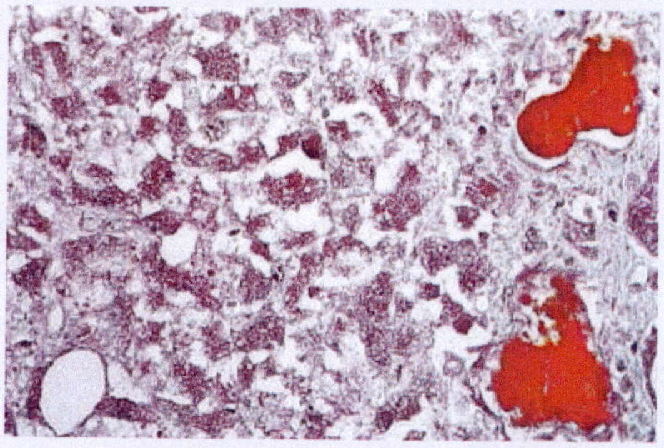

Figure 4.13. *Massive hepatocellular necrosis with marked periportal cholestasis (PAS ×200).*

Extensive analysis of clinical and pathological data strongly suggests that this is most likely a case of severe liver cell death caused by drug toxicity, possibly due to the use of orlistat. This drug has been previously linked to a case of hepatitis that did not result in death.

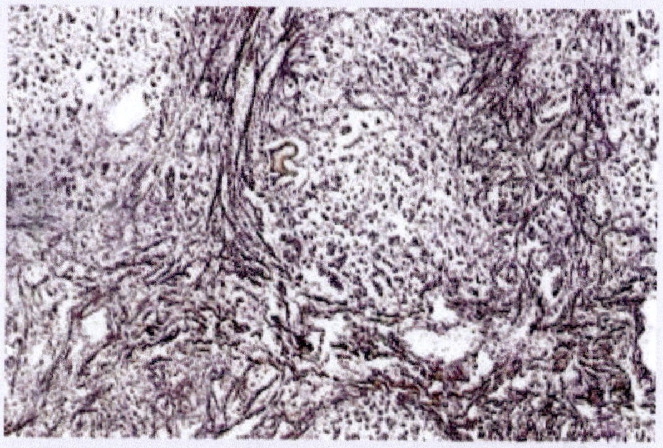

Figure 4.14. *Collapse of the hepatic reticulin framework (Gordon & Sweet's ×200).*

4.4.4. Adulteration of a Slimming Herbal Combination by Nitrosofenfluramine

A 42-year-old woman died from sudden and severe liver failure, followed by failure of multiple organs, after consuming an unknown amount of a herbal product for about four months before her illness began. The product included extracts of Herba Gynostemmae, Folium Camelliae Sinensis, Succus Aloes Folii Siccatus, Semen Raphani, and Fructus Crataegi. It was claimed to possess slimming, energizing, and cleansing properties. She ultimately underwent a complete removal of her liver, along with the creation of a connection between the portal vein and the inferior vena cava, in preparation for a liver transplant from a different donor. Regrettably, her state worsened and she passed away within 48 hours of the surgery, approximately three weeks after being admitted.

The autopsy revealed that the deceased had a pronounced case of jaundice and was extremely obese, with a BMI of 47.1. There were signs of widespread bleeding, including the presence of 1,350 mL of blood in the peritoneal cavity, which was likely caused by medical intervention. The liver was excised and subsequently retrieved as a specimen preserved in formalin. The structure was significantly reduced, consisting of numerous small nodules scattered among large regions of dense fibrotic tissue.

Microscopy revealed the total absence of the typical structure of the liver, characterized by extensive damage to the liver tissue and the breakdown of the reticulin framework (Figure 4.15). The remaining liver cells were arranged in nodules, showing varying degrees of cellular regeneration and ballooning degeneration, surrounded by large areas of densely fibrous tissue (Figure 4.16). The specimen exhibited excessive growth of ductal cells and a combination of mild to moderate inflammation, consisting of T-lymphocytes ($CD3^+$, $CD20^-$). There was a noticeable concentration of cholestasis, primarily located within the bile canaliculi and bile ducts, as shown in Figure 4.17. No significant accumulation of copper or iron was observed. These characteristics were found to be in line with the process of repairing and limited regrowth of liver tissue after extensive death of liver cells.

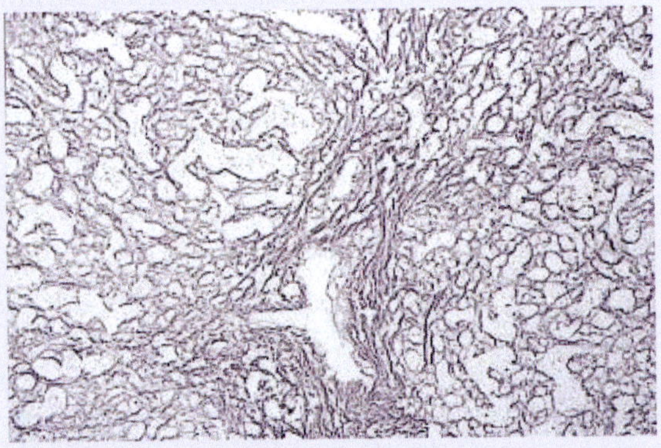

Figure 4.15. *The liver's microarchitecture exhibits the collapse of the reticulin framework. Gordon & Sweet's ×100).*

Source: Lau G, Lai SH. 2008, Creative Commons License.

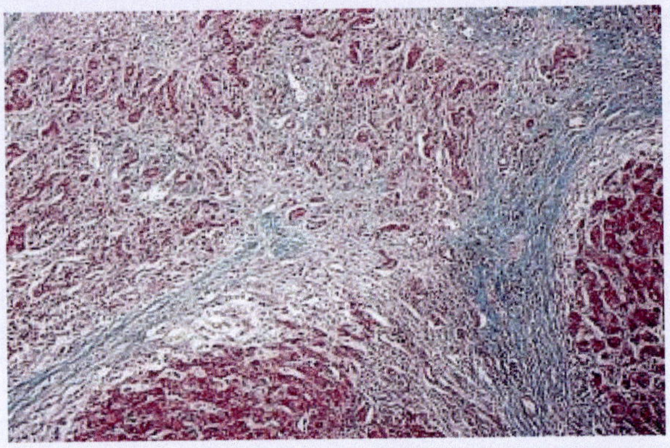

Figure 4.16. *Massive hepatocellular necrosis with marked architectural distortion and dense stromal fibrosis (Masson Trichrome ×100).*

Source: Lau G, Lai SH. 2008, Creative Commons License.

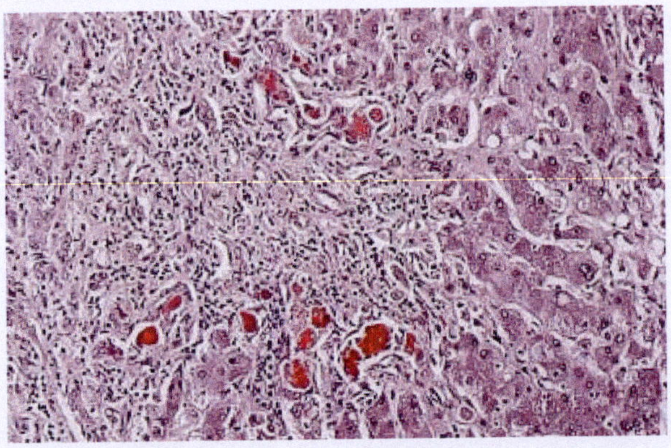

Figure 4.17. *N-Nitrosofenfluramine-induced liver pathology: ductal proliferation, mixed inflammatory infiltrates and prominent cholestasis (PAS ×200).*

Source: Lau G, Lai SH. 2008, Creative Commons License.

An examination of a blood sample taken after death revealed both effective and insufficient levels of various medications that were given to the patient during her final illness. Further examination of a residual herbal capsule sample indicated that it had been contaminated with fenfluramine, N-nitrosofenfluramine, nicotinamide, and thyroid extract. Currently, there is no evidence to suggest that any of the herbal ingredients mentioned are harmful to the liver. In fact, Succus Aloes Folii Siccatus is believed to have a protective effect on the liver. Similarly, fenfluramine, nicotinamide (unless taken in very high doses), and thyroid extract are also not known to be hepatotoxic. Due to the variable hepatotoxicity of nitrosamines, and in the absence of any other likely cause of liver damage, it was concluded that N-nitrosofenfluramine was the probable cause of the extensive hepatocellular necrosis in this case.

4.4.5. A Patient with an Ectopic Pregnancy Experienced Postanaesthetic Respiratory Distress Due to a Mediastinal Large B-Cell Malignant Lymphoma That Had Not Been Diagnosed Clinically

A 32-year-old woman was diagnosed with an ectopic pregnancy at six weeks of not having a menstrual period and underwent a laparoscopic salpingectomy. During a preoperative anesthetic review, the patient reported a mild, persistent productive cough that had been present for a month. The cough was determined to be caused by an upper respiratory tract infection. She experienced a serious respiratory complication after the removal of the breathing tube and passed away on the second day after the surgery.

The autopsy discovered a significant mediastinal tumor that was not anticipated before the surgery, but was indicated by a chest X-ray taken after resuscitation. The lesion, which was firm and fleshy, surrounded the ascending thoracic aorta, aortic arch, and the proximal portions of the brachiocephalic and subclavian arteries (Figure 4.18). It also resulted in partial compression of the airway from the outside.

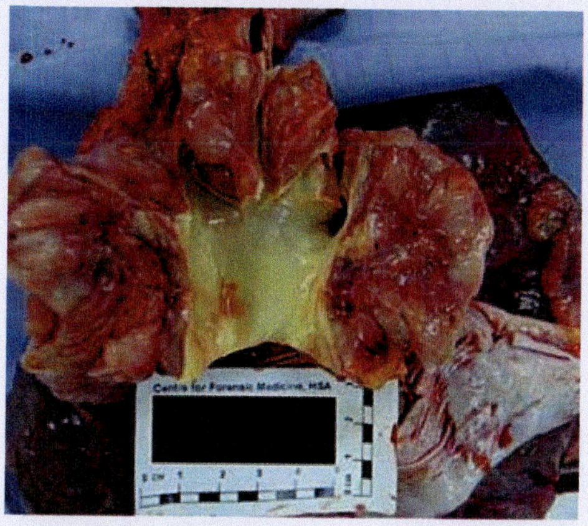

Figure 4.18. *A sizable, flesh-like tumor located in the mediastinum surrounds the aortic arch as well as the initial portions of the brachiocephalic and subclavian arteries.*

Source: Lau G, Lai SH. 2008, Creative Commons License.

The tumor was composed of large lymphoid cells that were malignant. These cells lacked CD1a and CD3 markers, but expressed CD20, CD45, and CD68 markers. The cells had pleomorphic, vesicular nuclei with prominent nucleoli and a relatively high amount of cytoplasm. Please refer to Figure 4.19A, B for visual representation. There was a lack of Reed-Sternberg cells. The immunohistochemistry tests for AE1/3, EMA, and PLAP showed negative results. There were regions of tissue death as well as widespread infiltration of nerves and blood vessels. The presence of cancerous cells invading the outer layer of blood vessels and the superficial layers of the middle layer was observed (Figure 4.20). The presence of these characteristics strongly indicated a diagnosis of mediastinal diffuse large B-cell lymphoma, while effectively ruling out the possibility of a thymoma or a germ cell tumor. Subsequent analysis revealed the presence of micrometastases in the tracheo-bronchial lymph nodes and the right adrenal gland (Figure 4.21), but not in the bone marrow.

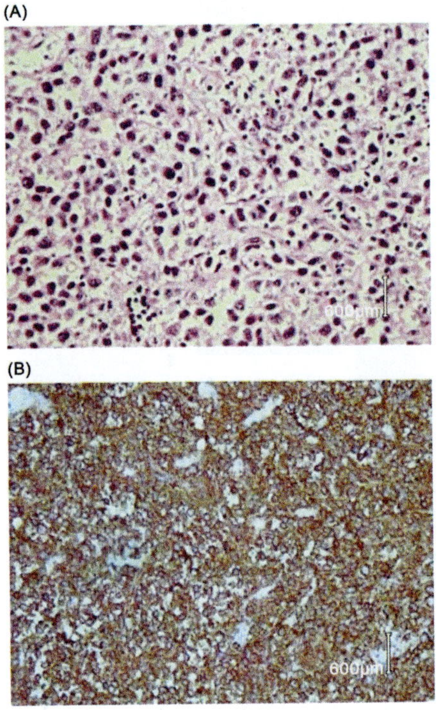

Figure 4.19. *Malignant, large lymphoid cells with pleomorphic vesicular nuclei, prominent nucleoli, abnormal mitoses and abundant cytoplasm (H&E ×400).* ***B****. Intense positive staining for CD20 (×200).*

Source: Lau G, Lai SH. 2008, Creative Commons License.

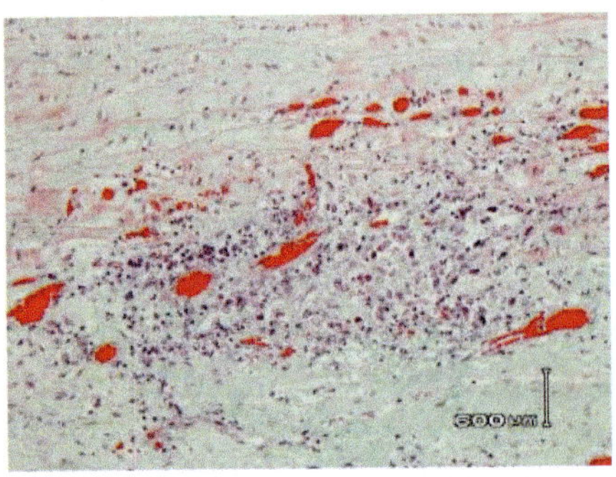

Figure 4.20. *Malignant lymphoid cells infiltrating the aortic adventitia and the superficial layers of the media (Masson-Trichrome ×200).*

Source: Lau G, Lai SH. 2008, Creative Commons License.

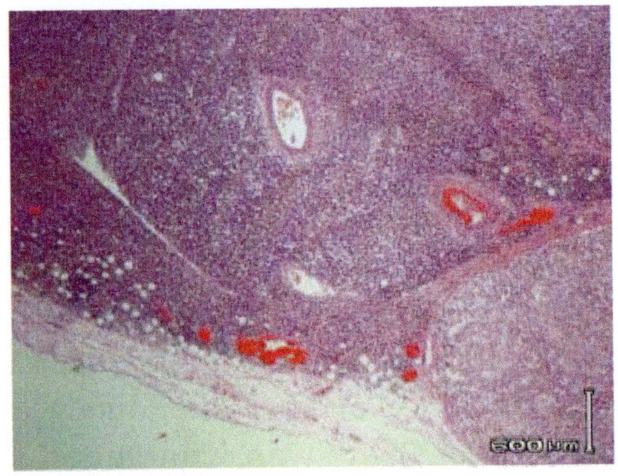

Figure 4.21. *Right adrenal metastatic malignant lymphoma (H&E ×4).*

Source: Lau G, Lai SH. 2008, Creative Commons License.

Most likely, the advanced mediastinal tumor's mechanical effects on the airways and thoracic cage, combined with the respiratory movement and airway patency disruptions caused by general anesthesia, resulted in the patient's sudden and unexpected death during early pregnancy (Sacco et al., 2022; Zapico & Adserias-Garriga, 2022).

4.4.6. An 8-Year-Old Girl Experienced a Cerebral Infarction as a Complication of Therapeutic Embolization for a Facial Cavernous Hemangioma

An 8-year-old girl developed left-sided hemiparesis approximately 2 hours after receiving elective angiographic embolization for a large right facial hemangioma while under general anesthesia. The computerized tomography scan showed a cerebral infarction in the right fronto-parietal region, along with significant cerebral edema and signs of hypoxic-ischemic encephalopathy. Following her initial condition, the patient experienced a series of medical complications including neurogenic ventricular arrhythmia, pulmonary edema, recurrent episodes of cardiorespiratory arrest, diabetes insipidus, and progressive neurological deterioration. These complications ultimately led to brain death two weeks later.

Facial soft tissue microscopy revealed the existence of a cavernous hemangioma (Figure 4.22) with intermittent areas of blood clotting and sudden bleeding, but no signs of cancer. The presence of foreign body emboli was observed, consisting of reticulated material that exhibited strong birefringence. This material is likely to be polyvinyl-alcohol particles that have been denatured by heat. It was stained intensely black using Verhoeff van-Gieson stain, as shown in Figure 4.23.

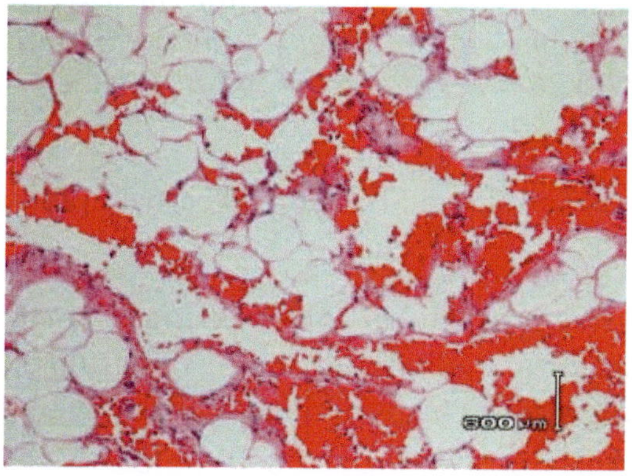

Figure 4.22. *The specimen consists of enlarged blood vessels with thin walls, which are surrounded by fully developed fatty tissue (H&E ×100).*

Source: Lau G, Lai SH. 2008, Creative Commons License.

(A)

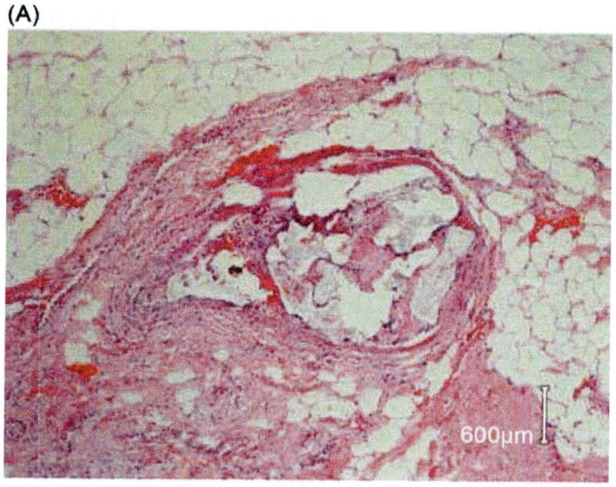

(B)

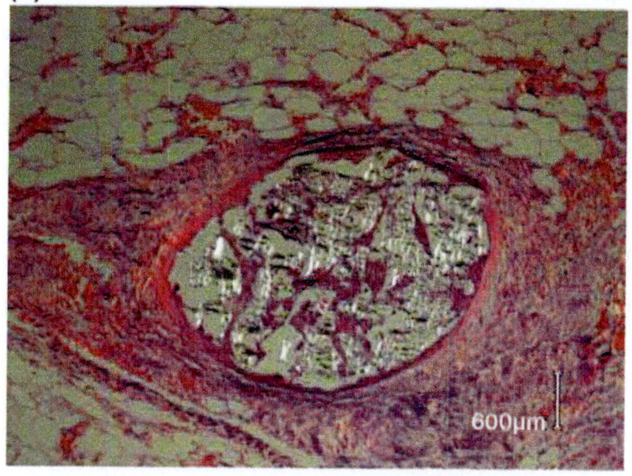

(C)

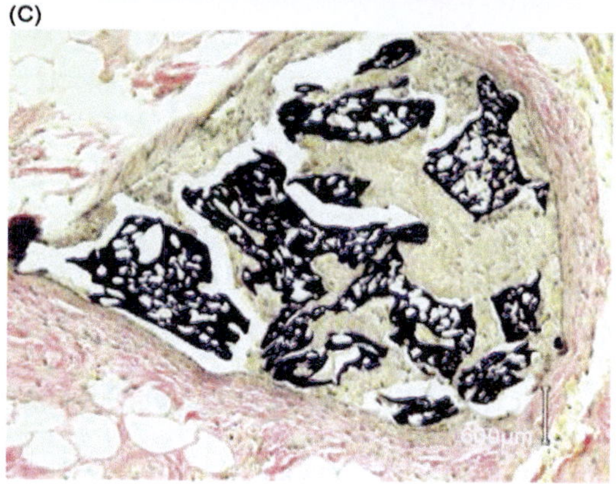

Figure 4.23. *Foreign body emboli within the cavernous hemangioma (H&E ×100); B Case #8: Marked birefringence (polarized ×100); and Case #8: Reticulated appearance (Verhoeff van-Gieson ×200).*

Source: Lau G, Lai SH. 2008, Creative Commons License.

Microscopically, the brain exhibited signs of autolysis, appearing pale when stained. Additionally, there was evidence of congestion and localized blood clot formation in the vessels of the cortex. Cortical infarction (Figure 4.24) primarily affected both temporal lobes, resulting in neuronal liquefactive necrosis primarily in the outer layers. This was accompanied by the presence of inflammatory infiltrates consisting of polymorph leukocytes and some foamy macrophages, as well as early astrocytosis.

Foreign objects that resemble the ones found in the facial cavernous hemangioma (as shown in Figure 4.25) were discovered in these regions, as well as in the occipital cortex and the basal ganglia. The cerebellar cortex exhibited widespread liquefactive necrosis of the Purkinje cells, indicating hypoxic-ischemic encephalopathy, while the hippocampus was mostly in a state of autolysis.

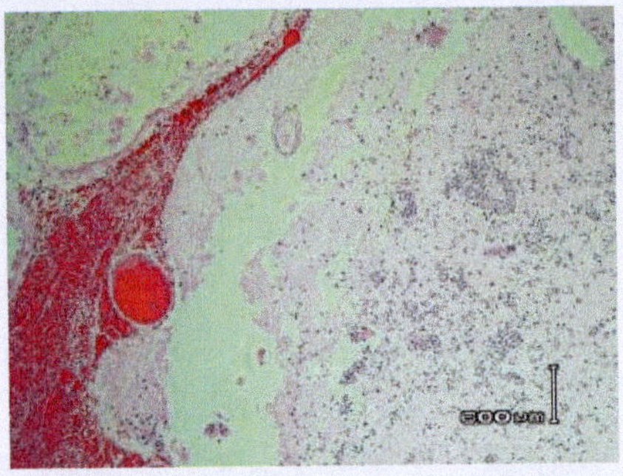

Figure 4.24. *Cerebral infarction (H&E ×100).*

Source: Lau G, Lai SH. 2008, Creative Commons License.

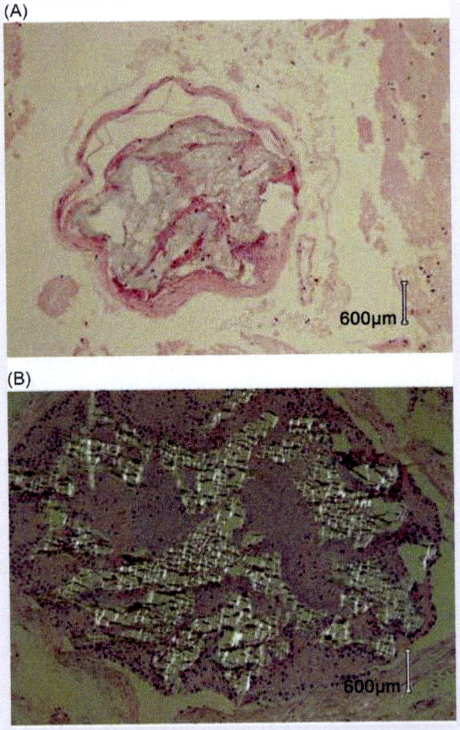

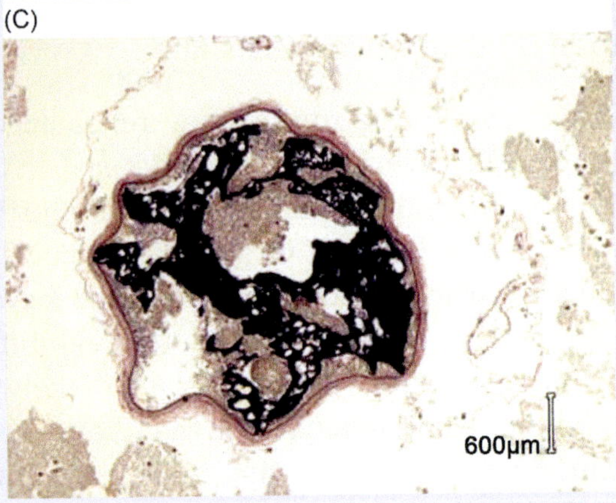

Figure 4.25. *Foreign body emboli, virtually identical to those found within the cavernous hemangioma, in the cerebral microvasculature. A H&E ×200. B Polarised ×400.* ***C*** *Verhoeff van-Gieson ×200.*

Source: Lau G, Lai SH. 2008, Creative Commons License.

The procedure for treating the facial hemangioma involved using angiographic embolization. This was done by selectively and sequentially catheterizing the right internal maxillary and facial arteries through the right external carotid artery, using a femoral approach. The purpose of this procedure was to introduce a combination of polyvinyl-alcohol particles (ranging in size from 150–250 µm) and gelfoam, suspended in a radiocontrast medium, into the main arterial feeders of the hemangioma. The goal was to achieve therapeutic occlusion of the relevant blood vessels. From a pathological standpoint, some of these particles could likely have entered the blood vessels in the brain through connections between the right external and internal carotid arteries, such as the middle meningeal and ophthalmic arteries. These particles may have then moved from the same side to the opposite side of the brain's blood vessels through the Arterial Circle of Willis, resulting in fatal outcomes (Sacco et al., 2022; Zapico & Adserias-Garriga, 2022).

4.4.7. Accidental Intraventricular Administration of Vincristine

A 27-year-old woman with acute lymphoblastic leukemia, which has spread to the central nervous system (CNS), was scheduled to undergo a more intense chemotherapy treatment. This treatment involves the use of intrathecal methotrexate (administered directly into the spinal fluid) and intravenous vincristine. The decision to proceed with this intensified treatment was made after the initial course of chemotherapy failed to achieve remission.

A right frontal Ommaya reservoir was implanted to provide access to the cerebral ventricles. Regrettably, a junior doctor mistakenly administered vincristine (2 mg) intrathecally, directly into the Ommaya reservoir, instead of the intended method. The error was discovered the next day, and a CNS washout was conducted, but it was ineffective. The patient developed progressive ascending paralysis, complicated by a persistent respiratory infection, eventually lapsing into a coma to die approximately 10 days after the lethal injection.

During the autopsy, the brain exhibited swelling and displayed widespread discoloration of the outer layer, along with significant and widespread softening. The spinal cord was necrotic almost throughout its entire length, and particularly along the cervical, thoracic and upper lumbar segments, where necrotic brain tissue was present within the spinal subdural space (Figure 4.26).

The cerebellar tonsils also exhibited necrosis. Microscopically, there were signs of inflammation in the brain and its covering membranes, known as meningoencephalitis, with significant damage to nerve cells and an increase in the number of astrocytes (Figure 4.27). Leptomeningitis was observed in the cerebellum, along with a specific area where Purkinje cells were lost. The brainstem exhibited various forms of neuronal damage, including ischemic-hypoxic alterations, necrosis, astrocytosis, and localized perivascular hemorrhage. These changes were particularly prominent in the pons and medulla. Leptomeningitis was observed in the spinal cord, along with extensive neuronal necrosis, especially in the anterior horn cells. This was accompanied by florid myelitis. Please refer to Figure 4.28 for visual representation. Fragments of necrotic cerebellar tissue were present along the cervical and thoracic segments and around the nerve roots. No signs of demyelination were found. There was also histological evidence of bronchopneumonia with heavy leukemic infiltrates within the myocardium, spleen, bone marrow, kidneys, and the portal tracts of the liver.

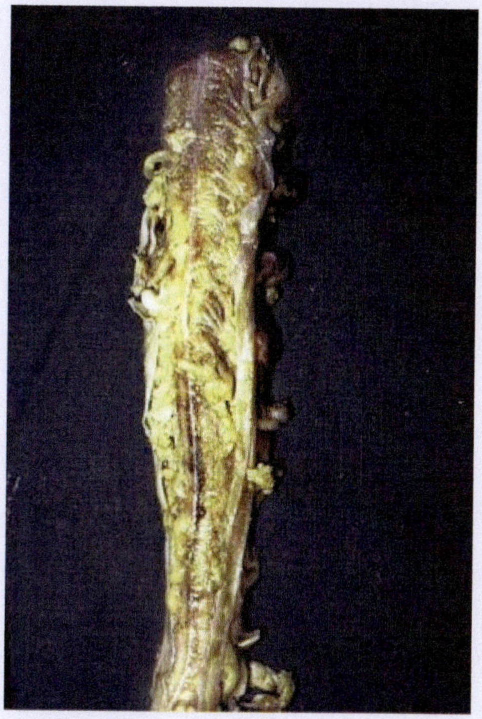

Figure 4.26. *The cervical spinal cord is necrotic, and there are fragments of cerebellar tissue present next to it.*

Source: Lau G, Lai SH. 2008, Creative Commons License.

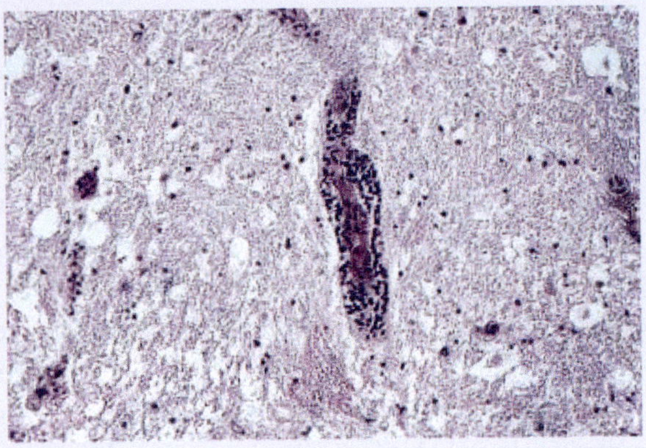

Figure 4.27. *The individual is experiencing inflammation of the brain and meninges, characterized by the presence of lymphocytes forming a cuff around blood vessels (H&E ×200).*

Source: Lau G, Lai SH. 2008, Creative Commons License.

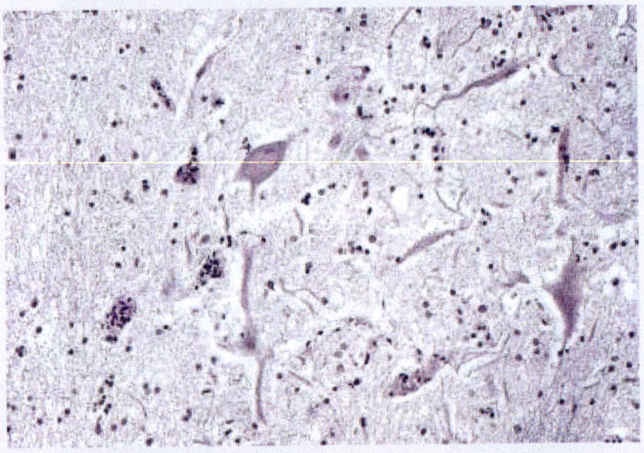

Figure 4.28. *Neuronal necrosis and degeneration of the anterior horn cells of the spinal cord (H&E ×200).*

Source: Lau G, Lai SH. 2008, Creative Commons License.

This case is just one of many similar, if not identical, instances of a completely preventable medication error. Specifically, it involves administering the correct drug through the incorrect route, resulting in irreversible and fatal consequences.

- **As a Permanent Record of Lesions:** It is important to note that, even in cases where there is no doubt about the cause of death or any of the autopsy findings, taking samples of the main organs' tissues can still provide permanent evidence of the presence or absence of any significant abnormality that is relevant to determining the cause of death. This is especially crucial for states and countries where cremation is the customary and favored method of laying the deceased person to rest.
- **As an Invaluable Resource for Teaching, Training, and Research:** Lastly, histological sections and materials are invaluable assets for teaching, training, and education. Nevertheless, the degree to which this ultimate benefit can be implemented organically differs among jurisdictions (Sacco et al., 2022; Zapico & Adserias-Garriga, 2022).

4.5. The Scope of Forensic Histopathology

Forensic pathology, in contrast to surgical pathology, serves the distinct purpose of investigating the mechanism, cause, and manner of death, and supplying pertinent information for legal proceedings. Although there may be some similarities, specific conditions observed in medicolegal autopsy practice are unlikely to be encountered in routine surgical pathology. Forensic pathology practice involves several key areas of histology, including the identification of specific disorders that necessitate the use of microscopy for their detection, such as myocarditis, amniotic fluid embolism, and fat embolism. Some medical conditions can only be diagnosed through autopsy histology, including hypothermia (Figure 4.29), electrocution, drowning, and fire deaths (Figure 4.30). These conditions have histological characteristics that can help with their diagnosis to varying degrees.

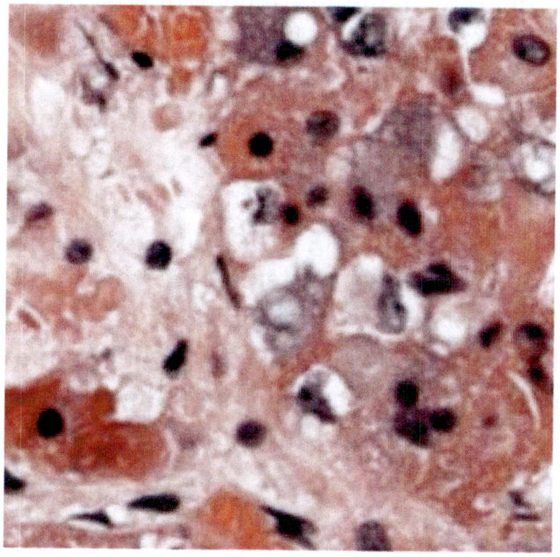

Figure 4.29. *Vacuolation of cells in the pituitary in hypothermia (H&E, x200).*

Source: Lau G, Lai SH. 2008, Creative Commons License.

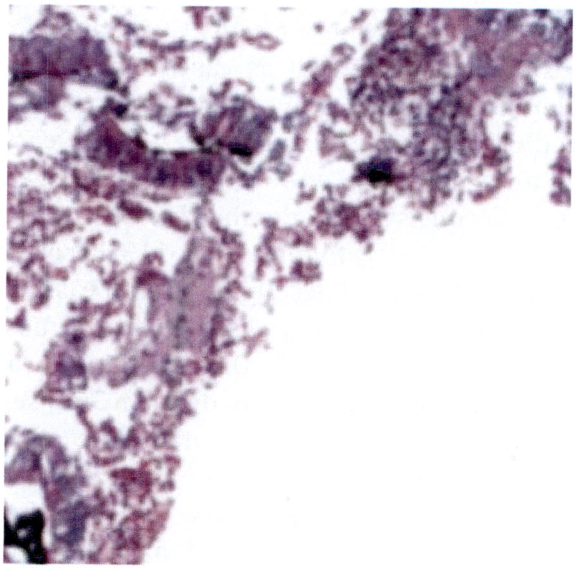

Figure 4.30. *Soot in the airway in fire death (H&E, x100).*

Source: Lau G, Lai SH. 2008, Creative Commons License.

Injuries such as bruising, lacerations, and fractures exhibit distinct microscopic characteristics. Considerable time and effort have been dedicated to attempting to determine the timing of injuries using histological methods. However, the practical application of these methods in real cases has been more limited than initially expected. Microscopic examination can also provide support for systemic responses to injury, such as pulmonary embolism, ischemia, and sepsis.

4.5.1. Utility of Histopathology in Forensic Pathology Practice

There are specific investigations that, due to tradition and established procedures, necessitate thorough histological examination. These encompass fatalities that occur unexpectedly during infancy and deaths that occur during childbirth or shortly after. However, these deaths are relatively uncommon in most forensic pathology cases, and the usefulness of microscopy in other investigations is subject to further discussion. Studies on the utility of microscopy in medical autopsies have demonstrated notable disparities between macroscopic and microscopic diagnoses. Benardi and his colleagues conducted a study on 1,273 medical autopsies and discovered that the lungs had the highest percentage of discrepancies at 38.7%, followed by the liver at 35.1%, and the kidneys at 30.3% (4). Hunt and colleagues demonstrated that there were frequent inconsistencies between the macroscopic and microscopic diagnoses of bronchopneumonia (5). Roulson and colleagues conducted a meta-analysis of the existing literature to examine the disparity between clinical and autopsy diagnoses, as well as the significance of postmortem histology. Their analysis revealed that more than 20% of autopsy findings that were not anticipated based on clinical information could only be diagnosed through histological examination. This included 5% of significant findings.

Research has investigated and documented the significance of regular histopathology in the field of forensic pathology. A study conducted in 2006 by Molina and colleagues from Bexar County, Texas determined that routine histopathology in medicolegal cases was unnecessary. Out of the 189 cases examined, only one case of leukemia showed a change in the cause of death as a result of histology. There were no alterations made to the cause of death in any of the seven cases. The chosen cases were characterized as those in which both the cause and manner of death were clearly indicated by visible observations, and where microscopic examination was not typically performed. The average age was 41 years. 25% of cases were attributed to natural deaths, while accidents constituted the largest group at 36% and homicides accounted for 27%. Gunshot wounds and blunt force injuries were the primary causes of death, each accounting for 22% of cases. They claimed that their discoveries and methodology adhered to the guidelines put forth by the College of American Pathologists and the National Association of Medical Examiners. These guidelines essentially grant professionals the authority to decide whether or not to examine histology based on their own judgment.

In a separate 2006 study conducted in Sydney, Australia, Langlois examined 638 adult medicolegal autopsies to determine the significance of histology (8). The age range spanned from 16 to 98 years, with a mean and median age of 53 years. This series involved a substantial amount of histology blocks collected. Specifically, there were 3,088 blocks of lung obtained from 638 cases, 3,392 blocks of left ventricle obtained from 636 cases, and 1,260 renal blocks obtained from 636 cases, among others. He observed a significant discrepancy between the macroscopic and microscopic diagnoses of the lungs, specifically regarding the diagnosis of pneumonia. Additional matters investigated encompassed the correlation between the visual assessment of coronary artery constriction and the microscopic analysis, revealing only a moderate level of concurrence. He asserted that histology was considered to be in some manner contributory to the cause of death in 53% of cases, either by providing, altering, or confirming the cause of death. Out of 203 cases where the cause of death was not specified following a thorough examination, histology was able to determine the cause of death in 49 cases, accounting for 24% of the total. The primary disparities between the macroscopic and microscopic examination were observed in the heart and lung sections.

In a 2010 study, de la Grandmaison et al. conducted a prospective examination of 1,786 autopsies from Garches, France (9). The researchers conducted thorough sampling, which involved examining the nervous tissue and two pathologists carefully assessed the slides of 428 cases that were chosen at random. They omitted cases of sudden infant death syndrome (SIDS) and cases where organs were taken for transplantation, as well as cases where only skeletons remained. The population consisted of individuals ranging in age from 5 to 91 years, with an average age of 46.2 years. The largest category consisted of deaths due to natural causes (n = 130), followed by 113 cases of suicide, 104 cases of accidents, and 40 cases of homicides. Cardiovascular disease was the most prevalent cause of death. Only histology was able to determine the cause of death in 36 cases, accounting for 8.4% of the total. Nine cases were diagnosed with ischemic heart disease, six cases with acute myocardial ischemia, five cases with cardiomyopathy, and six cases with myocarditis. Six cases were diagnosed with acute pneumonia. They reported that the cause of death was determined in 40% of cases and that how the body tissues were affected influenced the manner of death in 13% of cases. 22% of cases had more comprehensive documentation of traumatic lesions. Their findings regarding the usefulness of histology aligned with those of Langlois.

During an analysis of 100 instances of hanging, histology revealed some additional information, but microscopic examination did not offer any insights into the mechanism, cause, or manner of death (10). Fronczek and colleagues analyzed 500 coronial autopsy cases (11). The cases involved 113 deaths from natural causes, 65 homicides, 60 suicides, 160 accidents (mostly road traffic accidents), complications of medical therapy in seven cases, and 95 deaths that were classified as undetermined. The average age of the cases was 49 years. Histology was preserved in 287 cases. Out of these 287 cases, it was discovered that only five (2%) were diagnosed solely based on histology. The histology contributed to the medical cause of death in 8% of cases. 61% of cases confirmed the cause of death, while in 30% of cases, histology did not contribute to determining the cause of death. In 16% of cases, inconsistencies were identified between the macroscopic and microscopic observations.

In general, the studies that have been published on the usefulness of histology in forensic pathology demonstrate varying outcomes and reflect the diverse practices that exist in various medicolegal jurisdictions. It is widely acknowledged that there are substantial variations in autopsy rates among countries (12). Consequently, it is unsurprising that there are varying perspectives on the importance and usefulness of histology in establishing the cause of death.

An article in the journal "Forensic Science, Medicine and Pathology" examined the significance of forensic histology (13–18). All of the authors were seasoned forensic professionals. Overall, the authors expressed a positive stance towards the utilization of histology, with certain individuals strongly advocating for an increased emphasis on histology rather than reducing its importance. The primary opposing viewpoint is in favor of exercising professional discretion based on the specific circumstances of the case. Standards that have been officially released may differ across different jurisdictions. The authors of the study also emphasized the importance of adhering to legal obligations, which could potentially limit the ability to perform histology procedures.

4.5.1.1. Histology

Histology refers to the examination of the microscopic composition of tissues, while histopathology specifically focuses on the microscopic alterations in tissue resulting from disease (1, 2). Standard textbooks (2) contain detailed explanations of the procedure and the stains that were utilized. In summary, the conventional approach for creating microscopic slides involves taking tissue and immersing it in a fixative, typically formaldehyde solution (formalin) (2). The concentration of the solution is typically 4% formaldehyde, which is obtained by diluting a 40% formaldehyde solution 10 times. This is why it is commonly known as a 10% formalin solution. A solution containing 20% formalin is commonly employed for brain fixation. Formaldehyde can be adjusted to a neutral pH of 7 by buffering it with a phosphate buffer. The duration for fixation varies based on the tissue type and its dimensions, with smaller fragments typically undergoing fixation within a timeframe of four to six hours. After the tissue is stabilized, it can undergo dehydration in ethanol, usually with a small quantity of methanol, to begin the transformation into a microscopic slide. Subsequently, the process involves the removal of any remaining substances, usually accomplished by employing a solution such as xylene or toluene. After being impregnated with paraffin wax, the sample is embedded to facilitate cutting on a microtome and the creation of a slide. This process is referred to as microtomy. Currently, these processes exhibit varying levels of mechanization, although certain processes like microtomy still require significant manual labor. After the production of a tissue slide, it can undergo staining using histochemical or immunohistochemical stains. An alternative to using paraffin embedding is to utilize frozen sections. This enables prompt diagnosis, albeit with subpar histology. However, it is necessary to detect specific substances that are eliminated during the paraffin embedding process, particularly fat stains in forensic practice.

4.5.1.2. Histochemical Stains

Hematoxylin and eosin (H&E) is the most commonly employed stain in microscopy, including in the field of forensic pathology. Hematoxylin is obtained from the *Hematoxylon campechianum* tree and is used to color nuclei in a blue-black shade. There are multiple types of hematoxylins available. Hematoxylin is not a substance used for staining, but its primary result of oxidation, hematin, is. Eosins are a type of xanthene dyes that can color the cytoplasm in a pink-red shade. Some laboratories employ alternative stains, such as hematoxylin phloxine saffron (HPS), although this particular stain is more costly.

The standard protocol involves staining all collected sections with H&E, followed by any additional stains as needed. Forensic practice commonly employs a restricted range of histochemical stains, as indicated in Table 4.1. These encompass connective tissue stains, iron stains, membrane stains, and stains for microorganisms.

Table 4.1. Histochemical Stains Commonly Used in Forensic Histopathology

Stain	Tissue	Example of Case
Hematoxylin and eosin	All tissues	
Masson trichrome	Connective tissue	Fibrosis (e.g., alcoholic liver disease, vascular dissection)
Movat's pentachrome	Connective tissue – elastin highlighted	Vascular dissection
Perls' Prussian blue	Hemosiderin	Aging injury, liver disease
Periodic acid-Schiff	Basement membrane tissue carbohydrates, fungi	Fungi, glycogen
Gram	Bacteria	Bacterial endocarditis, necrotizing fasciitis
Ziehl–Neelsen	Mycobacteria	Tuberculosis
Grocott	Fungi	Fungal infections
Congo red	Amyloid	Senile cardiac amyloidosis, congophilic angiopathy

Source: Adapted from Bucholz, T. A., & Sobel, D. (2011). Histopathological techniques in forensic pathology. In: Spitz, A., & Fisher, D., (eds.), Forensic Pathology: Principles and Practice (2nd edn., pp. 211–227) Academic Press.

4.5.1.3. Connective Tissue Stains

Several connective tissue stains are accessible, such as Van Giesson, Masson trichrome, Martius scarlet blue (MSB or Lendrum's stain), phosphotungstic acid hematoxylin (PTAH), periodic acid-Schiff (PAS), methanine silver, and reticulin (2). Masson trichrome, a frequently employed stain in our field, produces a blue-black coloration in nuclei, a red coloration in cytoplasm, and a blue coloration in collagen (Figure 4.31). Another beneficial dye is Movat's pentachrome. Collagen is stained yellow, mucin is stained blue, fibrin is stained an intense red, muscle is stained red, and elastin is stained black. Therefore, it is highly useful for studying vascular tissue (Figure 4.32). Elastin can be detected using other staining techniques, such as Verhöeff's method. Martius scarlet and blue are valuable dyes for the purpose of staining fibrin. Periodic acid-Schiff (PAS) staining is a valuable technique for visualizing basement membranes and tissue carbohydrates.

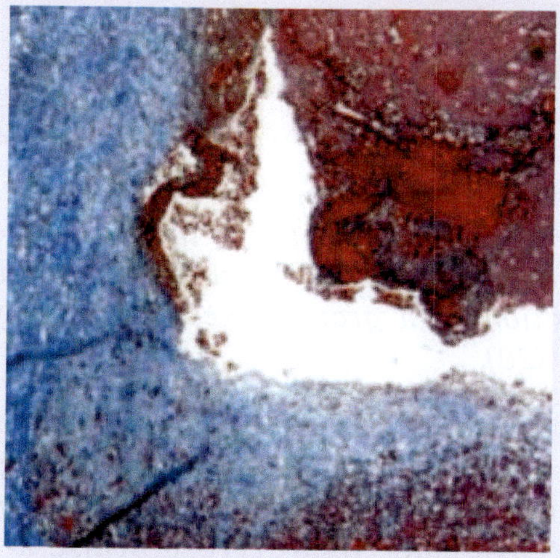

Figure 4.31. *Coronary artery atheroma with plaque hemorrhage and thrombus (Masson trichrome, x25).*

Source: *Adapted from J. E. McLendon and W. G. Darby, "Cardiovascular Pathology," in Atlas of Forensic Pathology, 3rd ed., edited by M. L. DiMaio and S. P. DiMaio, Cambridge University Press, 2016, pp. 178–180.*

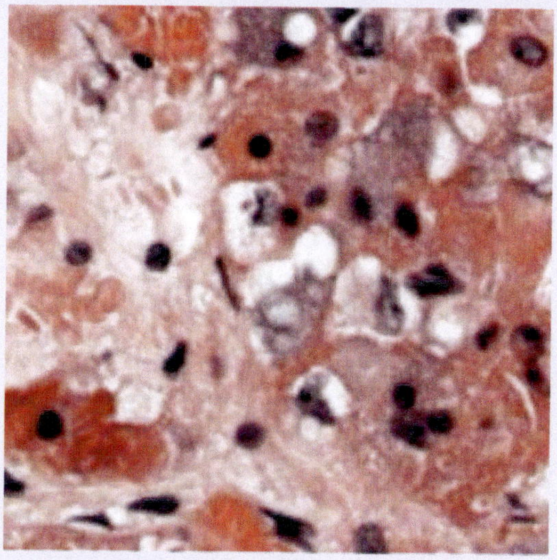

Figure 4.32. *Carotid artery dissection (Movat stain, x100).*

Source: *Adapted from S.J. Sheppard and K.M. Simpson, "Vascular Pathology in Forensic Medicine," in Forensic Pathology: A Comprehensive Guide, 3rd ed., edited by R. Saukko and B. Knight, CRC Press, 2015, pp. 352–367.*

4.5.1.4. Periodic Acid-Schiff Stain (PAS)

The Periodic acid-Schiff stain, also known as PAS, is a valuable stain used to detect glycogen, making it a useful tool in the diagnosis of glycogen storage diseases. Pretreatment with diastase can eliminate glycogen. In cases of alpha-1 antitrypsin deficiency, hepatocytes may exhibit a positive reaction, as intrahepatic globules can be stained with periodic acid-Schiff (PAS) and are resistant to diastase. Periodic acid-Schiff stains fungi, specifically viable hyphae, while Grocott stains both living and dead hyphae as well as the basement membrane. This staining technique is commonly used to detect fungi in tissues, such as in the kidney. The PAS stain is a valuable tool for detecting glycogen in the Armanni-Ebstein lesion, a condition that can manifest in cases of diabetic ketoacidosis.

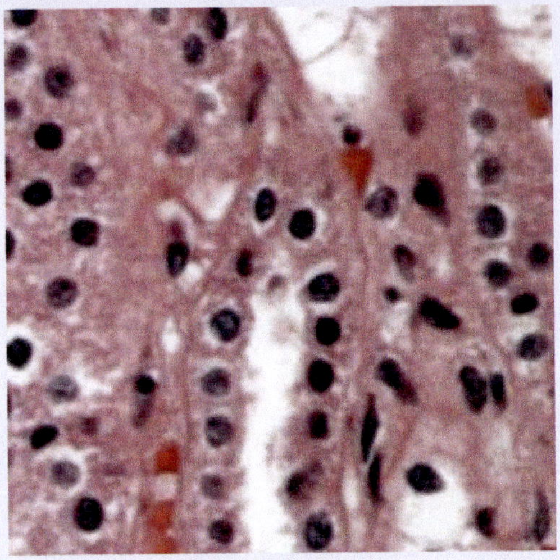

Figure 4.33. *Armanni-Ebstein lesion in the renal tubules (H&E, x200).*

Source: Adapted from M. Roggin and J.P. Siegel, "Renal Pathology in Forensic Histopathology," in Essentials of Forensic Medicine, 2nd ed., edited by R. Honig and L. Clark, Elsevier, 2018, pp. 287–298.

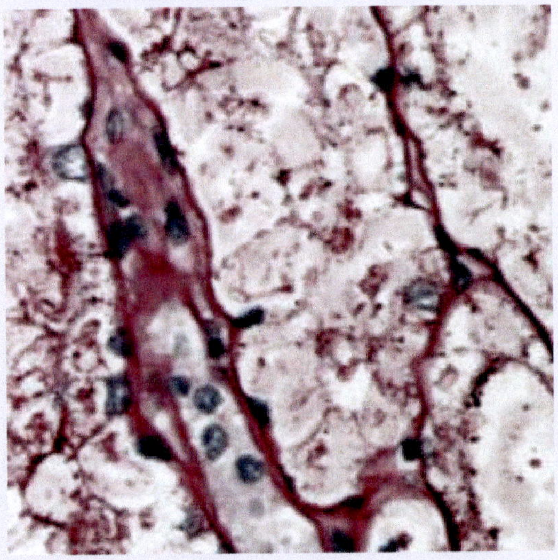

Figure 4.34. *Armanni-Ebstein lesion in the renal tubules (PAS, x200).*

Source: Adapted from J.M. Crawford and S.B. Taylor, "Renal Pathology in Forensic Medicine," in Principles of Forensic Pathology, edited by J.A. Prahlow and R.M. Byard, Humana Press, 2017, pp. 185–198.

4.5.1.5. Iron Stain

Iron is observed in the aftermath of hemorrhage during a period of survival. Additionally, it can build up in cases of liver cirrhosis and hemochromatosis. The presence of hemosiderin can assist in determining the age of injuries, as it typically takes 48–72 hours to appear (Figures 4.35 and 4.36). Hemosiderin can be observed on H&E-stained slides, but it is more prominently identified using the Perls' Prussian blue stain. Perls' method is widely regarded as the inaugural and seminal histochemical reaction, with its origins dating back to 1867.

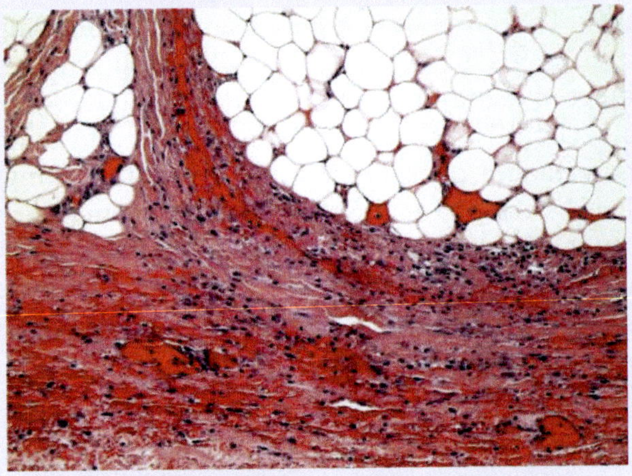

Figure 4.35. *Fresh bruise, a few hours old. The microphotography shows the bleeding area (fibrous septum in the hypodermis) with initial infiltration with granulocytes (Haematoxylin-eosin, X20).*

Source: Histological Characteristics of Bruises with Different Age – Scientific Figure on ResearchGate. Available from: https://www.researchgate.net/figure/Fresh-bruise-a-few-hours-old-The-microphotography-shows-the-bleeding-area-fibrous_fig3_320561842 [accessed 8 Jul, 2024].

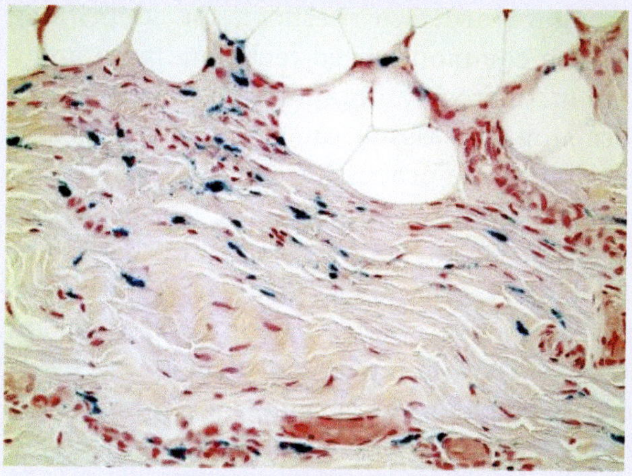

Figure 4.36. *Five days old bruise. The microphotography shows macrophages filled with hemosiderin, as well as hematoidin granules between erythrocytes in the bleeding area (Pearls Prussian Blue, X 100).*

Source: Histological Characteristics of Bruises with Different Age – Scientific Figure on ResearchGate. Available from: https://www.researchgate.net/figure/Five-days-old-bruise-The-microphotography-shows-macrophages-filled-with-hemosiderin-as_fig5_320561842 [accessed 8 Jul, 2024].

4.5.1.6. Fat Stains

The demonstration of fat is crucial in identifying fat embolism, although alterations in blood vessels, especially in the lungs, can indicate fat embolism when examined using routine staining (Figures 4.37 and 4.38). Adipose tissue can also be found in other organs, such as the renal tubules during ketoacidosis and in the liver during various conditions (Figures 4.39 and 4.40). As part of our medical procedure, we apply a staining technique to detect the presence of fat in the liver, kidney, and myocardium of deceased infants.

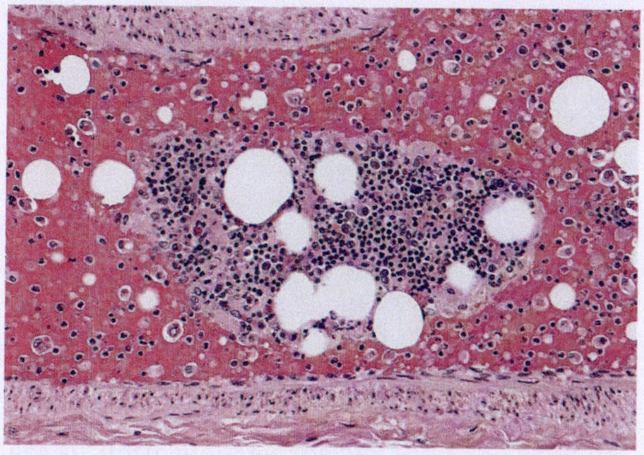

Figure 4.37. *Histopathology of a pulmonary artery with fat embolism (seen as multiple empty globular spaces on this H&E stain since its processing dissolves fat), seen on autopsy.*

Source: Wikimedia commons, Creative Commons license.

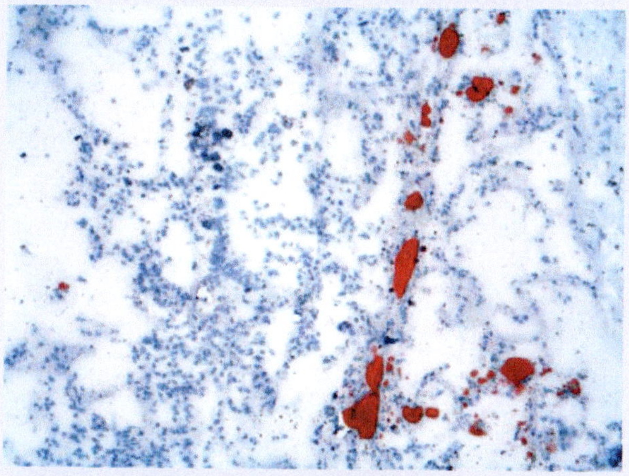

Figure 4.38. *Histopathological section of lung tissue stained with oil red O. Fat is seen as half-moons and globules, which probably cause incomplete and complete obstructions of capillaries and slightly larger vessels.*

Source: A young trauma patient with five fractures and multi-organ failure – Scientific Figure on ResearchGate. Available from: https://www.researchgate.net/figure/Histopathological-section-of-lung-tissue-stained-with-oil-red-O-Fat-is-seen-as_fig2_325030245 [accessed 8 Jul, 2024].

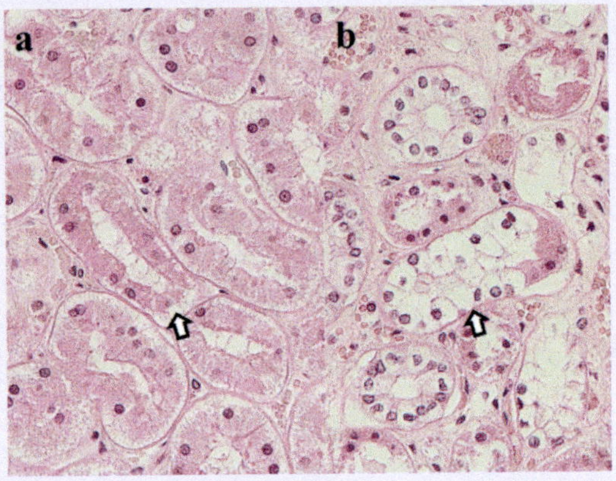

Figure 4.39. *A subnuclear vacuolization in the renal tubule epithelium (arrow) was observed (Hematoxylin and eosin staining, 400×). b Armanni-Ebstein lesion (arrow) was detected (Hematoxylin and eosin staining, 400×).*

Source: Prominent black esophagus, Wischnewsky spots, and black duodenum in a fatal hypothermia case with an underlying diabetic ketoacidosis – Scientific Figure on ResearchGate. Available from: https://www.researchgate.net/figure/Histopathology-of-the-kidney-a-Subnuclear-vacuolization-in-the-renal-tubule-epithelium_fig4_381400969 [accessed 8 Jul, 2024].

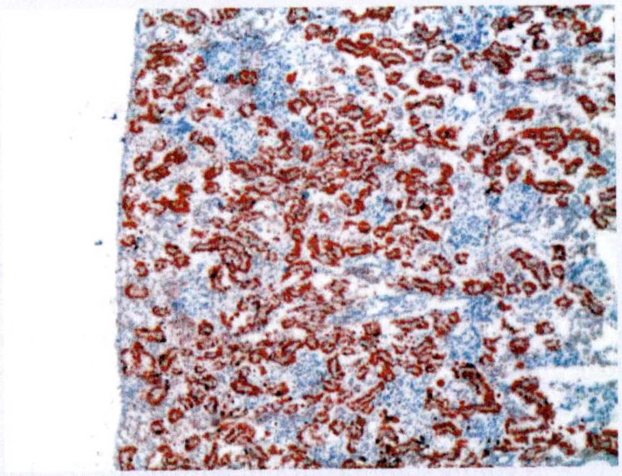

Figure 4.40. *Kidney with subnuclear vacuolation in ketoacidosis due to fat accumulation (oil red O, x25).*

Source: Lau G, Lai SH, 2008. Creative Commons License.

There are two methods for identifying fat. One commonly used technique is to apply a stain to freshly obtained, unaltered tissue. Formalin-fixed tissue can be utilized, if it has not undergone processing, as this would result in the removal of fat. Next, the frozen section is subjected to staining using oil red O or Sudan black. Osmium tetroxide possesses post-fixation characteristics and exhibits excellent fat visualization; however, it is hindered by its toxicity and high cost, leading most laboratories to opt for oil red O instead (Sacco et al., 2022; Zapico & Adserias-Garriga, 2022).

4.5.1.7. Amyloid

Amyloid refers to a collection of interconnected proteins that have the potential to cause diseases in humans. Staining for amyloid can sometimes provide useful information during postmortem examinations. Congo red and Sirius red are dyes employed for visualizing amyloid deposits, which exhibit apple-green birefringence under polarization. There are also immunohistochemical stains available for detecting amyloid. Amyloid can be found in vascular diseases such as congophilic angiopathy (Figure 4.41).

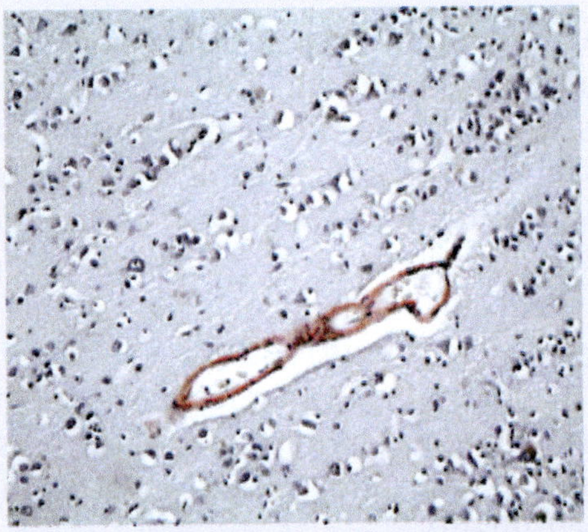

Figure 4.41. *Congophilic angiopathy (Congo red, x200).*

Source: Lau G, Lai SH, 2008. Creative Commons License.

In cases of senile cardiac amyloidosis, the staining with Congo red is not very strong and shows better results when using immunohistochemistry with transthyretin (Figures 4.42 and 4.43).

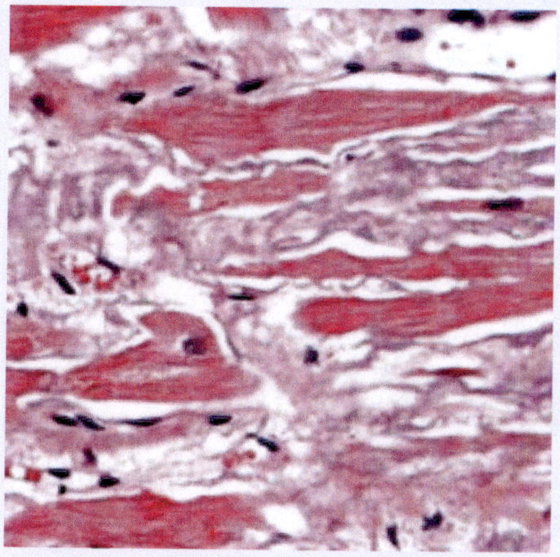

Figure 4.42. *Senile cardiac amyloidosis (H&E, x100).*

Source: Lau G, Lai SH, 2008. Creative Commons License.

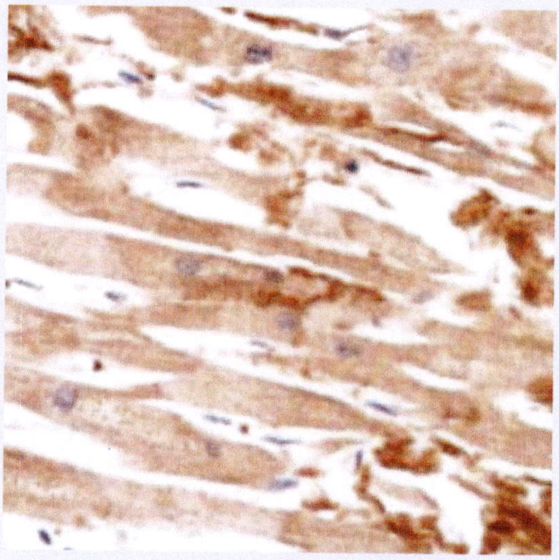

Figure 4.43. *Senile cardiac amyloidosis (transthyretin immunohistochemistry, x100).*

Source: Lau G, Lai SH, 2008. Creative Commons License.

4.5.1.8. Microorganisms

Infections are frequently responsible for mortality. Not all cases necessitate detailed examination, as the presence of pneumonia or meningitis can typically be observed through macroscopic analysis. Microbiological investigations can then be used to determine the specific organism(s) responsible. A routine Gram stain is employed to visualize bacteria in tissue. Fungi can be visualized using a PAS or Grocott stain. The latter stain also detects organisms such as *Pneumocystis jiroveci* (Figures 4.44 and 4.45). Mycobacteria can be stained using the Ziehl–Neelsen staining method.

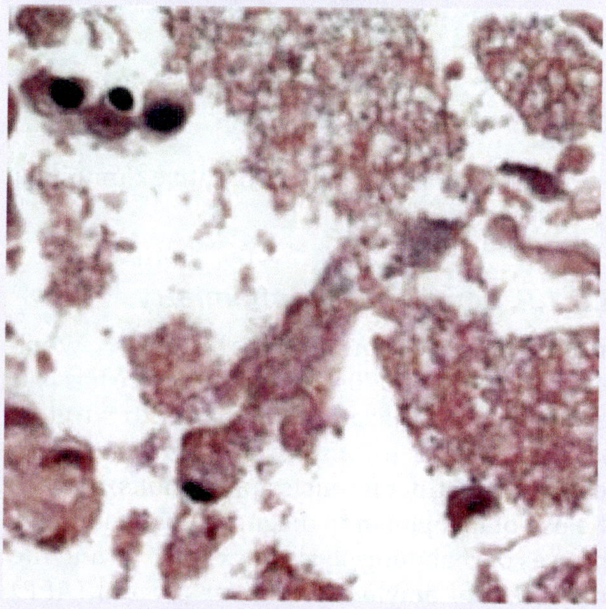

Figure 4.44. *Lung with pneumocystis pneumonia (H&E, x100).*

Source: Lau G, Lai SH, 2008. Creative Commons License.

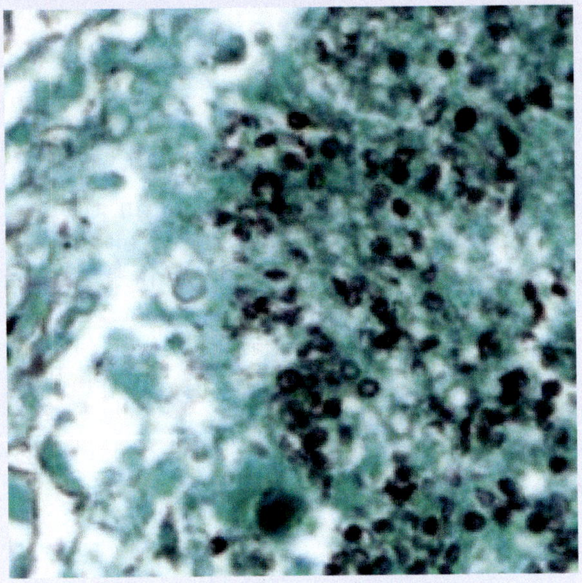

Figure 4.45. *Lung with pneumocystis pneumonia (Grocott, x100).*

Source: Lau G, Lai SH, 2008. Creative Commons License.

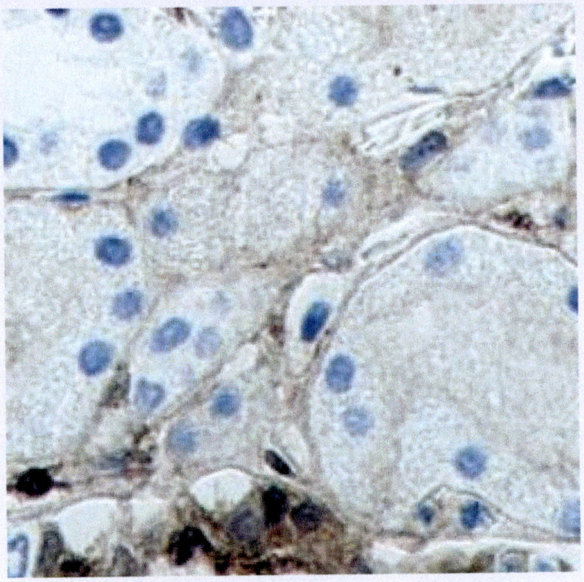

Figure 4.46. *Kidney. Myoglobin in rhabdomyolysis (myoglobin, x200).*

Source: Lau G, Lai SH, 2008. Creative Commons License.

4.5.1.9. Immunohistochemistry

Immunohistochemical techniques were pioneered in the 1970s. Forensic practice has had less extensive utilization compared to surgical pathology (refer to Table 4.2). However, certain tests have distinct forensic applications, such as the use of myoglobin to diagnose myoglobinuria in cases of rhabdomyolysis (Figure 4.46), and the utilization of amyloid precursor protein (APP) to identify damaged axons. CD 68 is used to detect and identify macrophages, which can be helpful in determining the age of injuries. Tumor markers can assist in identifying the specific type of cancer, but their medicolegal significance is generally limited. However, in some rare instances, there may be genetic implications associated with them. Immunohistochemistry using cytokeratin is highly valuable for diagnosing amniotic fluid embolism.

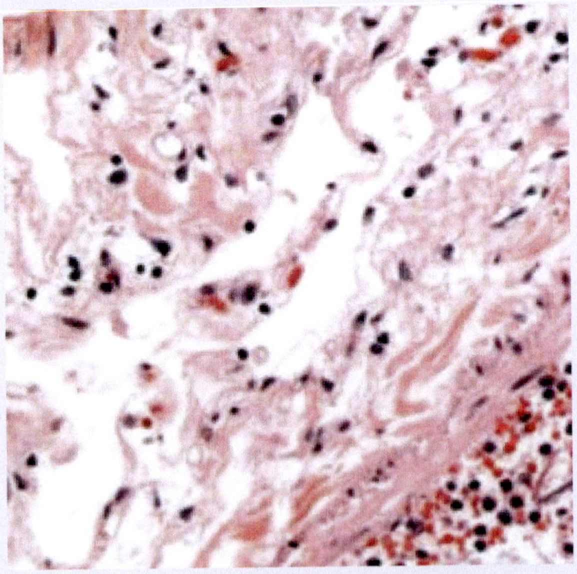

Figure 4.47. *Lung. Amniotic fluid embolism (H&E, x100).*

Source: Lau G, Lai SH, 2008. Creative Commons License.

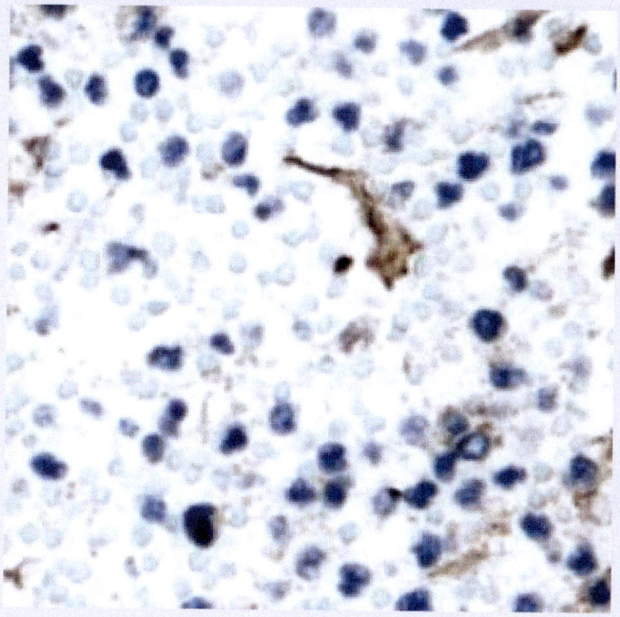

Figure 4.48. *Lung. Amniotic fluid embolism. Immunohistochemistry for cytokeratins (AE1/AE3, x200).*

Source: Lau G, Lai SH, 2008. Creative Commons License.

Table 4.2. Some Immunohistochemical Stains Used in Forensic Pathology Practice

Stain	Tissue	Example of Case
Myoglobin	Myoglobin	Myoglobinuria
Amyloid precursor protein (APP)	Damaged axons	Head injury, cerebral hypoxia
Cytokeratins	Multiple	Undifferentiated cancer, amniotic fluid embolism
Amyloid	Multiple	Cardiac amyloid
CD 68	Macrophages	Dating injuries

Source: Parai JL, Milroy CM, 2018.

4.5.1.10. Decomposed Tissue

While autolysis and putrefactive changes can negatively impact the quality of histology, it is still feasible to identify relevant changes in less advanced stages. Therefore, histology can be valuable in decomposed bodies (Figure 4.49). Rajapaksha and Pollanen provide an example of a decomposed body where liver emboli were found in the lung, suggesting that there was trauma to the liver during the person's life.

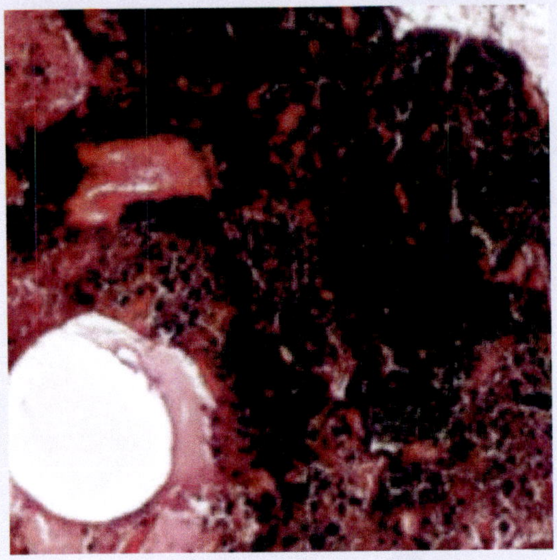

Figure 4.49. *Decomposed lung showing features of crack cocaine use with prominent black areas (H&E, x25).*

Source: Parai JL, Milroy CM, 2018.

4.6. Looking Ahead – the Future of Forensic and Autopsy Histopathology

In the future, the use of immunohistochemistry and other molecular diagnostic techniques may be further extended in the field of forensic pathology. While tissue quality is frequently the primary constraint in utilizing these techniques, significant progress can still be made in instances where autolysis is not significantly advanced. The above illustration demonstrates the successful identification of the SARS coronavirus using in-situ hybridization, which serves as a noteworthy example.

Colleagues from various parts of the world are currently making progress in refining post-mortem and forensic diagnosis methods, leading to numerous areas of research interest. The subsequent section provides a concise overview, which is not intended to be exhaustive or all-encompassing, of select research conducted in this field.

4.6.1. Immunohistochemistry and Forensic Neuropathology

Immunohistochemistry for ß-APP in the brain has led to new insights into the pathology of axonal injury, whether caused by trauma or other factors, in recent years. Immunohistochemistry analysis of ß-APP revealed that traumatic axonal injury is significantly more prevalent than previously acknowledged. It became evident that axonal injury was not exclusively limited to trauma. For example, it has been demonstrated that ischemia is also linked to axonal injury.

4.6.2. Immunohistochemical Diagnosis in Cardiac Pathology

Accurate and precise techniques for detecting acute damage to the heart muscle are especially valuable in forensic investigations due to the high prevalence of cardiac disease as a leading cause of sudden death. Several applications of histochemistry have previously been mentioned in relation to the dating of myocardial infarcts.

A recent study has examined the importance of elevated levels of complement C9 in the damaged myocardium caused by ischemia. The authors observed a progressive and varying increase in the expression of complement C9 in individuals with histological evidence of acute myocardial infarctions, individuals with only electrocardiographic evidence of acute myocardial infarctions, and individuals with severe coronary artery disease but no evidence of acute myocardial ischemia.

The TUNEL method has been used to investigate the detection of apoptosis in the myocardium in cases of sudden cardiac death, as compared to a control group. Nevertheless, there was no notable disparity in the ratio of apoptotic myocardial nuclei between instances of myocardial infarction caused by coronary artery disease and instances of sudden cardiac death in the absence of coronary artery disease.

The authors proposed utilizing the technique as a screening tool for the postmortem diagnosis of sudden death resulting from cardiac causes.

Immunohistochemical detection of cardiac troponin-C (cTnC) and cardiac troponin-T (cTnT) can be used as a method to identify acute myocardial damage. In cases of myocardial infarction, the expression of cTnC was found to be highly positive, widespread, and more common than cTnT.

Dettmeyer et al. sought to distinguish dilated cardiomyopathy caused by inflammation from idiopathic/alcoholic dilated cardiomyopathy by using immunohistochemistry to detect markers of T-lymphocytes (LCA, CD3), macrophages (CD68), and tenascin. The suggested criteria for inflammatory cardiomyopathy involve visually quantifying more than 2 CD3 positive lymphocytes per high-power field and more than 7 CD3 lymphocytes per square millimeter.

4.6.3. Immunohistochemical Diagnosis of Sepsis

The identification of sepsis is crucial in forensic practice, particularly in cases of sudden deaths and certain instances of hospital deaths. An investigation has been conducted on the increased levels of different cellular adhesion molecules, growth factors, and proteins in the lungs of patients who died as a result of sepsis or had sepsis at the time of death. E-selectin, which was absent in the unstimulated endothelium of the pulmonary microvasculature, was observed to be increased in sepsis. ICAM-1 expression increased in the endothelium and leukocytes in the lungs, while lactoferrin and VLA-4 were also up-regulated in pulmonary leukocytes. On the other hand, sepsis-induced lung injury causes a decrease in the expression of vascular endothelial growth factor (VEGF), which is typically highly expressed in the healthy alveolar and bronchial epithelium of individuals.

4.6.4. Wound Pathology

The histological aging of wounds continues to be a challenging area. Research has long been focused on the process of wound aging and determining the vitality of wounds. Grellner et al. observed that the expression of transforming growth factors (TGF)-alpha and transforming growth factor-beta1 increased in damaged skin, peaking within 30–60 minutes after the injury. It was noted that both factors, particularly TGF-beta1, remained measurable at increased levels in injured tissues for several days to weeks. The authors proposed that the expression patterns of the two factors could be utilized as a tool to assist in the assessment of wound age.

ICAM-1 was found to be a valuable indicator of both the extent of skin wound inflammation and an early indication of wound healing. Furthermore, the level of VEGF expression in aging wounds has been documented, but it is only reliable in identifying wounds that are at least seven days old. The significance of detecting p53, however, remained uncertain in this domain.

4.6.5. The Challenges Ahead

In the field of forensic examination, the supplementary methods exhibit a significant amount of potential. On the other hand, additional research is necessary to reproduce and replicate some of the observations to refine them for application. The field of forensic diagnosis may one day be able to make use of molecular diagnostic techniques that will be more advanced in the future (Sacco et al., 2022; Zapico & Adserias-Garriga, 2022).

A Closer Look

Forensic Pathology of Liver Trauma

The forensic pathology of liver trauma is a critical area within forensic medicine that examines injuries to the liver resulting from various forms of trauma. This field is essential in understanding the severity, mechanism, and implications of liver injuries, which can range from minor lacerations to life-threatening ruptures. An in-depth analysis of liver trauma involves recognizing the anatomical and physiological aspects of the liver, identifying the common causes and types of liver injuries, and assessing the implications for forensic investigations.

The liver, a vital organ located in the upper right quadrant of the abdomen, performs numerous functions, including detoxification, protein synthesis, and the production of bile. Its vascular structure, characterized by a rich supply of blood vessels and the hepatic portal system, makes it particularly vulnerable to traumatic injury. Forensic pathologists must consider the liver's unique anatomy when evaluating trauma cases, as the severity of injury can be influenced by the location and extent of damage to its blood vessels and parenchyma.

Common causes of liver trauma include blunt force trauma, penetrating injuries, and iatrogenic injuries. Blunt force trauma, often resulting from vehicular accidents, falls, or physical assaults, can cause liver contusions, lacerations, or even ruptures. Penetrating injuries, such as those from stab wounds or gunshot wounds, can lead to direct disruption of liver tissue and blood vessels. Iatrogenic injuries, occurring during medical procedures, can also result in liver damage if not carefully managed.

The classification of liver injuries is based on their severity and impact on liver function. The American Association for the Surgery of Trauma (AAST) provides a grading system for liver injuries, ranging from Grade I (minor contusions or lacerations) to Grade V (liver ruptures or large devascularized areas). This grading system helps forensic pathologists categorize the extent of trauma and assess its implications for both immediate and long-term health outcomes.

In forensic investigations, the examination of liver trauma involves a thorough autopsy and pathological assessment. During autopsy, forensic pathologists look for evidence of liver injury, such as hemorrhage, lacerations, or necrosis. They also evaluate the liver's vascular structures to determine if there has been significant bleeding or disruption of blood flow. Histological examination of liver tissue can reveal details about the injury's timing and severity, including the presence of cellular damage, inflammation, and necrosis.

Determining the cause and manner of death in cases involving liver trauma requires careful consideration of the injury's impact on overall health. Forensic pathologists must differentiate between traumatic liver injuries and other potential causes of liver damage, such as pre-existing liver disease or infections. Additionally, they must assess the potential for complications, such as internal bleeding or shock, which can influence the outcome of the trauma.

Liver trauma has significant implications for forensic investigations and legal proceedings. Accurate documentation and analysis of liver injuries can provide crucial information in cases of homicide, accidents, or medical negligence. Forensic pathologists' findings can help establish the sequence of events leading to the trauma, assess the severity of injuries, and contribute to determining the cause of death.

Summary

- Forensic histopathology is a specialized field within forensic medicine that focuses on the microscopic examination of tissues to determine the cause of death, disease processes, and other pathological conditions in a legal context. This discipline combines traditional histological techniques with modern forensic science to analyze tissue samples obtained during autopsies or from living individuals in cases of suspected abuse or poisoning.
- The primary role of forensic histopathology is to provide crucial evidence that can aid in criminal investigations, legal proceedings, and public health interventions. It involves the study of tissue morphology, cellular patterns, and the identification of pathological changes that may indicate trauma, disease, or toxic exposure. Forensic histopathologists work closely with forensic pathologists, toxicologists, and law enforcement agencies to ensure accurate and thorough investigations.
- Key applications of forensic histopathology include determining the time and mechanism of death, identifying signs of injury or disease, detecting toxic substances, and differentiating between natural and unnatural causes of death. Advances in immunohistochemistry, molecular pathology, and digital imaging have enhanced the precision and scope of this field, making it an indispensable tool in modern forensic science. Through meticulous tissue analysis, forensic histopathology contributes significantly to the pursuit of justice and the advancement of medical knowledge.

References

1. Bonicelli, A., Mickleburgh, H. L., Chighine, A., Locci, E., Wescott, D. J., & Procopio, N. (2022). The 'ForensOMICS' approach for postmortem interval estimation from human bone by integrating metabolomics, lipidomics, and proteomics. *eLife*, *11*, e83658. https://doi.org/10.7554/eLife.83658.
2. Boroumand, M., Grassi, V. M., Castagnola, F., De-Giorgio, F., D'aloja, E., Vetrugno, G., Pascali, V. L., Vincenzoni, F., Iavarone, F., Faa, G., et al. (2023). Estimation of postmortem interval using top-down HPLC–MS analysis of peptide fragments in vitreous humor: A pilot study. *International Journal of Mass Spectrometry*, *483*, 116952. https://doi.org/10.1016/j.ijms.2023.116952.
3. Broadbelt, K. G., Rivera, K. D., Paterson, D. S., Duncan, J. R., Trachtenberg, F. L., Paulo, J. A., Stapels, M. D., Borenstein, N. S., Belliveau, R. A., Haas, E. A., et al. (2012). Brainstem deficiency of the 14-3-3 regulator of serotonin synthesis: A proteomics analysis in the sudden infant death syndrome. *Molecular & Cellular Proteomics*, *11*(12), M111.009530. https://doi.org/10.1074/mcp.M111.009530.
4. Choi, K. M., Zissler, A., Kim, E., Ehrenfellner, B., Cho, E., Lee, S. I., Steinbacher, P., Yun, K. N., Shin, J. H., Kim, J. Y., et al. (2019). Postmortem proteomics to discover biomarkers for forensic PMI estimation. *International Journal of Legal Medicine*, *133*(4), 899–908. https://doi.org/10.1007/s00414-019-02163-w.
5. Hernández-Romero, D., Sánchez-Rodríguez, E., Osuna, E., Sibón, A., Martínez-Villanueva, M., Noguera-Velasco, J. A., & Pérez-Cárceles, M. D. (2020). Proteomics in deaths by drowning: Diagnostic efficacy of apolipoprotein A1 and α-1 antitrypsin, pilot study. *Diagnostics*, *10*(11), 747. https://doi.org/10.3390/diagnostics10110747.

6. Sacco, M. A., Cordasco, F., Scalise, C., Ricci, P., & Aquila, I. (2022). Systematic review on post-mortem protein alterations: Analysis of experimental models and evaluation of potential biomarkers of time of death. *Diagnostics*, *12*(6), 1490. https://doi.org/10.3390/diagnostics12061490.

7. Zapico, S. C., & Adserias-Garriga, J. (2022). Postmortem interval estimation: New approaches by the analysis of human tissues and microbial communities' changes. *Forensic Sciences*, *2*(2), 163–174. https://doi.org/10.3390/forensics2020012.

Chapter 5

CARE OF DETAINEES

Contents

Introduction

This chapter discusses the various treatment options that are available to jail inmates who are incarcerated for relatively short periods of time and who suffer from substance use disorders. An examination of what constitutes a jail, who is incarcerated in jail, how and when substance abuse treatment can be provided, and what types of treatment are effective in this setting are some of the topics that are covered in this chapter to discuss treatment issues that are specific to jails. Finally, recommendations are made regarding the treatment interventions that are most suitable for brief, short-term, and long-term periods of jail treatment. These recommendations pertain to the treatment services that can be provided within the confines of a jail, which include the physical restrictions, the legal restrictions, and the policy restrictions. An overview of the larger systems that have an impact on treatment in a correctional facility comes next. The chapter provides an overview of the research, illustrates some of the programs that are currently in place, and offers some suggestions for the treatment of substance abuse in correctional facilities and detention centers.

Orientation and Directional Terms

Term	Definition	Illustration
Jail inmates	Individuals who are confined in a jail, usually serving short-term sentences or awaiting trial.	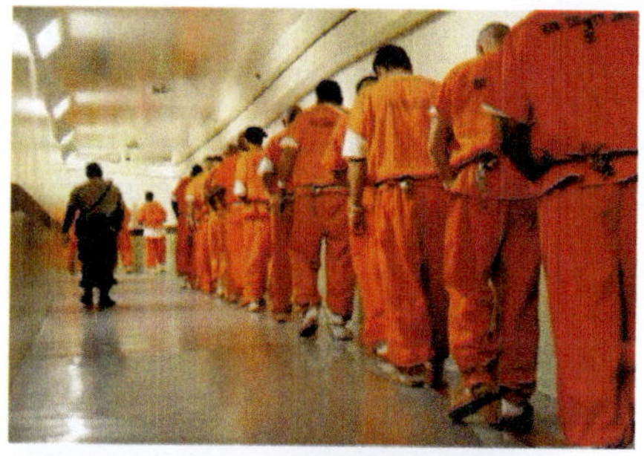
Detention centers	Facilities designed to house individuals who are awaiting trial, sentencing, or serving short-term sentences, often for juvenile or pre-trial detainees.	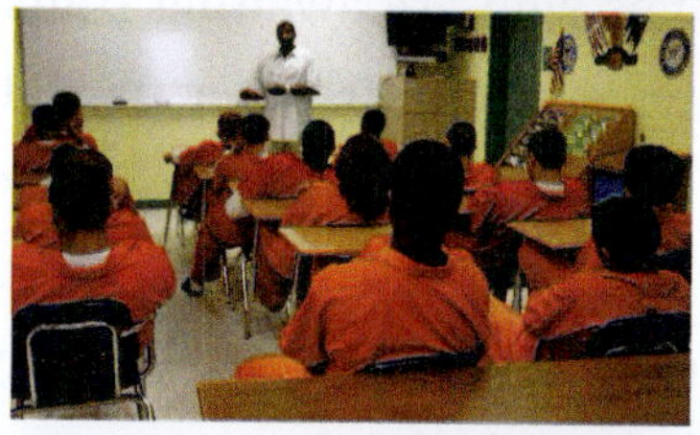
Juveniles	Individuals who are under the age of 18 and are subject to the juvenile justice system rather than the adult criminal justice system.	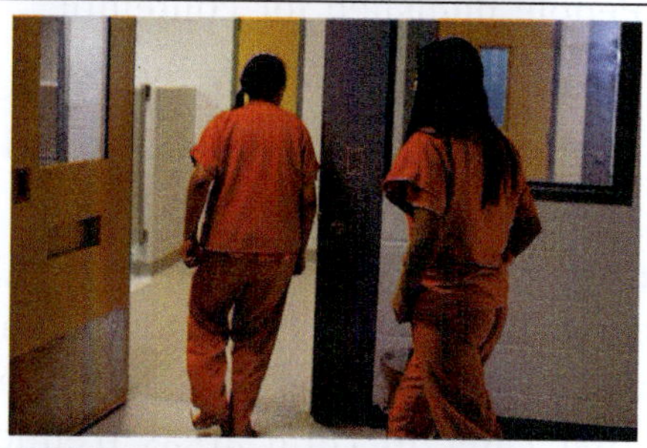
Drug offenses	Criminal activities related to the possession, distribution, manufacture, or trafficking of controlled substances or illegal drugs.	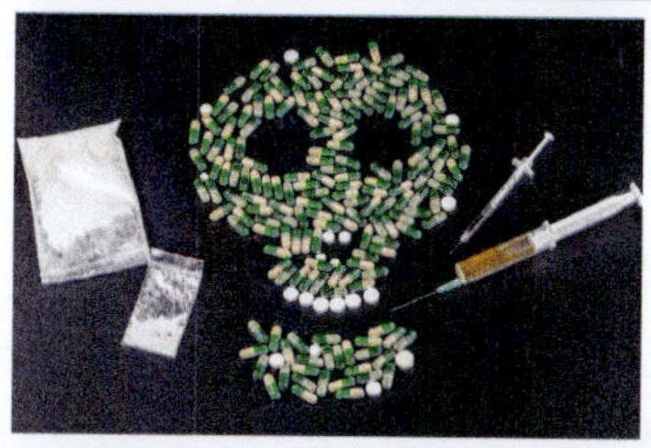
Domestic violence	Physical, emotional, or psychological abuse directed at a partner or family member within a domestic setting, often involving ongoing patterns of control or intimidation.	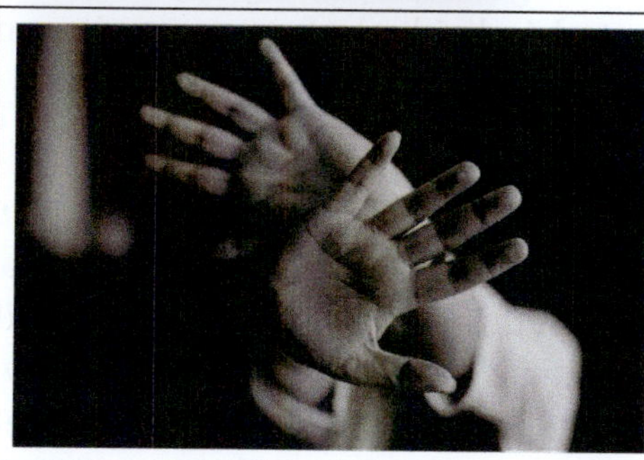

5.1. Definitions

Correctional facilities, commonly known as jails or detention centers, accommodate heterogeneous populations of individuals who are detained for a multitude of reasons. Jails are facilities that detain individuals while they are going through the legal process, which includes arraignment, criminal court, grand jury, hearings, trial, and sentencing. These individuals are commonly known as detainees and are currently awaiting sentencing. Jails also confine those sentenced to short-term incarceration (usually 1 year or less) and serve as a holding facility for:

- Individuals who have allegedly violated probation, parole, or bail conditions
- Those who are absconding from court-ordered programs or other community placements
- Juveniles who are awaiting transfer to juvenile authorities or adult State prisons
- Inmates awaiting transfer to State, Federal, or other local authorities
- Inmates transferred from overcrowded Federal, State, or other prisons
- Individuals detained by the military
- Those held for protective custody
- People punished for contempt
- Witnesses detained by the court
- People with mental illness pending transfer to appropriate mental health facilities (Harlow, 1998).

Defining a Jail There are around 3,365 jails in the United States (Stephan, 2001), which vary in size from small jails in rural areas to large jails usually found in or near big cities. The sociodynamics of jails differ based on their size. For instance, prisoners residing in correctional facilities that cater to rural areas frequently have acquaintances among their fellow inmates, whereas those confined in expansive and complex prison systems have a lower likelihood of being housed with familiar individuals.

5.2. Trends

Various recent trends have resulted in alterations in the incarcerated population. The implementation of more stringent sentencing laws for drug offenses has resulted in a rise in the population of incarcerated individuals from minority and female demographics. Simultaneously, a substantial decrease in funding for the mental health care system has resulted in a rise in the population of inmates with multiple problems (Peters 1993; Peters et al. 1997; National GAINS Center 2002).

Due to these changes, prisons are now accommodating an increasing number of individuals who have been excluded from conventional societal support systems, such as State hospitals. Jails have expanded their role to include identifying and addressing various psychosocial issues in the community, such as HIV/AIDS, domestic violence, educational deficiencies, homelessness, mental illness, and substance use disorders (Peters & Matthews, 2002).

The prevalence of substance use disorders among incarcerated individuals has increased since the 1980s. In 1989, a majority of jail inmates, specifically 67%, were incarcerated either for committing a drug offense or for engaging in regular drug use. As of May 1998, the percentage had risen to 70%, which is roughly equivalent to 7 out of every 10 jail inmates. Approximately 16% of individuals committed their offense intending to acquire funds specifically for the purchase of drugs (Wilson 2000). The growth of jail substance abuse treatment programs has not kept pace with this trend (Belenko & Peugh, 1998; Peters & Matthews, 2002). Recently, there has been a stabilization or slight decrease in levels of substance use and abuse, varying depending on the specific substance. According to James (2004), in 2002, 66% of jail inmates reported consuming alcohol regularly, which was a slight decrease from 66.3% in 1996. Additionally, 68.7% of inmates reported regular use of illicit drugs, which was an increase from 64.2% in 1996. Regular use was defined as using these substances at least once a week for a month or longer.

Prisons frequently act as the initial chance for criminals to have their substance use disorder and other issues (such as other mental disorders) recognized, to have their immediate needs stabilized (such as detoxification from alcohol or opioids), and to be referred to in-house or community services (Peters & Matthews, 2002). Indeed, a significant number of individuals begin their participation in treatment programs while incarcerated (Mumola, 1999). Therefore, jail administrators face a dual challenge: acknowledging the necessity of treatment and comprehending that treatment should be tailored to the specific population, taking into account factors such as culture, average length of stay, type of crimes, and psychosocial needs.

5.3. Treatment Services in Jails

Multiple studies have shown that in-jail substance abuse treatment programs are effective in reducing criminal recidivism (Peters & Matthews, 2002). Treated inmates experience a decrease in rearrest rates ranging from 5 percent to 25% compared to untreated inmates, during follow-up periods lasting from 6 months to 5 years. Incarcerated individuals who receive treatment also experience a longer period of time before being arrested again after their release, compared to those who do not receive treatment. Additional favorable results linked to in-jail treatment include decreased relapse rates among individuals receiving treatment (Tucker, 1998), decreased levels of depression (San Francisco County Sheriff's Office Department 1996), and a decrease in disciplinary infractions (Tunis et al., 1997). The cost savings linked to jail treatment programs range from $156,000 to $1.4 million per year, as reported by the Center for Substance Abuse Research in 1992 and Hughey and Klemke in 1996.

According to the Substance Abuse and Mental Health Services Administration (SAMHSA) in 2000, even though in-jail treatment has shown positive results, two-thirds of jails do not provide treatment, excluding additional services like assessment, self-help groups, and educational programs. Approximately 66% of the facilities offer self-help programs, while around 30% provide detoxification programs. Out of the jail inmates who admitted to using drugs, only one out of eight had received any form of treatment since their admission. The majority of those who did receive treatment reported participating in self-help programs (Wilson, 2000).

5.4. Description of the Population

As of midyear 2003, there were 762,672 individuals under the custody or supervision of local jails. Approximately 10% of these individuals (71,371) were not physically present in the jail facility. Instead, they were either under electronic monitoring, participating in outside treatment programs, or on work release. This number represented a 3.9% increase compared to the number of inmates held in jail in midyear 2002. From 1995 to 2003, the incarceration rate rose from 193 to 238 inmates per 100,000 residents, representing a growth of more than 23%. According to Harrison and Karberg (2004), a majority of the adult jail inmates, specifically 60.6%, were still awaiting trial and had not been found guilty of the crime they were being detained for. Based on a survey conducted in 1999, it was found that 5% of jail inmates were identified as noncitizens (Stephan, 2001).

5.4.1. Crimes

The crimes committed, or purportedly committed, by incarcerated individuals are roughly equally distributed among violent offenses (24.4%), property offenses (24.4%), drug offenses (24.7%), and public-order offenses (24.9%). According to James (2004), the most prevalent criminal activities are drug trafficking, accounting for 12.1% of offenses, assault, accounting for 11.7% of offenses, and drug possession, accounting for 10.8% of offenses. According to Maruschak (1999a), individuals who drive while intoxicated and end up in jail are typically older, have a higher level of education, and are more likely to be Caucasian and male compared to other inmates.

5.4.2. Income and Education

Based on data from 2002, around 44% of individuals incarcerated in jails had not obtained a General Educational Development (GED) certificate or completed high school. At the time of their arrest, 29% of jail inmates were unemployed, while only 57.4% were engaged in full-time employment. According to James (2004), a significant majority of jail inmates had meager incomes, as 59% of them reported earning less than $1,000 per month.

5.4.3. Gender

From midyear 1995 to midyear 2003, the proportion of male prisoners decreased from 89.8% to 88.1%, while the proportion of female prisoners increased from 10.2 to 11.9%. In 2003, men had a per capita likelihood of being in jail that was eight times higher than that of women. Between July 1, 2002, and June 30, 2003, the population of female inmates in jail experienced a 6.3% growth, while the number of male inmates saw a 3.7% increase (Harrison & Karberg, 2004).

According to James (2004), more than 55% of incarcerated women have experienced physical or sexual abuse before being imprisoned. Of these, 44.9% have reported physical abuse and 35.9% have reported sexual abuse. Women exhibit a higher probability of being diagnosed with mental illness. According to Ditton's study in 1999, around 22.7% of female inmates and 15.6% of male inmates were diagnosed with mental illness. According to a survey conducted among inmates in State prisons and jails, it was found that men with mental illness were twice as prone as other men to disclose a past experience of abuse (Ditton, 1999).

Gender influences the types of offenses committed. Women exhibited a higher likelihood of being detained for drug possession rather than trafficking, while the opposite was true for men. Additionally, women were more prone to being detained for property offenses rather than violent offenses, whereas men showed the opposite pattern. Nevertheless, a higher proportion of incarcerated women are serving sentences for drug-related crimes. In 2002, the primary offenses for which women were incarcerated included drug possession (14.5%), fraud (14%), drug trafficking (10.9%), and larceny/theft (10.3%). According to James (2004), the primary crimes committed by men were drug trafficking (12.3%), assault (12.2%), drug possession (10.3%), and burglary (7.2%).

5.4.4. Race and Ethnicity

In midyear 2003, the majority of jail inmates consisted of Caucasians (43.6%) or African Americans (39.2%). According to Harrison and Karberg (2004), African Americans had a 5-fold higher likelihood of being incarcerated compared to Caucasians, and a 3-fold higher likelihood compared to Hispanics/Latinos. According to Ditton's study in 1999, Caucasian jail inmates had a higher prevalence of mental illness (21.7%) compared to African Americans (13.7%) and Hispanics/Latinos (11.1%). According to James (2004), a higher percentage of Caucasians who were convicted jail inmates were found to be using alcohol (38.5%) and/or illicit drugs (33.2%) at the time of their offense compared to African Americans (29.3% and 27.3% respectively) or Hispanics/Latinos (30.1% and 23.8% respectively).

5.4.5. Substance Abuse

The jail population commonly exhibits a history of drug use, although there have been some alterations in usage patterns in recent years. In comparison to incarcerated individuals in 1996, inmates in 2002 reported a higher prevalence of marijuana, depressants, stimulants (excluding cocaine), and hallucinogen use in the month leading up to their offense. Conversely, they reported a lower incidence of cocaine and heroin/opioid use. In 2002, it was observed that 66% of jail inmates engaged in consistent alcohol consumption, while 68.7% engaged in regular use of illegal drugs. According to James (2004), around 35% of male convicts and 31% of female convicts stated that they were under the influence of alcohol at the time they committed their crimes. According to Wilson's study in 2000, 72% of inmates who were found guilty and involved in drug-related activities were under the supervision of the criminal justice system at the time of their arrest. This means they were either on probation, parole, awaiting trial, released on bail, or had escaped.

The rate of participation in substance abuse treatment programs in jails exhibits significant variation. The average population consists of predominantly young males, with a relatively equal distribution of African Americans (42%) and Caucasians (39%), similar to the overall jail population. According to Peters and Matthews (2002), a significant proportion (58%) of the participants are mandated to undergo treatment programs as a requirement of their sentence, and the majority of them have previous felony convictions. The proportion of incarcerated individuals who engaged in regular alcohol or drug use and subsequently received some form of substance abuse treatment, including participation in self-help groups, rose from 12.3% in 1996 to 15.1% in 2002 (James, 2004). Out of the inmates incarcerated for driving while intoxicated (DWI) offenses, only 17% participate in programs focused on self-help and educational groups for alcohol abuse. In contrast, 62% of probationers receive these services. According to Maruschak's research in 1999, only a mere 4 percent of individuals who are incarcerated for driving while intoxicated (DWI) are provided with any form of alcohol abuse treatment, such as detoxification or counseling.

5.4.6. HIV Status

In 2002, 1.3 percent of jail inmates who disclosed their test results were confirmed to have HIV, which is significantly higher than the rates in the general population. From 1998 to 1999, AIDS-related deaths constituted 8.5 percent of all deaths in jails, ranking it as the third most common cause of death in jails. The leading cause of death was natural causes, followed by suicide (Maruschak, 2001). Nevertheless, there was a decline in the number of deaths caused by AIDS in prisons, dropping from 9 per 100,000 incarcerated individuals in 2000 to 6 per 100,000 in 2002 (Maruschak, 2004).

The participation rate in substance abuse treatment programs in jails exhibits significant variation. In 2002, the prevalence of HIV-positive tests was 3 percent among African-American women, 2.9 percent among Hispanic/Latino inmates (both male and female), 1.6 percent among Caucasian women, 1 percent among African-American men, and 0.6 percent among Caucasian men. Among jail inmates who tested positive for HIV, African-American men constituted the highest count, with a total of 163,219 individuals (Maruschak, 2004).

5.4.7. Co-Occurring Mental Disorders

According to data from 1998, approximately 16% of individuals incarcerated in jails reported having either a mental disorder or having spent a night in a mental hospital. Offenders between the ages of 45 and 54 had the highest prevalence of mental illness, with 23% of them being identified as mentally ill (Ditton, 1999). A significant number of individuals with mental illness experience a recurring pattern of being incarcerated in jails. The rate of admission for individuals with mental illness in jails is approximately eight times higher than the rate of admission in public psychiatric hospitals. Consequently, the number of individuals suffering from severe mental illness incarcerated in U.S. correctional facilities exceeds the number of patients in State hospitals (Torrey et al., 1992). An analysis of administrative data on individuals held in jails and prisons in New York City revealed that around 15,000 individuals with mental health issues go through the correctional system and return to the community annually. A considerable number of these individuals also have co-occurring disorders (Lamon et al., 2002). According to the Urban Justice Center, a New York City advocacy group, individuals who have mental illness and are detained or imprisoned spend a considerably longer period of time incarcerated. On average, they spend 215 days in custody, whereas those who are not identified as mentally ill spend only 42 days (Winerip, 1999). A study conducted by Michaels et al. in 1992 revealed a significant correlation between homelessness and mental illness among inmates in the New York City correctional system. Specifically, half of the inmates who had experienced homelessness in the past responded affirmatively to at least one question in a mental illness screening. A significant proportion, if not the majority, of those individuals are habitual offenders.

Based on the research compiled and documented by the National GAINS Center (2002), it was found that 6.4 percent of male jail detainees and 12.2% of female jail detainees suffer from severe mental illness. Out of the male detainees who are admitted, 2.7 percent are diagnosed with schizophrenia/schizophreniform disorder, 1.4 percent with mania, and 3.9 percent with major depression. Out of the female detainees, 2.0 percent have schizophrenia/schizophreniform disorder, 1.4 percent have mania, and 10.5% have major depression. According to the National GAINS Center in 2002, 29% of male jail detainees and 53% of female jail detainees suffer from a substance use disorder. Additionally, both male and female detainees have a 72% rate of co-occurring mental illness and substance use disorders. Individuals who have both disorders are considerably more prone to experiencing various difficulties in terms of employment, family relationships, and health. They are also at a higher risk of not adhering to treatment, being rearrested, becoming homeless, engaging in violent behavior, and exhibiting suicidal tendencies, when compared to those who do not have this combination of disorders (Peters et al., 1992; Borum et al., 1997; Steadman et al. 1998; RachBeisel et al., 1999; Swartz and Lurigio 1999).

A research study conducted on 204 pretrial jail detainees undergoing substance abuse treatment in a Chicago jail revealed that over 50% of them fulfilled the criteria for at least one mental disorder throughout their lives. Additionally, the rates of severe mental illness experienced by these individuals throughout their lives were higher compared to the rates reported in the general jail population. Individuals who have co-occurring disorders also have a higher likelihood of being arrested for property offenses. They are also more likely to be dependent on alcohol, marijuana, or PCP, and to have multiple psychiatric disorders. Furthermore, the study uncovered a connection between profound mental illness, antisocial personality disorder, and substance abuse (Swartz & Lurigio, 1999).

Prisons can play a crucial role in involving family members, peers, and community organizations in supporting the rehabilitation efforts of prisoners.

5.5. Key Issues Related to Treatment

Various factors influence the accessibility and efficacy of treatment within correctional facilities. Consensus panel members have observed that treatment may not be provided to those who require it due to inadequate screening and selection methods for treatment participants. For certain prisoners, the duration of their incarceration may not be sufficient for implementing effective measures to address substance abuse issues. Some individuals, particularly those who are awaiting trial, may choose not to take part. Despite the presence of services, they often fail to adequately address the psychological, social, medical, and mental health needs of inmates. Additionally, certain inmates have highly complex special needs that cannot be fully addressed through brief or short-term treatment.

This section discusses specific factors related to jails that the consensus panel believes can influence the availability and effectiveness of treatment.

5.5.1. Public Perceptions About Jails

While jails are intended to enhance public safety and administer punishment by temporarily detaining defendants and convicted inmates, they are occasionally viewed unfavorably by the public. An unfavorable perception can have a detrimental impact on the morale and attitudes of prison personnel, especially in regard to treatment services. It is important to note that a considerable proportion of individuals held in jails are arrested for minor, nonviolent offenses. Furthermore, many of the offenses committed by inmates in jails are directly linked to their substance abuse and/or mental health issues. It is also worth mentioning that the majority of these individuals will be released back into their community relatively quickly.

Treatment staff can help dispel misperceptions and enhance the jail's sense of inclusion within the community's network of services by collaborating with local community agencies. Jails, due to their interaction with individuals who frequently utilize various community services and agencies, are in an advantageous position to establish collaborations aimed at enhancing community services. Several correctional facilities have made efforts to establish strong footholds to provide healthcare services, prevention and education programs, and vocational services, specifically targeting vulnerable populations such as the homeless, individuals with HIV/AIDS, and inmates with co-occurring mental disorders. Jails play a crucial role in involving family members, peers, and community organizations in supporting substance abuse treatment and the recovery efforts of inmates who are participating in treatment services. Prisons can also aid in fostering collaborations between community organizations and local correctional facilities to identify, treat, and direct inmates with substance use disorders toward appropriate care, either through diversion programs or aftercare. This helps to reinforce the notion that "treatment is effective."

5.5.2. Time Constraints

A significant obstacle faced by substance abuse treatment in correctional facilities is the limited time frame, both in terms of scheduling treatment and the duration of jail incarceration (Leukefeld & Tims, 1992). A significant number of pretrial inmates are temporarily detained in jail. Time limitations are a notably important aspect, as research indicates a connection between the efficacy of treatment and the duration of time spent in treatment (Swartz et al., 1996).

A correctional facility must adhere to a predetermined timetable that includes designated time periods when prisoners are confined to their cells to conduct inmate counts, provide meals, or engaging in other organized activities such as work. Therefore, although the amount of time spent in treatment is crucial, programs must vie for the inmate's time. Certain correctional facilities provide evening programming, although it can be challenging to organize and significantly raises the expenses associated with staffing. Because of scheduling limitations in correctional facilities, incarcerated individuals may be required to choose between participating in a treatment program or an educational program.

Furthermore, individuals who have committed crimes are restricted to the confines of the jail for a restricted duration, which is frequently uncertain. This is especially applicable to unsentenced, pretrial inmates who may be unpredictably released from jail after a court hearing. Optimally, treatment programming can be designed based on a modular framework that can adapt to various time durations and objectives, ranging from initial involvement and education to skill development and task completion.

5.6. Environmental Issues

There is a significant influx of individuals who enter correctional facilities, either as visitors or as service providers. Although it is important to welcome support from the community and visits from family members, it is essential to acknowledge that managing and supervising these activities can be burdensome for staff. This is because they may have to allocate time to handle and accompany visitors, which could otherwise be utilized to attend to clients. External treatment providers may also experience a substantial amount of time spent waiting and processing while visiting clients at the institution.

Jails also maintain a classification-based system that is typically based on security needs and bed/space availability, and which may or may not coincide with an inmate's treatment needs. Many small, rural, or older jails in particular have environments and structures that are not conducive to treatment: They were built to detain, house, and process inmates, and not to provide screening, assessment, or treatment services. Individual interview or treatment rooms may be limited, and there may also be a shortage of space for group treatment. When there is available activity space, educational, work, religious, and treatment programs frequently vie for this space, resulting in a compromised amount of treatment programming. Architecturally, jail activity rooms and housing units are not soundproof. Excessive noise can serve as a hindrance to treatment activities and can induce stress for both clients and treatment providers.

Discovering a location that offers both confidentiality and protection for both employees and prisoners poses a difficulty. It is crucial to inform clients about the limitations even though corrections and treatment staff may come up with collaborative solutions. The counselor should also be cognizant of the constraints that may arise when discussing specific topics or working with certain groups (e.g., detainees facing specific charges, individuals who have experienced certain traumatic events, individuals with severe mental illness), or even when conducting a comprehensive evaluation. Privacy is compromised by the constant presence of electronic surveillance, security personnel, and fellow inmates, which prevents inmates from being alone.

5.6.1. Gang Affiliation

The counselor must possess knowledge of the jail's policies and programs concerning gang affiliation, including regulations pertaining to the eligibility of individuals for specific groups and activities, as well as the consequences that may result in an administrative or new criminal charge while in detention. Familiarity with the prison gangs enables the counselor to anticipate potential actions that may provoke rival gangs. This allows the counselor to establish explicit guidelines for group activities and define their role in maintaining both security and proper treatment practices. By doing so, the counselor can avoid sending conflicting messages to inmates and prevent any conflicts with the correctional system.

5.6.2. Stress Related to Incarceration

Several factors, apart from the individual's preparedness for treatment, can influence their involvement in the treatment process while in jail. Several stressors can be found in jails, such as trauma resulting from the recent arrest, uncertainty regarding the legal situation, and the potential loss of employment or custody of children. Counselors can help clients develop strategies to deal with substance abuse problems while considering various internal and external sources of stress. They can also determine which issues can be addressed during incarceration within specific time limits. Additionally, counselors can refer clients to other jail or community services to address non-substance abuse-related problems and ensure a smooth transition from jail to the community. These services may include assistance with legal and medical issues, education, vocational training or work programs, as well as diversion or aftercare programs.

5.7. Issues Related to Justice System Processing and Legal Representation

The legal process can understandably confuse detainees, and either this disorientation can persist for a lengthy period (e.g., during adjournments, plea bargaining, competency processes, or diversion planning), or the status of the case can rapidly shift and the detainee may be suddenly released from jail. Often there is little communication between the court, jail staff, and treatment staff, which has a direct impact on the therapeutic relationship, as the detainee's legal status is a major concern.

Defense attorneys frequently refrain from visiting clients during their incarceration, opting instead for brief encounters at court before the demanding and occasionally bewildering legal proceedings. Moreover, when detainees seek assistance from their peers, the information they receive is frequently incorrect, which can intensify their feelings of urgency and despair. Given the diverse range of populations held in jails, detainees may acquire knowledge about situations that are unrelated to their own legal proceedings.

Attorneys do not always recognize the benefits of treatment and may not encourage the inmate's involvement in treatment. Due to the substantial workload, numerous public defenders fail to provide clients with guidance on the potential benefits of treatment. In certain legal jurisdictions, the assigned defense counsel may not necessarily come from the public defender's office and may lack knowledge about diversionary or alternative treatment options. In certain instances, defense attorneys may hesitate to recommend that their clients willingly undergo treatment for substance abuse due to the conditions of supervision that are likely to result in penalties and imprisonment. The exchange of information between legal and treatment professionals can present challenges, particularly regarding the specific types of information that counselors are permitted to disclose to their clients' attorneys, the admissibility of counselors' testimony in court, and the specific legal information that treatment providers require for counseling purposes.

5.7.1. Confidentiality

Substance abuse treatment programs ought to establish unambiguous guidelines concerning the permissible disclosure of information after an offender's execution of a valid consent form. The Federal laws and regulations regarding confidentiality protect any information pertaining to an individual who has sought or received substance abuse-related services from a program that falls under the purview of these laws. The programs included are specifically designed to provide treatment, counseling, assessment, and referral services for offenders who have alcohol or other drug-related issues. In small, rural jails, a distinct confidentiality concern may arise due to the familiarity between inmates and officers. The existence of residents with substance use disorders is widely recognized, and maintaining the confidentiality of their treatment is challenging.

5.7.2. Counselor-Client Issues

Considering the complex nature of the environment and the issues that require attention, it is beneficial for the counselor to explicitly explain their responsibilities and the boundaries associated with their role, the framework of the suggested treatment, and the different alternatives that are accessible. For example, the counselor should clarify their level of involvement in legal, family, medical, disciplinary, or other matters. The counselor should provide a comprehensive explanation of the available treatment options, including their potential effects on the client's issues. Additionally, they should discuss any alternative treatments or interventions that may be necessary to address the client's problems, which are not available in a jail setting. Although the client's responses to this information may initially range from anger to apathy to relief, providing strategies to manage constraints and sources of stress is more beneficial than simply appeasing the client at first. The counselor should possess knowledge regarding the safeguards and boundaries associated with informed consent.

5.7.2.1. Supervision and Training

Supervision and continuous involvement in training are crucial for jail treatment counselors, considering the complex nature of issues, symptoms, and behaviors exhibited by the inmate population, as well as the constraints imposed by the physical structure and environment of the jail. Supervision can assist the counselor by helping them understand and navigate the various demands of different systems, potential personal reactions to these demands, and personal reactions to the clients they work with. These clarifications aid in determining the appropriate inclusion or exclusion of these issues in the treatment process, as well as identifying which issues should be addressed on a systemic level. Providing support and ongoing opportunities for professional growth can help mitigate therapist burnout and enhance the effectiveness of treatment.

5.8. What Treatment Services Can Reasonably be Provided in a Jail Setting?

Various initiatives have been undertaken to establish guidelines for jail-based treatment programs that outline exemplary treatment methods and essential benchmarks for quality care. An instance of this is when the Office for Treatment Improvement, which is now known as the Center for Substance Abuse Treatment (CSAT), organized a meeting called the "Criminal Justice Treatment Evaluation Meeting" in 1992. The purpose of this meeting was to determine the essential components of substance abuse treatment programs in jails and establish guidelines for treatment in jail settings (SAMHSA 1996). However, local jails still require more specific guidelines that can be implemented effectively. The American Correctional Association (ACA) and the National Commission on Correctional Health Care (NCCHC) have standards about jails, but their coverage of substance use is notably restricted, and significantly less comprehensive and precise compared to the standards established for mental health services in jail. There are currently no established guidelines for addressing substance abuse treatment in jail, and the existing standards do not consider the complex contextual and environmental factors that influence treatment in jail settings.

Currently, there is no standardized model for jail substance abuse treatment programs. Instead, there are various programs available that differ in their content and intensity based on the duration of inmates' stay (Leukefeld & Tims, 1992; Peters & Matthews, 2002). Certain detainees spend less than a week in jail, during which they may only undergo assessment and referral, while others are incarcerated in a jail environment to serve a sentence. This section explores various treatment durations to analyze the different treatment options that could potentially be offered in a correctional facility. This section proposes a framework for determining which treatment services should be given priority, based on the limited time available to provide treatment for inmates. In this section, the term "brief" treatment refers to a period of up to 30 days, "short-term" treatment refers to a period of 1 to 3 months, and "long-term" treatment refers to a period of 3 months or more. Irrespective of the length of treatment, the primary objective should always be to actively involve clients, ensuring that treatment and recovery can be sustained upon their release from jail.

The intensity and duration of treatment are augmented in proportion to the length of stay, which also expands the range of topics that can be addressed. Given the lengthy development of the substance abusing lifestyle, it is often necessary to provide more intensive treatment services that cannot be changed within a short period of a few weeks.

Irrespective of the length of treatment, individuals in jail face various challenges such as having multiple medical issues alongside histories of physical and sexual abuse, unstable relationships and social support systems, poverty, homelessness, gender, and cultural disparities, among other factors. The interaction of various factors with different subpopulations can have diverse implications for treatment strategies and significantly influence treatment outcomes. Hence, when formulating or modifying treatment programs, it is crucial to consider these variables in conjunction with the substance preference patterns of consumption and the types of prior treatment and services. Providing support and ongoing opportunities for professional growth can help mitigate therapist burnout and enhance the effectiveness of treatment.

5.8.1. Level I: Brief Treatment

Certain perpetrators may be promptly identified during their brief incarceration in jail for their involvement in community diversion programs, which encompass their participation in treatment. Case management, referral, and brief interventions can be offered to other inmates who are incarcerated for a duration of 30 days or less. Concise therapy typically concentrates on providing information and offering recommendations for further assistance.

5.8.1.1. Motivational Enhancement Therapy and Motivational Interviewing

Motivational enhancement approaches assist clients in confronting their conflicting feelings about participating in substance abuse treatment and in finding strategies to manage these conflicting feelings. The objective of this process is to actively involve incarcerated individuals in a conversation about the treatment process and their underlying motivations for altering their substance abuse patterns. The aim is to assist inmates in formulating their own justification for modifying this behavior. This approach is specifically tailored to assist counselors in working with clients who exhibit ambivalence towards treatment, deny their circumstances, and display resistance toward change.

Project MATCH, the most extensive clinical trial ever conducted to compare various alcohol treatment approaches, found that a four-session motivational enhancement therapy produced long-term overall outcomes that were comparable to those of other, more intensive outpatient methods. Moreover, the findings of this study strongly indicated that motivational interviewing has the potential to be utilized among diverse cultural and economic populations.

Improving detainees' motivation for change and increasing their openness to substance abuse treatment can also be effective in this context. One instance of materials created at Texas Christian University (TCU) is a board game called Downward Spiral. This game assists individuals in exploring the outcomes of substance abuse. Another beneficial exercise is the Decision Matrix, which assesses the pros and cons of ongoing substance use from the client's viewpoint and evaluates the advantages of opting to stop using. This aids in identifying the functional aspects of their substance use, such as socialization and the reduction of negative emotions, which maintain the patterns of use. These aspects may also act as obstacles to achieving continued abstinence and engagement in treatment.

5.8.1.2. Substance Abuse Education

An educational component can be effective in informing and potentially altering risky behaviors among inmates who may not have previously considered the adverse health consequences associated with substance abuse. This education can be conveyed through the use of films, presentations, and literature. The primary objective of treatment is complete abstinence. However, individuals with a history of prolonged substance abuse often struggle to effectively address challenges such as monotony, unease, social uneasiness, and exclusion from their family and social circle.

5.8.1.3. Information on Available Community Resources

Community resource information encompasses a wide range of topics, including the process of acquiring a restraining order and the availability of substance abuse treatment services provided by community organizations. Pretrial counselors must possess knowledge of the available resources within their community to effectively support their clients upon their release. A significant number of these individuals will be reintegrated into the community without their multiple needs being addressed or fulfilled. Individuals can be directed to Alcoholics Anonymous (AA) and Narcotics Anonymous (NA) support groups, while counselors can offer assistance in locating vocational training programs, educational programs, clothing, food, and public aid. Before presenting this information to inmates, counselors must verify that an agency is willing to receive referrals from the criminal justice system and evaluate the eligibility criteria. Several programs have created resource directories containing detailed descriptions of community service programs and pertinent contact details.

5.8.1.4. Facilitating Access to Community Services

It is possible to create incentives for substance abuse treatment personnel to enter correctional facilities and collaborate with incarcerated individuals who are participating in treatment programs. One necessary action is to create contractual terms that designate incarcerated individuals as a high-priority population eligible for publicly funded substance abuse treatment services. Another option is to secure funding for health benefits. For instance, in New York City, an incarcerated individual's eligibility for Medicaid in a community program can be restored while they are still in jail, ensuring that the necessary paperwork is prepared for their release. Additionally, a comparable system has been devised to establish temporary Medicaid coverage. Community organizations may be more receptive to accepting former inmates as clients if they are receiving Medicaid assistance. If a health issue or mental disorder is diagnosed, Medicaid may be necessary to provide coverage for community-based treatment for affected individuals.

5.8.1.5. Community Linkage and Transition Services

Substance-abusing offenders are particularly susceptible to harm when reintegrating into society. The treatment system needs to plan for an inmate or detainee who is leaving the jail, and the community needs to be prepared to receive the individual. Case managers or other types of "boundary spanner" staff are particularly trained to manage these transitions. They are cross-trained in issues related to the mental health, substance abuse, and criminal justice systems, and will help to facilitate aftercare or diversion (Steadman et al., 1995; Taxman, 1998) (see also TIP 30, Continuity of Offender Treatment for Substance Use Disorders From Institution to Community [CSAT 1998b]).

These staff members can handle multiple tasks—from being advocates to understanding the available community resources and linking exiting inmates to those resources. The most common types of linkage and transition services provided by jail substance abuse treatment programs are assessment of aftercare needs, discharge planning, placement planning, and coordination with community treatment agencies (Peters & Matthews, 2002). Jail aftercare coordinators or treatment counselors, community resource coordinators, or case managers often provide these services.

Specialized reintegration programs are often helpful in developing postrelease plans related to housing, aftercare, relapse prevention, and employment.

While the goal of treatment is to help an inmate abstain from substance use, the reality is that inmates are at high risk for relapse and in some cases overdose upon their release from jail. Overdose prevention efforts before release can prevent deaths, especially for inmates who have been off the streets for a period. Counselors should provide inmates with information about the decreased tolerance that results from abstinence.

5.8.1.6. Psychotropic and Other Medications: Education and Adherence

Providing education to inmates about psychoactive medications can be highly beneficial. This education should cover topics such as the mechanisms of action of these medications, the rationale behind specific medication schedules, the flexibility in dosage, the potential side effects, and strategies for managing them. Additionally, inmates should be informed about the connection between mental and substance use disorders, noncompliance with medications, and the reduced effectiveness of these medications. Clients need to comprehend the difference between psychotropic medication and substances of abuse, as well as to be aware of which medications have the potential for addiction. This form of education also offers an opportunity to explore the connection between symptoms of mental disorders and the possible feeling of shame linked to mental health issues and the continuous use of medication.

For a considerable proportion of incarcerated individuals with a past of opioid addiction, it would be highly beneficial to assess the efficacy of current opioid substitution medications, such as methadone, levo-alphaacetyl-methadol, buprenorphine, and other drugs employed in the detoxification or reduction of opioid consumption. The limited adoption of these medications in correctional facilities is mainly due to concerns about their potential for contraband, the potential to prolong physical dependence on opioids, and the need for specialized medical supervision.

5.8.2. Level II: Short-Term Treatment

Level II, short-term treatment (lasting approximately 4–12 weeks) allows for a more profound engagement in the treatment process. The short-term treatment is based on the fundamental Level I services that were previously described. Level II or short-term treatment interventions primarily emphasize the development of coping mechanisms to prevent substance use and maintain long-term recovery.

5.8.2.1. Substance Cravings, Urges, and Relapse Prevention

Prisoners are educated about the specific behaviors that can provoke their desire for drugs or alcohol, as well as how these cravings and urges are connected to preventing a relapse. Additionally, individuals have the option to engage in exercises aimed at recognizing their own "substance use triggers" and examining techniques for both avoiding and managing these triggers. For instance, during a group discussion, the topic may revolve around the potential challenges that inmates might encounter when reintegrating into their families, particularly if their family members do not fully endorse their commitment to recovery. Although non-substance-using family members can provide significant support to help the client maintain sobriety after release, reuniting with family members often leads to stress due to the family's lack of trust and anger towards the offender's previous substance use, unresolved conflicts with the partner or spouse, changing parental responsibilities, and increased financial obligations (Peters, 1993). Residing with family members who engage in substance abuse or support substance use at home exposes the offender to more dangerous circumstances. Returning to the home environment can, in certain instances, provoke a relapse. Counselors should evaluate the domestic circumstances and potentially explore alternative housing options. Counselors may advise clients that specific areas of the city, such as drug-infested neighborhoods, are off-limits and that visiting those areas would be considered a breach of their treatment program and/or supervision requirements.

5.8.2.2. Self-Help Programs

Level II treatment provides inmates with the chance to acquire knowledge about self-help programs and their accessibility in the community. Although not commonly regarded as a form of substance abuse treatment, groups like NA (Narcotics Anonymous) and AA (Alcoholics Anonymous) offer a valuable and easily accessible form of peer support for inmates reintegrating into society.

Recent legal precedents have determined that AA and NA are fundamentally religious-oriented treatment programs. Although numerous states still impose AA or NA as sentences for offenders, the court in New York has determined that such practice constitutes a breach of the first amendment. The issue at hand could potentially be resolved by the authorities through the elimination of these coercive requirements or by integrating nonreligious alternatives (Cohen, 2000).

Certain correctional facilities provide alternative forms of peer support groups, including SMART Recovery, which is rooted in the cognitive-behavioral principles of Rational Emotive Behavioral Therapy. Although licensed professionals in the community may occasionally coordinate such groups, it is individuals who are in the process of recovery who take on the role of leading them.

5.8.2.3. Basic Cognitive Skills

Inmates can benefit from cognitive skills training, which aims to address thought patterns that may contribute to criminal behavior and substance abuse. These interventions assist incarcerated individuals in comprehending the connection between thoughts, emotions, and actions, as well as techniques to tackle harmful thought patterns that may result in conflicts with others, emotional instability, and aggressive and violent conduct. The cognitive skills acquired in correctional rehabilitation programs can often be applied to various contexts, such as employment, education, and interpersonal relationships with partners and family members.

5.8.2.4. Strengths Building

The strengths-based approach focuses on identifying and utilizing the resources and abilities that clients possess to enhance their likelihood of achieving successful recovery in the treatment program. Counselors can explore interactive methods to help participants identify their strengths, such as having inmates write positive statements about each group member, recognizing their own positive traits, and contemplating how they can further develop these strengths in the future.

TCU researchers have created a set of interventions for readiness and induction that include a strategy to enhance strengths (Dees et al., 2000). These interventions provide participants with distinct opportunities to determine their roles in treatment and uncover their positive personal strengths and latent cognitive abilities. During the Tower of Strengths intervention, participants analyze their existing strengths as well as the ones they desire the most. These activities are appropriate for implementation in either custody or community settings, and can be utilized in groups of up to 35 participants or in one-on-one counseling sessions.

The TCU readiness and induction interventions were specifically formulated to address the challenges commonly faced when working with individuals who are required to undergo treatment. The authors tackle the distorted and pessimistic assumptions regarding treatment that are prevalent among clients in criminal justice programs, as well as their low self-esteem stemming from personal setbacks, educational and vocational shortcomings, and inadequate coping abilities.

5.8.2.5. Communication Skills

This intervention has the potential to enhance interpersonal skills and bolster assertiveness when interacting with important family members, significant others, and colleagues. Key activities often address effective means of expressing anger and other negative emotions, dealing with conflict situations, and dealing with problems that arise in personal relationships, whether at work or in the home.

5.8.2.6. Anger Management

These activities can assist incarcerated individuals in developing self-awareness of their anger, identifying underlying triggers, and acquiring alternative problem-solving strategies to effectively regulate their anger. These interventions are beneficial for comprehending the correlation between anger and substance abuse, as inadequately controlled anger frequently leads to substance abuse.

5.8.2.7. Domestic Violence

In such instances, immediate measures are devised to ensure the personal safety of domestic violence victims and safeguard children, while also exploring long-term resolutions that encompass legal and law enforcement intervention. It is beneficial to have staff members who are knowledgeable about the community shelter and domestic abuse counseling services that are accessible.

5.8.2.8. Problem Solving

These skills enable individuals to effectively tackle and resolve their own daily issues by clearly defining those problems and carefully analyzing possible solutions. Prisoners can initiate discussions by addressing past challenges, describing their attempted solutions, and evaluating the outcomes of their endeavors. Subsequently, they can analyze the problems they have successfully resolved optimistically. Prisoners acquire the ability to make logical decisions by carefully evaluating options, rather than being driven by emotions or impulsively reacting. It is necessary for them to acquire the skill of carefully examining a problem, evaluating the benefits of different solutions, and predicting their consequences.

Engaging in conversations about actual instances of problem-solving can assist prisoners in expressing effective problem-solving techniques that usually lead to positive outcomes. For instance, a customer could recount a dispute with their employer and deliberate decision to arrive at work 15 minutes behind schedule the following day. If the response of that person did not enhance the situation, other members of the group may express their course of action when confronted with a similar scenario: "I would evade the situation," "I would attempt to disregard him," "When he inquired about something, I would become defensive." The objective of this exercise is to ascertain efficient approaches to proceed. A potentially efficacious approach that could lead to favorable responses and outcomes would involve politely requesting a brief conversation with one's supervisor, expressing remorse, providing a justification for the lateness, and pledging to avoid any future occurrences. The efficacy of this approach is maximized when counselors employ practical situations, enactments, and collective engagement.

5.8.2.9. Social Skills Training

Social skills training can be administered autonomously or as components of modules pertaining to problem-solving and anger management. This training can assist incarcerated individuals in effectively managing their interactions with colleagues, relatives, and acquaintances. The process entails acquiring and practicing drug-free and prosocial skills to effectively address interpersonal challenges encountered during the recovery process. Key components include communication skills, assertiveness, skills for developing and sustaining interpersonal relationships, and specific drug coping skills to handle high-risk interpersonal situations. Additional domains encompass conflict resolution and the acquisition of interpersonal competencies on professional, familial, and communal contexts.

Strengths-based approach involves recognizing and utilizing the positive qualities and resources that clients possess to enhance their likelihood of achieving successful recovery in the treatment program.

5.8.3. Level III: Long-Term Treatment

When inmates are imprisoned for a period exceeding 90 days, they have a greater opportunity to receive additional treatment to enhance the skills acquired during short-term treatment and assist them in reintegrating into the community. Level III or long-term treatment approaches incorporate elements that are comparable to those present in residential treatment within various community-based programs. These interventions aim to explore personal values, belief systems, and cultural and family background issues that have contributed to a substance abuse lifestyle.

5.8.3.1. Employment Counseling

Employment counseling, which entails assessing an inmate's job-related abilities and conducting skills assessments, can be integrated into work release or furlough programs. Counselors should offer pre-employment training, which includes instruction in communication skills with employers, responsibility, punctuality, and résumé writing. Clinicians can enhance their résumés by asking clients about their contributions as volunteers, community members, or during their time in jail that could positively impact their employment prospects, instead of solely focusing on conventional work experience. Counselors can assist their clients in formulating strategies to secure employment upon their release.

5.8.3.2. Building a Therapeutic Community

Some jail programs have implemented time-limited therapeutic communities.

5.8.3.3. Family Mapping and Social Networks

Family mapping is a systematic method for analyzing the familial connections and history. The objective is to examine the familial background and gain insight into any criminal or substance abuse history, as well as analyze the family's ability to adapt over time to preserve stability. Inmates often extend their focus beyond their immediate family to include grandparents, aunts, and uncles. This is because criminal and substance-using behaviors tend to be prevalent within families and can be passed down through generations. This thorough analysis enables individuals to comprehend the underlying causes and mechanisms behind substance abuse and other maladaptive behaviors within their familial context.

Female inmates, specifically, remain connected to their community even during their incarceration and actively cultivate social connections and maintain social support systems. Nevertheless, during their incarceration, individuals face considerable challenges in maintaining familial connections and receiving support. These difficulties include subjecting their children to contraband searches, restrictions on visitation, the presence of glass barriers separating mothers from their children, and the monitoring of visits by staff members. These circumstances frequently have an adverse effect on family relationships. Having the family present is crucial for addressing certain familial matters.

There exist pioneering prison programs that collaborate with inmates and child welfare agencies to establish designated visitation schedules for fathers or mothers, caseworkers, and children, to simplify visitation procedures for the agencies involved (City of New York, 2001). These models have the potential to be applied to other categories of family gatherings.

5.8.3.4. Co-occurring Disorders

Extended-duration treatment offers the chance to gain knowledge about the interconnectedness of substance abuse and mental disorders, including the factors that contribute to the recurrence of mental disorders, such as stopping a psychiatric medication. Additional crucial interventions encompass psychiatric consultation for medication assessment, education on mental disorders, and formulation of transition plans for subsequent mental health and substance abuse services in the community.

5.8.3.5. Criminal Thinking

A significant number of prisoners have developed deeply rooted cognitive patterns that contribute to their inability to form healthy relationships with others and ultimately result in conflicts and engagement in criminal activities. Many inmates often fail to recognize the correlation between their criminal actions and these cognitive patterns or belief systems. Through the process of recognizing and confronting dysfunctional criminal thought patterns, such as making broad assumptions, using extreme language, magnifying situations, and being dishonest, individuals who have committed crimes can develop a more analytical mindset and scrutinize the thoughts that contribute to their unlawful actions. Several structured curricula have been created to blend cognitive and behavioral approaches that align with other skills approaches utilized in substance abuse treatment programs within jails.

5.9. Coordination of Jail Treatment Services

To effectively implement a jail drug treatment program, the consensus panel emphasizes the necessity of collaboration among various stakeholders, including funding sources, the community, substance abuse counselors, criminal justice personnel, outside agencies, and the offender. This section draws on the experiences of the consensus panel members and focuses on the potential obstacles in coordinating jail treatment services. It then explores various solutions to commonly encountered barriers during the implementation of these services.

5.9.1. Barriers to Treatment

- Several variables present in the jail environment can impede the efficacy of treatment:
- Inadequate financial resources for the provision of services

- Lack of administrative assistance in the development of comprehensive treatment programs
- The substance abuse and criminal justice systems experience tensions due to their overlapping yet distinct concerns. The substance abuse system focuses on rehabilitation and treatment, while the criminal justice system prioritizes safety, control, and punishment.
- Unfavorable physical space and environment for treatment
- Activities of different institutional programs that are in competition with each other.
- Challenges in establishing systems for exchanging information between healthcare providers and law enforcement personnel
- Concerns regarding the protection of sensitive information and the necessity of exchanging data
- Insufficient provision of case management or ongoing care
- Insufficient provision of detoxification services
- Detoxification symptoms often misinterpreted as manifestations of mental illness
- Insufficient provision of gradually reduced doses of methadone for prisoners participating in methadone treatment programs before experiencing a return to drug use.
- Introducing family members for family reunification or family therapy without thorough security screening
- The prevalence of HIV/AIDS and sexually transmitted diseases among incarcerated individuals.
- Lack of capacity to furnish HIV/AIDS educational resources
- Limitations imposed by the institution regarding the use of video equipment, televisions, and VCRs (to play back practice job interviews).
- Challenges in implementing community outreach for both supplementary and fundamental treatment services.
- The hesitancy of treatment providers to operate within correctional facilities

The divergent objectives of the criminal justice and treatment systems can occasionally present challenges, even though these systems have numerous shared goals.

5.9.1.1. Limited Resources

The insufficient allocation of funds for treatment in numerous correctional facilities is indicative of the prevailing attitudes and beliefs within the community. These beliefs suggest that offering services, such as treatment, goes against a jail's primary objective of punishment and could disrupt its management. Furthermore, there is a widespread deficiency in understanding the influence that treatment can exert on criminal behavior. Many people are unaware of the numerous issues faced by individuals in jail, the frequent movement of this population between jail and the community, and the absence of systematic interventions that could break the costly cycle of jail and re-incarceration. Moreover, the challenge to obtain adequate resources for jail treatment may parallel the insufficient funding for treatment in the community. Treatment programs in correctional facilities may potentially rival or be perceived as rivals to community resources.

By conducting a needs assessment of its incarcerated population, a community can distribute limited treatment resources in the most efficient manner. Prisons that have sufficient resources are capable of establishing both specialized and comprehensive substance abuse treatment programs. Prisons that have limited resources may opt to allocate their resources towards two main areas: identifying and referring inmates with multiple disorders and issues (such as severe mental illness or homelessness) to community programs and providing traditional treatment services to inmates whose main problem is their substance use disorder.

To optimize the allocation of limited resources, the consensus panel recommends that jail-based substance abuse treatment programs establish explicit goals and objectives that are attainable within the constraints of the correctional environment. For instance, if the objective of jail treatment is to mitigate the adverse health effects that inmates experience due to their substance abuse (such as the risk of contracting HIV), the program would be designed differently compared to a program aimed at maintaining long-term abstinence after release from custody. Jail treatment programs have discovered the value of involving various stakeholder groups to provide extra resources within the institution and during the transition back to the community.

5.9.2. Solutions for Coordinating Jail-Based Treatment Services

There are several approaches that substance abuse treatment providers can take to improve services for people in jail and overcome the barriers described above. The sections that follow will go over these.

5.9.2.1. Prioritizing Substance Abuse Treatment for Traditional Versus Special Needs Populations

Because of limited resources, many jails must prioritize how to allocate treatment services to inmates with varying levels of need. One major issue is whether to target populations that require specialized care and are more likely to relapse, criminal recidivism, and high use of community services (e.g., chronically mentally ill, mentally retarded, or homeless inmates) or to focus resources on inmates with more traditional substance abuse treatment needs. Targeting one group over another has both advantages and disadvantages. The consensus panel recommends that jails assess their own treatment resources as well as the scope of subpopulations with special treatment needs to develop a plan that will ideally meet the needs of both groups.

5.9.2.2. Promote Understanding of Institutional Security Rules and Confidentiality Requirements

Insufficient comprehension of the regulations about the confidentiality of substance abuse treatment data and the security protocols within the institution can result in disputes between correctional and treatment personnel, thereby diminishing the efficacy and credibility of the treatment program. For instance, counselors may inadvertently introduce materials into the correctional facility for therapeutic reasons that security personnel may deem as contraband, or they may make commitments to inmates regarding scheduled activities, visitation, phone calls, or other privileges that are prohibited. An in-depth understanding of the regulations enables the treatment program staff to foresee these challenges and devise innovative solutions. It is important to extend an invitation to treatment counselors and ensure their willingness to engage in training sessions focused on security guidelines and methods. Treatment supervisors can provide support by offering guidance to counselors on strategies for addressing safety concerns and managing conflicts with security personnel. Ultimately, treatment and jail supervisory staff can collaborate through cross-disciplinary meetings and cross-training activities to effectively resolve potential conflicts regarding housing assignments, scheduling, reviewing responses to critical incidents (such as dealing with contraband), information sharing, and other aspects of program development.

5.9.2.3. Improve Coordination of Information Systems

Detainees who are involved in multiple systems may face difficulties due to a lack of synchronized information. Multiple open-source computerized management information systems have been created for this objective. This software enables the provision of effective, punctual, and uninterrupted healthcare by facilitating treatment matching and follow-up, and it may also incorporate information regarding drug test outcomes. A model, derived from the University of Maryland's High Intensity Drug Trafficking Area Automated Treatment Tracking Software (HIDTA-HATTS), allows substance abuse treatment and criminal justice professionals to access identical information when making decisions regarding the client (Taxman and Sherman 1998). Additional exclusive models derived from drug courts have broadened their scope to incorporate mental health screenings and evaluations. In addition, some jurisdictions have implemented systems to facilitate the exchange of mental health and substance abuse data between correctional institutions and community-managed care providers, such as the National GAINS Center in 1999. Every governing body involved in the development of these specific management information systems has resolved the matters of informed consent and differential confidentiality to facilitate the sharing of information. The mentioned models have also conducted their work within the framework of collaborative efforts involving multiple systems. They have, at times, utilized formal consensus-building processes involving the key stakeholders to ensure the uninterrupted provision of treatment (Broner et al., 2001b).

5.9.2.4. Educate Staff Regarding Pharmacotherapies

Certain jail administrators oppose the use of pharmacotherapy due to their philosophical objections to administering medication, such as methadone or psychiatric medications, to individuals with substance abuse issues. However, it is worth noting that most jails do provide a variety of psychiatric medications to inmates who have mental disorders. Most of these medications are non-addictive and do not pose a risk for being distributed as contraband within the institution. However, a small number of correctional facilities offer medication-assisted treatment for opioids and other substances.

There are valid concerns regarding the administration of certain medications in correctional facilities, especially when there is insufficient healthcare personnel to oversee and supervise their usage. Supervision of pharmacological treatments administered in correctional facilities should be carried out by a certified physician or nurse practitioner. Project KEEP is a program that combines pharmacological treatments with a jail setting.

5.9.2.5. Provide for Staff Development

Several frontline correctional facilities mandate that personnel possess solely a GED or high school diploma and possess no criminal history. Although correctional staff undergo comprehensive security training, they are not always provided with training specifically focused on working with particular populations and providing substance abuse treatment. Cross-training is a beneficial method for correctional and treatment staff to exchange knowledge and insights on important matters concerning institutional security and rehabilitation. Correctional officers can gain valuable insights by acquiring knowledge about the duration, curriculum, and constituents of substance abuse rehabilitation; employing effective communication techniques when interacting with treatment personnel regarding inmate conduct and attitudes; actively participating in treatment team, group sessions, and other unit events; and understanding their role in cultivating a therapeutic atmosphere. Treatment staff can gain advantages from receiving training on security protocols, proficiently communicating with corrections staff regarding inmate conduct, illicit items, and other security violations, and understanding their responsibility in upholding the security of the housing unit and the jail. Both corrections and treatment staff can actively participate in identifying critical incidents that may arise within the jail treatment unit, determining the specific information that should be exchanged between treatment and corrections staff, and devising strategies to resolve these situations.

Implementing treatment programs in correctional facilities offers a distinct opportunity for treatment personnel to cooperate with correctional staff in designing in-service training programs and promoting certification and degree training at nearby universities. New York City provides incentives and tuition reimbursement to its employees for undergraduate and graduate education, as well as a forensic certificate program offered by the New York University School of Social Work. Implementing a flexible job scheduling system could facilitate employees in enhancing their education. Additionally, offering coursework for academic credit at the workplace would enable jail personnel to pursue undergraduate or graduate degrees. Another alternative is to allocate dedicated time for career advancement while working, by devoting a few hours per week to attending a course that not only enhances job performance but also facilitates career growth.

5.9.2.6. Developing Community and Correctional Partnerships

Establishing collaborations between the correctional facility and the local community can facilitate the improvement and expansion of in-custody rehabilitation initiatives, as well as the effective coordination of offenders' integration into community diversion and post-release programs. Many correctional facilities have implemented a cooperative and collaborative approach in areas such as education, healthcare, diversion, and aftercare for individuals with substance use disorders or mental illnesses (Steadman et al., 1995; Broner et al., 2002). These partnerships enable the expansion, rather than repetition, of a wide range of community resources to address the substance abuse, mental health, medical, vocational, educational, and social service needs of this population.

However, managing the scheduling of numerous community volunteers to visit the jail can pose challenges in terms of security and staffing. Issues of concern encompass staffing arrangements, security measures, and contraband surveillance. This involves the coordination of schedules, allocation of staff time, as well as the task of escorting inmates to and from their designated group areas and accompanying visitors. Thus, procuring services from external sources creates an extra burden for jail administrators, which can potentially act as an obstacle. To address these issues, a possible solution would be to implement shared funding and allocate a budget from community organizations specifically for the time spent by jail officers. To achieve a harmonious balance between the requirements and worries of both parties, it is essential to establish a systematic framework that enables effective communication and problem-solving between community volunteers and jail administrators.

5.9.2.7. Creating Linkages Between Jail Treatment and Diversion and Reentry Court Programs

Drug treatment courts (DTCs), which are usually run by criminal courts, have established successful collaborations with local jails in numerous jurisdictions (Tauber & Huddleston, 1999). In certain drug court programs, the initial stage of treatment takes place in a correctional facility. During this phase, individuals receive intensive services that primarily involve a thorough evaluation of their psychological and social well-being, education on substance abuse, and active participation in and introduction to treatment. In alternative drug court programs, the inclusion of an initial in-jail treatment component is discretionary, contingent upon the level of drug treatment requirements and the significance of a controlled treatment environment. Jail treatment is also employed for inmates who are in the process of being placed in drug court treatment programs within the community.

Jail treatment programs also serve the purpose of offering more concentrated services for drug court participants who experience a relapse or engage in significant violations. In such instances, incarceration programs can function as a therapeutic measure to separate an individual from prominent triggers for relapse (such as peers who use drugs), to offer detoxification when necessary, and to reintegrate individuals into their rehabilitation programs. Several drug courts implement a system of progressive sanctions, wherein the number of days spent in jail for specific program infractions increases gradually (e.g., 2, 4, 7). Drug courts have occasionally resulted in extended periods of incarceration, although the therapeutic benefits of these penalties remain uncertain.

Several drug courts have established a coordinated reentry approach with in-jail treatment programs (Huddleston, 1998; Tauber & Huddleston, 1999). Each of these partnerships exhibits substantial adaptability in meeting the specific requirements of drug court participants. Several drug courts also maintain supervision over participants who are placed in both custodial and noncustodial settings. For example, two drug court and jail treatment collaborations (Los Angeles County and San Bernardino County, California, and Uinta County, Wyoming) enroll offenders in the jail treatment program as the initial stage of the drug court process.

Participants in the San Bernardino drug court are assigned jobs within the jail that enable them to attend treatment groups and classes. A distinct housing unit in Los Angeles County is specifically designated for drug court treatment and receives referrals from multiple drug courts within the county. One of the 11 drug courts in Los Angeles County is specifically intended for probation violators. As part of this program, individuals are required to undergo 3 months of treatment in jail before they can move on to the next stages of the program. Drug court participants in Uinta County, Wyoming, who have not succeeded in court-mandated treatment are enrolled in a 6-week incarceration treatment program as the initial stage of their involvement in drug court. During their enrollment in the jail treatment program, individuals in Uinta County must attend drug court once a week for status hearings.

Correctional programs can function as a therapeutic measure to separate an individual from prominent triggers that could lead to a relapse.

The DTC in Broward County, Florida, directs individuals to a 90-day incarceration-based treatment program if they have not successfully completed less intensive alternatives such as outpatient treatment (Tauber & Huddleston, 1999). Individuals who have been sentenced to jail before participating in the Broward County drug court are also directed to the jail treatment program to promptly involve them in treatment. The drug court then monitors their progress in the jail treatment program and provides a reentry mechanism upon their transfer to the drug court program.

In New Castle County, Delaware, the DTC has combined both short-term (6 months) and long-term (11–18 months) custodial substance abuse treatment with continued care upon rearrest for probation violators who have committed new felony-level offenses.

The court monitors the individual's progress through the prison- or jail-based treatment and develops a reentry treatment plan based on input from team members. The reduction of recidivism has been positively influenced by this (Statistical Analysis Center, 1998).

Several additional collaborations between drug courts and jails provide distinct features. In Los Angeles County drug courts, participants who are transferring from the jail treatment unit to community settings can use transition housing. In San Bernardino County, a comprehensive assessment is provided after 10 weeks of treatment in the jail program and is provided to the drug court judge before status hearings.

This assessment serves as the basis for the court's decision to order continued in-jail treatment, placement in a community residential treatment program, or placement in a community outpatient program. In New Haven, Connecticut, the drug court judge orders jail sentences as a sanction and requests on an individual basis that drug court participants receive priority access to drug treatment and self-help groups during the ensuing period of jail incarceration (Huddleston 1998).

5.10. Research Related to Jail Treatment

According to a survey of metropolitan jail treatment programs conducted by Peters and May in 1992, it was found that many jails have multiple treatment phases and support more than one therapeutic approach. The majority of the jail programs surveyed incorporated 12-Step groups, cognitive-behavioral groups, and relapse prevention programs. Several jail treatment programs have created specific programs for different groups, such as juveniles facing adult charges, individuals with co-occurring disorders, those arrested for driving under the influence, and blended groups for domestic violence and substance abuse (Peters & Mathews, 2002).

5.10.1. Outcomes of Jail Treatment

Treatment programs in jails often rely on local resources or knowledge, rather than consistent best practice models specifically designed for this setting. Although there are only a limited number of outcome studies available, the therapeutic community model demonstrates potential, even for individuals with short-term stays. The Amity/Pima County Substance Abuse Treatment Jail Project, which received funding from the U.S. Bureau of Justice Assistance in the late 1980s, provided evidence of the effectiveness of drug treatment in a correctional environment (Pima County Sheriff's Department 1988). Furthermore, several studies have shown that individuals who engage in in-jail drug treatment experience lower rates of rearrest and reconviction, longer periods of time before being rearrested, and fewer arrests during the follow-up period (Peters & Matthews, 2002).

5.10.2. Effects of Treatment Duration

Research examining the impact of the duration of substance abuse treatment in jail reveals that the likelihood of relapse is influenced by the length of treatment, with the most effective duration falling between 91 and 150 days (Swartz et al., 1996). Positive treatment results have been documented for jail programs lasting between 1.5 and 5 months. Participation in post-release aftercare treatment programs has been shown to decrease rates of criminal recidivism (San Francisco County Sheriff's Office Department 1996; Swartz et al. 1996). According to Taxman and Spinner (1997), individuals who have previously participated in a treatment program while in jail are more inclined to engage in aftercare treatment upon their release.

5.10.3. Predictors of Treatment Outcomes

Several studies have investigated factors that can predict the outcomes of jail treatment programs. These studies aim to identify the factors that contribute to successful completion of treatment (referred to as "completers") and the factors that hinder completion (referred to as "noncompleters"). In a study conducted by Peters et al. in 1993, it was found that the number of lifetime arrests was the most significant factor in predicting rearrests during a 1-year follow-up period. However, other psychological indicators and living arrangements were also identified as predictors. In a study conducted by Peters et al (1999), it was discovered that individuals who use cocaine were less inclined to successfully finish a treatment program compared to those who use alcohol or marijuana. Additional factors that were indicative of noncompletion included absence of a secondary education certificate, residing independently from one's parents, absence of full-time employment, and previous arrests for offenses unrelated to drug possession. There is a high probability that comparable factors could impact the retention of individuals in jail treatment programs, although further investigation is required to fully understand this phenomenon.

5.10.4. Importance of Aftercare

Regrettably, most individuals who are released from detention facilities do not have access to post-release support or treatment, and the majority of correctional institutions do not utilize alternative programs like drug courts. The implementation of treatment as required by drug courts has been found to be linked with a reduction in repeat offenses, an increase in the likelihood of completing treatment, and improved connections to post-treatment support services (Leukefeld & Tims, 1988). Tunis and colleagues (1997) discovered that drug treatment programs implemented in correctional facilities serve as an effective "behavioral management tool" that leads to a reduction in behavioral issues, particularly instances of physical violence. Nevertheless, the program had only a limited impact on recidivism rates in the year following release. Prisoners willingly engaged in the treatment programs, which involved counseling, self-help groups, and limited aftercare options in the community. Supplemental training for correctional staff could have enhanced their endorsement of aftercare.

5.11. Recommendations for Treatment Providers

To optimize the advantages of substance abuse services, treatment personnel who interact with clients in correctional facilities should take into account the following recommendations:

- It is important to acknowledge that there is a significant number of individuals in the community who frequently transition between the community and jail. In such cases, it is crucial to prioritize and refer these individuals to appropriate services.
- To better serve individuals in community treatment agencies, it is

recommended to have staff members who can offer services within jails and share their expertise through training and consultation with jail treatment staff.

- Offer continuous advisory services to jail administrators and other jail personnel regarding substance abuse matters, and strive to establish a comprehensive range of services within the jail and community for individuals grappling with substance abuse issues.
- Create treatment strategies specifically tailored to identified special populations, as outlined in this chapter.
- Provide support in carrying out regular evaluations of quality.
- Utilize evidence-based strategies such as motivational enhancement techniques, cognitive-behavioral interventions, relapse prevention, contingency management, and therapeutic communities.

A Closer Look

Drug offenses

Drugs of abuse encompass a wide range of substances that, when used recreationally, can lead to significant health problems, addiction, and societal issues. These substances are classified into several categories, each with distinct effects and potential for abuse.

Stimulants, including cocaine, methamphetamine, and ecstasy (MDMA), are known for their ability to increase energy, alertness, and euphoria. Cocaine, derived from the coca plant, can cause intense euphoria and increased physical stamina, but its use is associated with severe cardiovascular issues, neurological disturbances, and high potential for addiction. Methamphetamine, a synthetic stimulant, provides similar effects but with a higher risk of severe psychological and physical health problems, including violent behavior, dental decay, and long-term cognitive impairment. Ecstasy, while often associated with social and emotional closeness, can lead to dehydration, hyperthermia, and long-term effects on serotonin levels, impacting mood and memory.

Depressants such as alcohol, benzodiazepines, and opioids act to slow down the central nervous system. Alcohol, widely consumed and socially accepted, can impair motor functions and judgment, leading to accidents and risky behaviors, liver disease, and addiction. Benzodiazepines, prescribed for anxiety and insomnia, can cause dependence when used long-term, with withdrawal symptoms including seizures and agitation. Opioids, including heroin, morphine, and prescription painkillers like oxycodone and fentanyl, are highly addictive due to their powerful effects on the brain's reward system. Their misuse can lead to overdose, respiratory depression, and a significant increase in the risk of fatal outcomes.

Hallucinogens, such as LSD, psilocybin mushrooms, and PCP, alter perception, mood, and cognitive processes. LSD and psilocybin can induce profound changes in sensory perception and emotional state, but their use can also result in persistent psychological effects like paranoia and hallucinations. PCP, originally developed as an anesthetic, can cause severe dissociation, hallucinations, and aggressive behavior, posing risks of injury and self-harm.

Cannabis, derived from the Cannabis sativa plant, is used for its psychoactive effects, including relaxation, altered sensory perception, and euphoria. While cannabis is increasingly legalized for medical and recreational use in various regions, its abuse can lead to cognitive impairment, addiction, and mental health issues, including exacerbation of conditions like schizophrenia.

Inhalants, such as nitrous oxide and solvents like paint thinners and gasoline, are abused for their short-lived euphoric effects. Inhalant use can result in sudden death from asphyxiation, cardiac arrhythmias, or brain damage due to hypoxia. Chronic use can lead to severe neurological damage and organ failure.

The abuse of these substances not only affects individual health but also has broad social implications, including increased healthcare costs, crime, and loss of productivity. Addressing drug abuse requires a comprehensive approach, including prevention, education, treatment, and policy interventions to mitigate its impact on individuals and society. Understanding the diverse effects and risks associated with these drugs is crucial for developing effective strategies to combat addiction and promote public health.

Summary

- This chapter presents a comprehensive examination of the health and human rights of individuals held in detention. This chapter underscores the moral, ethical, and legal responsibilities of authorities to ensure detainees receive proper medical care. It highlights the vulnerability of detainees to physical and psychological abuse, exacerbated by overcrowded and unsanitary conditions. The chapter stresses the importance of medical neutrality, where healthcare professionals prioritize detainee well-being without interference or bias.
- The chapter advocates for standardized healthcare protocols tailored to the unique needs of detainees, including mental health support, access to necessary medications, and timely medical interventions. It emphasizes the role of independent monitoring bodies to oversee detainee treatment and uphold standards of care, ensuring compliance with international human rights laws.

References

1. Berlin, L. (2017). Medical errors, malpractice, and defensive medicine: An ill-fated triad. *Diagnosis*, *4*(3), 133–139. https://doi.org/10.1515/dx-2017-0016.
2. Bolcato, M., Fiore, V., Casella, F., Babudieri, S., Lucania, L., & Di Mizio, G. (2021). Health in prison: Does penitentiary medicine in Italy still exist? *Healthcare*, *9*(11), 1511. https://doi.org/10.3390/healthcare9111511.
3. Bourgon, G., & Guiterrez, L. (2013). The importance of building good relationships in community corrections: Evidence, theory and practice of the therapeutic alliance. In P. Ugwudike & P. Raynor (Eds.), *What Works in Offender Compliance: International Perspectives and Evidence-Based Practice* (pp. 256–275). Palgrave Macmillan.
4. Dermengiu, D., Hostiuc, S., Simionescu, M., Marcus, I., Asavei, V., Gherghe, E. V., & Badila, E. (2015). Is a full-fledged informed consent viable in prison environments? *Romanian Journal of Legal Medicine*, *23*(3), 143–150. https://doi.org/10.4323/rjlm.2015.143.
5. Emanuel, J. E., & Emanuel, L. L. (1992). Four models of the physician-patient relationship. *JAMA*, *267*(16), 2221–2226. https://doi.org/10.1001/jama.1992.03480160075038.
6. Giorgi-Guarnieri, D. (2019). Clinician liability in prescribing antidepressants. *Focus*, *17*(4), 372–379. https://doi.org/10.1176/appi.focus.170401.
7. Gostin, L. O., Vanchieri, C., & Pope, A. (2007). *Ethical Considerations for Research Involving Prisoners*. National Academies Press. https://doi.org/10.17226/11892.
8. Haney, C. (2003). Mental health issues in long-term solitary and "supermax" confinement. *Crime & Delinquency*, *49*(1), 124–156. https://doi.org/10.1177/0011128702239002.
9. Isailă, O. M., Hostiuc, S., Teodor, M., & Curcă, G. C. (2021). Particularities of offenders imprisoned for domestic violence from social and psychiatric medical-legal perspectives. *Medicina*, *57*(11), 1187. https://doi.org/10.3390/medicina57111187.
10. Jeng, F., Bonnell, A. C., O'Neil, E. C., Mehran, N. A., Kolomeyer, N. N., Brucker, A. J., & Kolomeyer, A. M. (2022). Vision-related malpractice involving prisoners: Analysis of the Westlaw database. *Retina*, *42*(5), 816–821. https://doi.org/10.1097/IAE.0000000000003376.

11. Kelk, C. (1999). Recommendation No. R (98) 7 of the Committee of Ministers to Member States concerning the ethical and organizational aspects of health care in prison. *European Journal of Health Law*, *6*(3), 265–266. https://doi.org/10.1163/157180999X00063.

12. Lv, H., Li, D., Li, C., Yuwen, P., Hou, Z., Chen, W., & Zhang, Y. (2021). Characteristics of the medical malpractice cases against orthopedists in China between 2016 and 2017. *PLoS ONE*, *16*(7), e0248052. https://doi.org/10.1371/journal.pone.0248052.

13. Pazart, L., Godard-Marceau, A., Chassagne, A., Vivot-Pugin, A., Cretin, E., Amzallag, E., & Aubry, R. (2018). Prevalence and characteristics of prisoners requiring end-of-life care: A prospective national survey. *Palliative Medicine*, *32*(1), 6–16. https://doi.org/10.1177/0269216317703135.

14. Tripathi, R., Rishabh, M., Ezaldein, H. H., Bordeaux, J. S., & Jeffrey, S. (2019). Prison malpractice litigation involving dermatologists: A cross-sectional analysis of dermatologic medical malpractice cases involving incarcerated patients during 1970–2018. *Journal of the American Academy of Dermatology*, *81*(4), 1019–1021. https://doi.org/10.1016/j.jaad.2019.01.029.

15. Vaughn, M. S., & Collins, S. C. (2004). Medical malpractice in correctional facilities: State tort remedies for inappropriate and inadequate health care administered to prisoners. *The Prison Journal*, *84*(4), 505–534. https://doi.org/10.1177/0032885504269170.

16. Watson, R., Stimpson, A., & Hostick, T. (2004). Prison health care: A review of the literature. *International Journal of Nursing Studies*, *41*(1), 119–128. https://doi.org/10.1016/j.ijnurstu.2003.07.010.

Chapter 6

FORENSIC AUTOPSY

Contents

Introduction

The term "autopsy" is derived from the combination of two Greek words, "autos" meaning "self" and "optos" meaning "seen." The word "Autos" means self, and the word "Optos" means seen. Autopsy refers to the act of observing one's own body. There are two types of autopsies. There are two types of autopsies: medicolegal autopsies and histopathological or clinical autopsies. This chapter primarily centers around the Medicolegal autopsy and its purpose. What are the necessary conditions or requirements for conducting an autopsy? Where can a medicolegal autopsy be performed? Who is qualified to perform the autopsy? What are the various methods of performing a medico-legal autopsy? In addition, we examine the specific organs that should be retained during various autopsy procedures, as well as the essential trace elements that should be gathered in typical forensic autopsies. The preservation of viscera and trace evidence obtained from a deceased body is achieved. We will also provide a concise overview of the preservatives employed. This chapter focuses on the evolutionary significance of autopsy, providing historical profiles, discussing the current state of the art, and outlining prospects for future development of the main techniques and methods used in related disciplines such as Radiology. These disciplines work in synergy with Forensic Pathology to conduct post-mortem assessments. The task can be accomplished by using the advanced molecular autopsy, which combines various skills to analyze the complex data generated by new technologies. This analysis requires a data mining approach guided by enhanced bioinformatics and computational biology tools. The advancement of scientific research and the improved precision of different fields will enable the justice system to assess the significance of evidence as both truth and proof.

Orientation and Directional Terms

Term	Definition	Illustration
Medico-legal autopsy	A medicolegal autopsy, also known as a postmortem examination, is an autopsy that's performed under the provisions of a state's medical examiners or coroners act and produces an evidentiary document that can be used in legal proceedings.	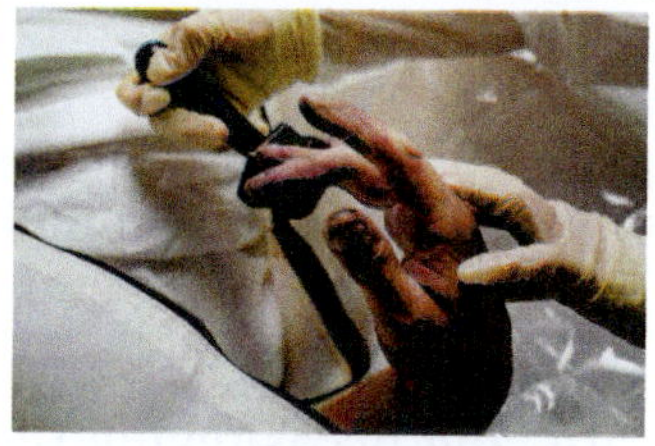
Adrenals	Glands located on top of each kidney that produce hormones such as adrenaline, cortisol, and aldosterone, which are involved in stress response, metabolism, and fluid balance.	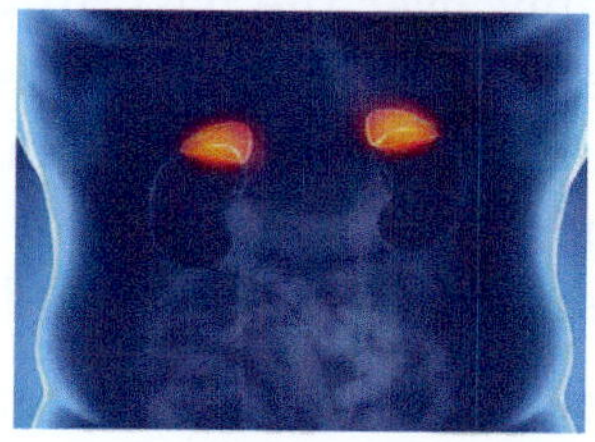
Neck	The part of the body connecting the head to the torso, containing vital structures such as the trachea, esophagus, major blood vessels, and cervical vertebrae.	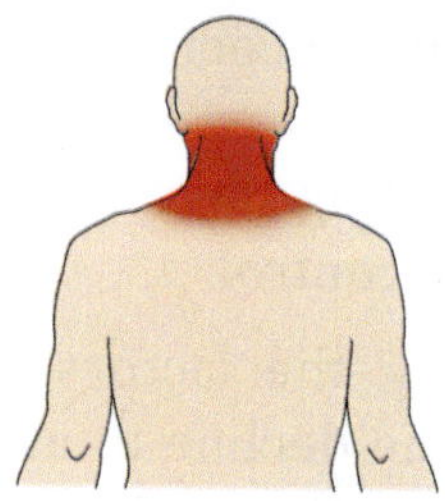
Lungs	Paired organs located in the chest cavity responsible for gas exchange; they oxygenate blood and remove carbon dioxide through the process of respiration.	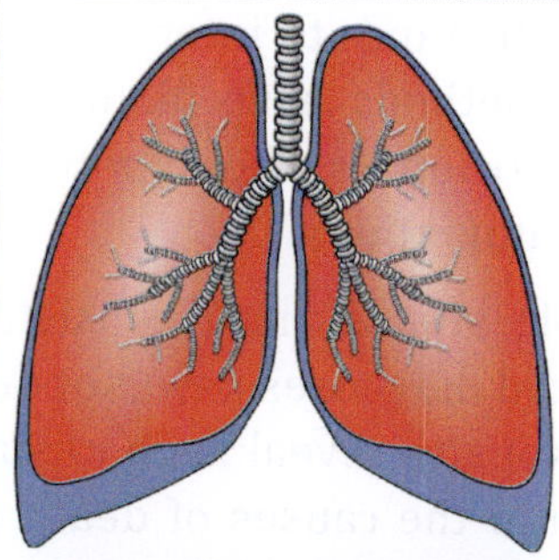
Heart	A muscular organ located in the chest cavity that pumps blood through the circulatory system, supplying oxygen and nutrients to tissues and removing carbon dioxide and other wastes.	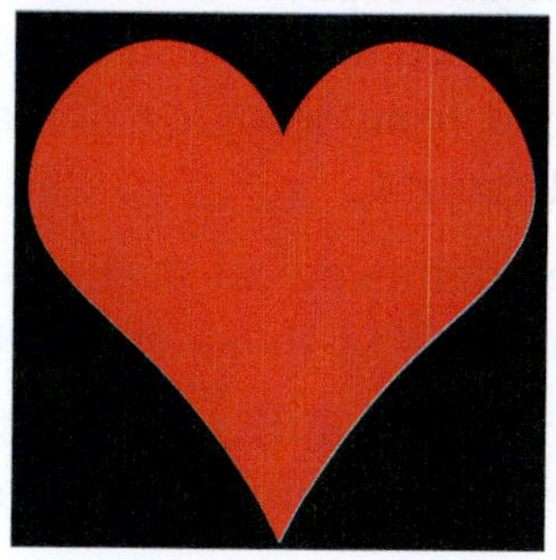

6.1. Autopsy

An autopsy is the postmortem examination of a deceased body to ascertain the cause of death or the characteristics of a disease.

Specifically, anatomical or anatomical-pathological autopsies are conducted to examine human morphology and enhance the understanding of medical students. Forensic autopsies are commissioned by law enforcement, prosecuting attorneys, coroners, or judges to address specific inquiries, encompassing not only the determination of the cause of death (whether natural or traumatic), but also the determination of the manner of death (homicide, suicide, accidental), the time of death, and occasionally the identification of the deceased.

Regrettably, over the past 50 years, there has been a significant decrease in the frequency of autopsies performed in many parts of the world. Historically, it was customary for the pathologist to disclose the anatomical abnormalities of patients. This activity served to validate or invalidate diagnoses, allowed for evaluation of the impact and suitability of treatment, and demonstrated the relentless progression of the disease.

The experience had the potential to be both humbling and reassuring, but it consistently served as a deterrent to medical hubris. Autopsies served as a comprehensive evaluation of the entire medical team, encompassing internists, surgeons, and radiologists. Due to a decreased focus on autopsies, there is a risk of losing the necessary skills for performing these procedures and accurately interpreting the related histopathology. This could result in the loss of a long-standing method of quality control.

Internationally, the factors contributing to reduced dependence on autopsies are varied. The reasons for the decline in autopsies include a focus on lowering healthcare and educational expenses, changes in the workload of pathologists who now spend more time on surgical pathology, a cultural reluctance to interfere with cadavers, the belief that advancements in imaging and other diagnostic methods have made autopsies unnecessary except for legal purposes, and concerns among practitioners about potential legal consequences if errors are discovered during post-mortem examinations.

Multiple studies have consistently shown that the rates of identifying diagnostic errors or unrecognized diagnoses have not decreased over time. It is commonly estimated that approximately 30% of autopsies reveal such mistakes. Several methods that involve less intrusion and narrower inquiries into the causes of death have been studied, but currently, we rely less on the complete examination of corpses. Estimates of total and cause-specific mortality are primarily obtained from data collected during individuals' lifetimes. However, there is a wealth of knowledge that can be gained from studying deceased individuals, which is valuable for both clinical and public health applications.

Some epidemiological studies showed in different countries a decline in autopsies for diagnostic purposes in favor of those of a judicial and, even, didactic nature.

It is therefore difficult to recognize autopsies conducted solely for medicolegal purposes, especially as the documentation on this subject is often dispersed in works, including those of a non-medical nature, that are difficult to uncover (Patowary, 2010; Smith et al., 2018; Norberti et al., 2019; Herath & Herath, 2021).

6.2. Autopsy Techniques

The 19th century in Germany saw the development of modern autopsy techniques, which involved observing individual organs and removing them in four distinct groups: 1) neck, lungs, heart, and thoracic aorta; 2) liver, spleen, stomach, duodenum, and pancreatic gland; 3) intestine; and 4) kidneys, adrenals, the abdominal part of the aorta, and pelvic organs. This novel technique enabled the examination of injuries in anatomical proximity to the adjacent organs and structures. Currently, this approach is commonly utilized and occasionally modified to suit the specific needs of each individual situation involving injury patterns. This includes instances such as neck trauma, traffic accidents, Sudden Infant Death Syndrome (SIDS), deaths of pregnant women, fatalities caused by air embolism, sexual homicides, and cases of medical malpractice.

Before conducting an autopsy, it is necessary to first examine the location where the death occurred. Following this, various radiological examinations such as X-rays, CT scans, and MRIs may be performed. Subsequently, a comprehensive external examination of the deceased's body is conducted, followed by a thorough internal examination by opening all three body cavities.

To maximize its effectiveness in convicting the guilty and protecting the innocent, the forensic autopsy should be conducted thoroughly ("a partial autopsy is even worse than no autopsy"). In fact, an incomplete autopsy may require a subsequent exhumation of the body, because what may seem initially not important could be it for the resolution of the case.

To conduct a thorough autopsy, it is necessary to take various measurements, such as body weight, body length, chest circumference, and the weights of different organs. These measurements help describe the overall health condition and, in the case of children, their development. As for the "report," the initial section should provide a detailed description of all the observations made during the external and internal examination, including both normal and abnormal findings. The second section comprises an initial evaluation of the outcomes. The inclusion of any necessary additional investigations, such as radiological examinations (e.g., X-ray, CT, and MRI), chemico-toxicological tests, or microbiological exams, must be explicitly stated.

Moreover, it is necessary to collect and preserve tissue samples obtained during an autopsy for subsequent histological and immunohistochemical examinations. This may include whole organs such as the brain, heart, and lungs, as well as wounds, body fluids, and tissue specimens for toxicology, genetics, and microbiology analyzes. All of these must be stored under special conditions, at different temperatures and for varying periods, guaranteeing an adequate chain of custody (Patowary, 2010; Smith et al., 2018; Norberti et al., 2019; Herath and Herath, 2021).

6.3. Microscopic Techniques

Microscopic examination is required in all instances where macroscopic examination yields contradictory findings.

The stains used for forensic purposes include hematoxylin-eosin (HE) for identifying hemorrhages, Prussian blue reaction and Quincke stain for detecting hemosiderin, Hematoxylin-Orange and Weigert stain for identifying fibrin in thrombosis, Sudan III for detecting fat embolism, Hematoxylin-Orange for identifying inflammatory cells (leucocytes), carmine or Gentian violet for mast cells, and Heidenhain iron hematoxylin stain and eosin for identifying fibroblasts.

In the field of forensic histopathology, numerous experimental studies have been conducted to discover novel staining techniques for identifying metal deposits on the skin caused by electric marks, studying gunshot entrance wounds and gunshot residues (such as Giemsa staining), and determining the presence of glycogen in cardiac tissue (using PAS – periodic acid Schiff staining).

The experimental enzymatic studies focused specifically on the cerebral injuries or sequence of lesions.

Recently, scanning electron microscopy (SEM) has expanded research opportunities in areas such as the heart, the identification of gunshot residue, and the study of electric and thermal injuries. Moreover, transmission electron microscopy (TEM) was capable of illustrating the presence of hemorrhages and edema in cases of asphyxia deaths, as well as the presence of silicon in cases of lung silicon embolism. The Laser scanning confocal microscope enables the simultaneous observation of multiple fluorochromes and allows for multidimensional analysis (2D, 3D, and 4D) of images. This capability facilitates the evaluation of the cell's activation stage and the detection of metals in tissues.

Environmental scanning electron microscopy has enabled the analysis of materials or tissues without the need for specimen preparation. This technique is used to identify saw or stab marks on bones, detect diatoms in cases of drowning, investigate forensic cases of intoxication, and estimate the firing distance in gunshot-related deaths.

Immunohistochemistry (IHC) is primarily employed to examine the viability and timeline of skin lesions or burned bodies, the timeline of cerebral hypoxia and myocardial ischemia, and the diagnosis and duration of asphyxia, hypothermia, or hyperthermia.

The technique of double-color immunofluorescence analysis, in conjunction with confocal microscopy, is employed to evaluate the sequence of lesions and determine the cause of death in cases of asphyxia.

In situ hybridization (ISH) is employed for gender determination and the detection of viral DNA, particularly in the investigation of sudden infant death syndrome (SIDS) diagnoses.

In the past, it was advised to examine microscopic sections of both normal and abnormal areas of each organ for histological analysis in the field of histology. However, more recently, it has become necessary to collect samples from the main organs for histological examination in all autopsies. This is because histology plays a crucial role in identifying and dating natural or traumatic diseases, determining the cause of death in cases of acute or chronic exposure to foreign substances, and reconstructing accidental or criminal events, including instances of medical malpractice (Patowary, 2010; Smith et al., 2018; Norberti et al., 2019; Herath and Herath, 2021).

6.4. Forensic Radiology

Forensic Radiology has become increasingly significant in the realm of Legal Medicine. However, it is important to note that each method has its own set of advantages and limitations, which are contingent upon the specific method employed and the expertise of the "legal radiologist." These examinations were employed to assess the age and stature of the individuals, primarily for identification.

6.4.1. Virtual Autopsy

In 2000, the renowned Virtopsy project initiated a collaboration between Legal Medicine and Radiology, integrating various fundamental techniques (such as conventional X-rays, CT scans, and MRI) and complementary methods (including imaging-guided sampling, post-mortem angiography, and ultrasound) to conduct systematic research in this field.

6.4.1.1. Conventional X-ray

It is the oldest technique of forensic imaging and has almost been eclipsed by CT in modern imaging.

6.4.1.2. Computed tomography

The post-mortem CT (PMCT) technique is utilized for the generation of two- and three-dimensional images, particularly in the analysis of the skeletal system. This method serves as a highly effective screening tool and supplement to the traditional autopsy due to its exceptional ability to provide detailed imaging, quick examination times (allowing for a full body scan in just a few minutes), user-friendly CT unit operation, ability to detect foreign objects (such as projectiles or surgical materials), and its usefulness in identifying the age and gender of victims in mass disasters. The straightforward and unambiguous images provide easily understandable information to judges, police officers, and other individuals working in the field of forensic medicine.

Nevertheless, the method's drawbacks lie in its low contrast for organ visualization and limited sensitivity for detecting organ findings. As a result, it is more appropriate to examine cases of traumatic death, such as firearm cases, rather than natural death.

6.4.1.3. Magnetic Resonance

MRI can surpass the constraints of PCMT, but its application in forensic imaging is infrequent due to its complex nature, necessitating specialized training and incurring high maintenance expenses. MRI's exceptional soft-tissue resolution makes it an ideal tool for identifying natural causes of death, such as those affecting the heart, as well as for investigating traumatic soft-tissue injuries, such as those occurring in the brain.

6.4.1.4. Imaging-Guided Biopsies

These additional methods enhance the sensitivity of the radiological examination by allowing for minimally invasive collection of various samples such as organ tissue, body fluids, or gas composition. These samples can then be subjected to histological, toxicological, or microbiological investigations. This combination of techniques, including imaging-guided biopsies or liquid aspiration, enables the differentiation of gas resulting from post-mortem decomposition, vital gas embolism, or other sources.

6.4.1.5. Angiography (PMA)

The method shows promise as it involves the injection of a contrast agent into the vascular system, either selectively (such as in the coronary arteries) or throughout the entire body. The use of PMA in conjunction with PMCT also results in enhanced contrast in the soft tissue, enabling the identification of pathological abnormalities. The predominant method utilized is multi-phase PMCT angiography (MPMCTA), which involves conducting a CT scan followed by the administration of a contrast agent (Angiofil®) using a perfusion device (Virtangio®). By utilizing PMCT, the sensitivity for identifying pathological findings in forensic cases can be enhanced from 65% to approximately 81%, which is comparable to a traditional autopsy. This method offers significant benefits in instances of sudden cardiac death, as it enables thorough examination of the coronary arteries. It also proves valuable in cases of fatal hemorrhage, as it allows for the detection of even the most minute sources of bleeding. Additionally, PMCT is advantageous in investigating stab and gunshot trauma, as well as suspected medical errors. The application of contrast agent externally to the blood vessels has been utilized to illustrate the ability to reconstruct the direction of stab wounds and estimate their depth.

6.4.2. Micro-Radiology and Future

Micro-radiology has the potential to serve as the link between histopathology and diagnostic imaging, emerging as a distinct subspecialty. Its application in forensic sciences is also expanding. The primary application is the analysis of calcified tissues, which enables the quantification and computation of mineral density, volume, and surface area. This analysis helps in identifying any abnormalities such as lesions, fractures, or dislocations in bones or calcified tissues. This technique can provide information about the shape of tool marks on bone, the vitality and timing of fractures, and the identification of age.

Micro-CT and micro-MRI can aid in the identification of fire victims and provide estimates of the age at death and the temperature at which human remains were cremated.

This technique can accurately analyze the three-dimensional spatial distribution of gunshot residue particles, even in wounds that are covered by textiles or have been altered by putrefaction, fire, or water. It is used to determine whether a wound is an entrance or exit lesion and to estimate the distance from which the firearm was discharged.

Micro-MRI imaging enables the assessment of neuronal loss associated with aging, cranial trauma, or degenerative diseases (Patowary, 2010; Smith et al., 2018; Norberti et al., 2019; Herath and Herath, 2021).

6.5. Specific Autopsy Procedures

In 2015, the European Council of Legal Medicine (ECLM) released a checklist aimed at identifying competent forensic experts who provide professional services of exceptional quality and have successfully completed official accreditation or certification.

The ECLM document serves to standardize the medico-legal examination process for determining the manner and cause of death. Specifically, the document stipulates that the specialists must possess substantial expertise in Legal Medicine, maintain autonomy from the police or prosecuting authorities, and possess all the requisite equipment to produce reports of exceptional quality. The document encompasses both broad aspects, such as administrative space, quality assurance, and statistical reports, as well as more specific aspects, including scene investigation, external examination, autopsy performance, radiological examinations, histological examinations, and toxicological examinations. Any institution can request accreditation from the president of the ECLM, who will then nominate two inspectors to conduct an assessment. The standards outlined in this document, which incorporate the previous recommendations of the Council of Europe, are the essential requirements for classifying the operations of a forensic pathology service.

6.6. Post-Mortem Interval (PMI)

The Post-Mortem interval (PMI) is one of the most important items in forensic investigation, above all in cases of homicide o traumatic deaths.

We can identify two different objectives of PMI at the scene of violent death (e.g., homicide):

1. To give a preliminary opinion of the time of an assault.
2. To check whether PMI is consistent or inconsistent with the alibi of a suspect.

For estimating the PMI, different sources are used:

1. Information from the environment in the vicinity of the body (e.g, date, and hour in a watch).
2. Anamnestic factors concerning the deceased's habits (e.g., work, activities).
3. Post-mortem changes.

All sources of information on PMI always should be kept in mind.

In forensic medicine, much research has been carried out on post-mortem changes. The progression of all post-mortem changes is influenced by many internal or external factors, mainly the ambient temperature. The longer the post-mortem interval, the less accurate is the estimation of the time since death based on post-mortem changes.

Various methods are proposed for estimating the PMI, in particular:

1. Physical processes, like body cooling and hypostasis.
2. Physicochemical processes, like rigor mortis.
3. Concentration changes of metabolites or substrates.
4. Autolysis with increase or decrease of analytes in various body fluids.
5. Putrefaction due to bacterial processes.

Furthermore, the methods for estimating the PMI are not only different but also have widely varying scientific value in terms of the underlying scientific background, the mode of investigation and the validation of the method.

Chemical and biochemical analysis of bodily fluids, including Vitreous Humor, after death is a crucial method for determining the Postmortem Interval (PMI).

The Vitreous Humor (VH) is a chemically complex liquid solution containing carbohydrates, proteins, electrolytes, and other small molecules found in living organisms. This biological fluid is valuable due to its isolated environment, which is protected from bacterial contamination, decomposition, autolysis, and metabolic reactions. VH has been utilized as a biofluid in various forensic studies. A recent review assessed the chemical and biochemical advancements, focusing on the endogenous compounds present at the time of death and their subsequent changes. These compounds are crucial for predicting the postmortem interval (PMI) and occasionally determining the cause of death. This review validates the utility of VH analysis, particularly in determining the dosage of its endogenous compounds, for accurately calculating the postmortem interval (PMI) and occasionally identifying the causes of death. However, additional studies are required to further support these findings. Vitreous humor (VH) possesses favorable attributes as a biological specimen for estimating post-mortem interval (PMI) due to its watery composition and low cellular content (Patowary, 2010; Smith et al., 2018; Norberti et al., 2019; Herath and Herath, 2021).

These qualities distinguish it from other biological samples, like blood, and provide some protection against post-mortem changes and bacterial contamination. Postmortem, there is a substantial increase in K^+ and NH_3 levels, whereas Na^+ and Cl^- levels exhibit a minor decrease. Additional research is required to investigate the marginal elevation of magnesium lactate, amino acids, and creatinine. Potassium ions (K^+), sodium ions (Na^+), chloride ions (Cl^-), and amino acids have a strong correlation with PMI. On the other hand, magnesium ions (Mg^+), chloride ions (Cl^-), and lactate have a weak correlation with PMI. There was no observed correlation between the decrease in glucose levels and PMI, or between the increase in creatinine levels and PMI.

The aforementioned methods currently in use are still inadequate in providing an accurate estimation of the PMI. Consequently, it is imperative to investigate novel approaches for more accurate PMI estimation. The post-mortem alterations of the body are thus utilized as "indicators" of the PMI, offering only a rough estimate of the time range. Advances in molecular biology have led to efforts to determine the PMI by analyzing the degradation pattern of biological markers such as DNA, RNA, and proteins. DNA has been demonstrated to be highly stable during extended post-mortem periods, whereas RNA is considerably more susceptible to degradation and is sensitive to tissue-specific factors. Recently, certain authors conducted a review that primarily examines the potential application of RNA markers in estimating the PMI. For this review, 47 studies were systematically evaluated based on the predefined criteria for inclusion and exclusion. Forensic scholars have made numerous attempts to accurately determine the PMI, but these attempts have relied on conventional and established methods. In their recent review, Sangwan et al. documented the utilization of RNA, DNA, and protein degradation to estimate the PMI. Several studies have been conducted to discover a more precise and dependable technique for estimating the PMI, but at present, none are capable of providing an accurate estimation of the PMI. The decay of DNA nucleic acids seems to be temporally correlated, making it valuable for estimating the PMI over extended durations. Various ante-mortem and post-mortem factors, such as environmental conditions, have a significant impact on the degradation of DNA. Prior research has primarily concentrated on animal models. However, the multiparametric mathematical model that relies on DNA degradation has not been successful in accurately assessing the error associated with a known PMI. Although RNA degradation has shown significant potential in estimating PMI through molecular techniques, it is not currently utilized in forensic practice. Out of the various studies conducted on RNA degradation, primarily using animal models, the multiparametric mathematical model stands out as the most dependable approach for estimating PMI.

Another novel approach to estimating PMI involves utilizing protein degradation. Experimental studies have been carried out on four types of animal tissues: lungs, kidneys, bones, and skeletal muscles. However, it is worth noting that studies on human tissue in the forensic field are rare, but of exceptional quality. One significant constraint, apart from the predominant reliance on animal models and the exclusion of the forensic field, is the utilization of biomarkers that pose challenges when applied to humans.

Undoubtedly, the future will prioritize the integration of various techniques, while also taking into account the impact of environmental factors when estimating the PMI.

To gain a more comprehensive understanding of the efficacy of these methods, it is imperative to conduct additional research using human samples and tissues. Although there have been many improvements in estimating PMI, the inaccuracies found in these methods necessitate additional research. In the future, advancements in more dependable and cost-effective methodologies will significantly impact the field of forensic science, particularly in the determination of PMI.

Researchers must employ cutting-edge methodologies that yield rapid and dependable outcomes to secure validation and acceptance, not solely within the forensic scientific community, but particularly within courtrooms.

6.7. Types of Autopsy

The term "Autopsy" is derived from the combination of two Greek words, "Autos" meaning "self" and "Optos" meaning "seen." The word "Autos" means self, while the word "Optos" means seen. Autopsy, therefore, refers to the act of observing oneself. It is frequently referred to as a postmortem examination. An autopsy is of two types:

1. medicolegal autopsy/forensic autopsy; and
2. histopathological autopsy/clinical autopsy.

Medicolegal Autopsy is performed in cases of death resulting from non-natural causes, as well as in cases where the cause of death is uncertain or involves deceased individuals. The primary purpose of the medicolegal autopsy is to assist law enforcement agencies in determining the deceased person's identity, cause of death, type of weapon involved, the time elapsed since death, and manner of death, and to gather any potential trace evidence. Only registered medical practitioners in India have legal authorization to perform autopsies in medicolegal cases. This can only be done upon the request of the investigating officer and must take place at an authorized location, accompanied by the necessary inquest papers. Relatives' consent is unnecessary. Before commencing a postmortem examination, it is necessary to have relatives present to identify the deceased. Once the postmortem examination is finished, the body of the deceased is transferred to the police or investigating officer. This is done along with numbered and initial inquest papers, as well as a medicolegal autopsy report. In the context of a Clinical Autopsy, the autopsy is performed by a Pathologist who obtains the consent of the deceased's relatives beforehand. If necessary, further investigation is conducted as part of the autopsy process. Before commencing a clinical autopsy, it is imperative to ensure or confirm that it is not a medicolegal case.

Autopsies are performed at the behest of medical professionals and with approval from the hospital administrator to understand the progression of the disease in the deceased body and enhance medical knowledge. The pathologist has the discretion to decide whether or not to disclose the autopsy report to the family members. In a medicolegal autopsy, the background information is minimal, maybe distorted or non-scientific as per the knowledge available with the investigating police official while in the histopathological autopsy, the detailed events of disease, and case sheets made by well-educated staff are available. The defense lawyer will scrutinize the medicolegal autopsy report during the court proceedings, while the histopathological autopsy findings will be subject to critical evaluation and discussion in peer review meetings.

The Medicolegal Autopsy is studied under the following heads

- Preliminary Examination of Inquest Papers.
- Gross/External Examination of the body
- Internal examination of the body.
    - o Skin incisions
    - o Methods of removal of organs
    - o Samples to be collected
- Preservatives used for various samples

6.8. Preliminary Examination of Inquest Papers

Medicolegal Autopsy is conducted pursuant to the directives of legal authorities such as the Police, Magistrate, or Coroner. In India, a Medicolegal autopsy is typically requested by the police, and is therefore referred to as a Police Inquest. In certain medicolegal cases, such as dowry death or custodial death involving armed forces, a Magistrate is authorized to order an investigation. This type of investigation is commonly referred to as a Magistrate Inquest. In the Western world, coroners are responsible for conducting inquests as well. Therefore, it is referred to as a Coroner Inquest.

An inquest refers to a formal process of conducting an inquiry or investigation. The individual who is granted the authority to conduct an official examination is referred to as the Investigation Officer. The individual responsible for conducting the investigation may vary depending on the specific circumstances and legal requirements of the case. This could include a law enforcement officer, a judicial official such as a magistrate, or a coroner, as dictated by the applicable local laws. A medicolegal autopsy is typically performed in cases of abrupt, inexplicable, or atypical deaths. In India, the investigating officer formally asks a Registered Medical officer (RMP) to perform an autopsy by submitting an application along with the necessary inquest papers. In India, cases of suicide and suspicious deaths are investigated by Police officials under section 174 and by a magistrate under Section 176 of the Criminal Procedure Code, 1973. Additionally, deaths related to dowry or cruelty by in-laws are investigated under Section 174.

Upon concluding the investigation, the Police officer must submit an Inquest report in Form 25.35 A, B, C for cases involving natural causes, violence, and poisoning, respectively. The inquest report should include the explicit cause of death, a detailed description of any visible signs of violence on the body, and a description of the suspected weapon used. The Inquest report should include the layout of the death scene, the detailed list of clothing, and other relevant information. The requested documents include a compilation of articles of the body, a compilation of articles submitted for medical examination (if applicable), and a copy of the police information (PI) obtained from the Hospital. Additionally, the Hospital record and a death summary should be included.

6.9. Gross/External Examination of the Body

Before commencing the postmortem examination, the registered medical practitioner (medical officer) records the initial information pertaining to the deceased in a computerized format. This includes details such as the name, father's name, age, gender, residence, report number, date, the name of the investigating officer along with their belt number and police station, as well as the names and signatures of two relatives who have identified the body of the deceased on the autopsy table before the commencement of the postmortem examination.

Performing a gross examination of the deceased is a crucial step in conducting an autopsy. In cases involving medical and legal matters, such as road traffic accidents, homicides, suicides, burns, vitriolage, and firearm incidents, a thorough examination of the external body provides important information to supplement the internal examination. During the gross or external examination, we record the following parameters from the body of the deceased.

1. Height
2. Weight
3. Clothes
4. Skin (injuries, tattoos, moles, and any disease)
5. Eyes (Injuries, Tardieu spots, Hemorrhages)
6. Mouth (externally) including lips
7. Nose (injury, deformity, blood, etc.)
8. Face, Ears, and neck (injuries, nail marks, ligature, injection marks)
9. Palpate Chest, abdomen and testis
10. Back of the body and lower and upper limbs (injuries, nail marks, ligature, injection marks)

Once the aforementioned parameters have been recorded, it is imperative to conduct photography prior to any manipulation or relocation of the body. Clothing is carefully taken off the body. It is necessary to preserve and photograph each piece of clothing individually. It is important to ensure that any cuts or tears on clothes are not altered or damaged when removing the clothes from the body. For instances of murder and situations where the investigating officer has requested the clothes to be sealed, they must be marked with the postmortem number, signed and dated, and securely enclosed in a packet with specified seals. The packet should be appropriately labeled, signed, and stamped before being handed over to the investigating officer. All trace evidence found while removing clothing from the body, such as nail fragments or loose firearm projectiles, should be carefully preserved in a separate packet. The packet should be labeled, sealed, signed, and stamped. After the autopsy is completed, the packet should be handed over to the investigating officer, who should provide a receipt to maintain the chain of custody of the evidence.

6.10. Internal Examination of the Body

Following the initial gross or external examination and removal of clothing, a subsequent examination of the deceased body should be conducted to identify any injuries, as well as the presence of biological materials such as semen, saliva, or any foreign objects. Through the process of Gross examination, we had already developed an initial plan to continue our work. The body contains three cavities: the abdominal or peritoneal cavity, the thoracic cavity, and the cranial cavity. Based on the characteristics of the case, we proceed to expose the cavity where we observe additional injuries. However, as part of our standard procedure, we begin by opening the skull, followed by the abdomen and chest. Upon initially opening the skull, the entirety of the blood was extracted from the neck. Consequently, we obtained a distinct and non-bleeding visual of the tissues in the neck. The phenomenon of asphyxia, such as hanging and strangulation, is widely understood and recognized.

However, during a thorough examination, we observed injuries to the abdomen and thorax. Consequently, we proceeded to open the abdomen and thorax before moving on to the cranial cavity.

6.11. Skin Incisions Used for Opening Cavities During an Autopsy

A cranial incision is a frequently performed surgical cut made on the scalp, beginning at the mastoid process of one side of the skull and extending upwards through the vertex of the cranial cavity, ultimately ending at the mastoid process of the opposite side. The scalp is elevated to the frontal eminence on the anterior side and the occipital protuberance on the posterior side of the skull. Next, the cranial vault is accessed using a skull opening machine, which involves making a V or Z-shaped incision on the exterior of the skull. The presence of V and Z-shaped incisions in the cranial vault facilitates a secure closure when suturing the scalp after positioning the cranial vault.

There are mainly three conventional skin incisions used in most of the world on the thorax and chest while doing the autopsy. These are as follows:

6.11.1. I-Shaped Incision

This surgical cut is commonly employed when accessing the abdominal and thoracic cavities. The incision follows an I-shaped pattern, beginning below the chin and extending down to the pubic symphysis, with a lateral curve around the umbilicus. The umbilicus is preserved intact to preserve the aesthetic appearance. It is composed of dense fibrous tissue, which makes it challenging to incise and suture during the procedure (Figures 6.1–6.3).

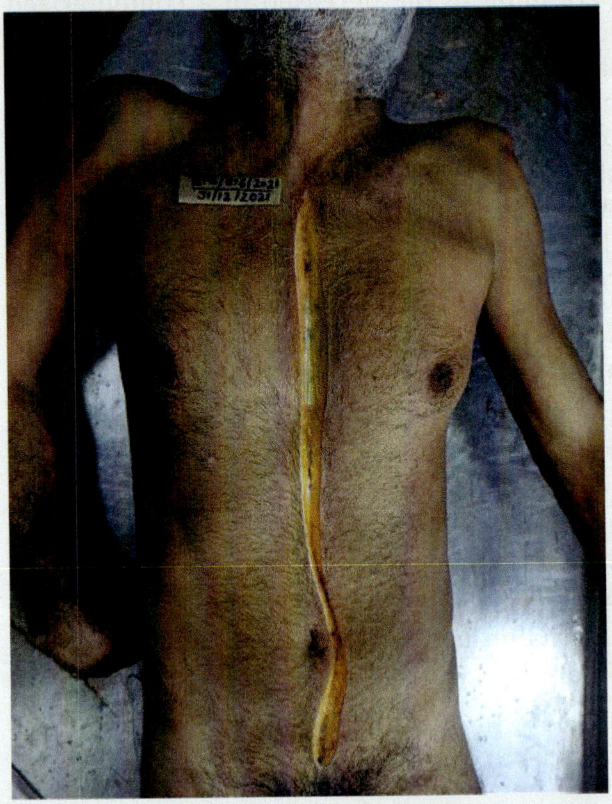

Figure 6.1. *An I-shaped incision was observed on the anterior aspect of the deceased's body while lying in the supine position. The diagram depicted a surgical cut beginning at the suprasternal notch of the manubrium and descending along the midline, curving around the umbilicus, and extending to the symphysis pubis while the person is lying on their back. The incision is extended vertically from the midline up to the chin to complete the I-shaped incision.*

Source: *https://www.researchgate.net/figure/Showed-I-shaped-incision-on-the-body-of-the-deceased-in-the-supine-position-The-figure_fig2_365065214 [accessed 8 Jul, 2024].*

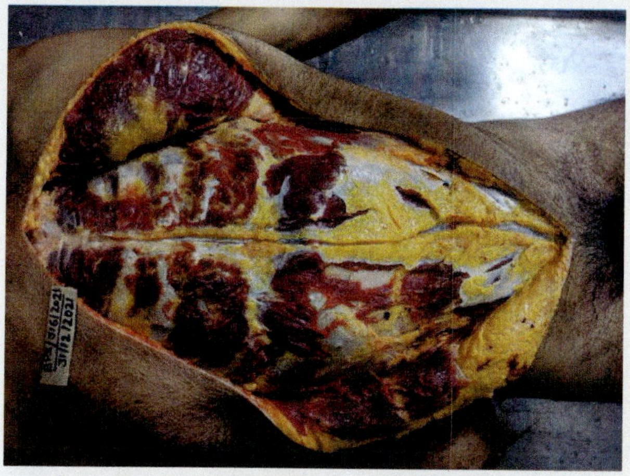

Figure 6.2. *An I-shaped incision was observed on the body of the deceased while they were lying face up. The diagram depicted an I-shaped surgical cut, beginning at the suprasternal notch of the manubrium and extending to the symphysis pubis. This incision was made to allow for the separation of soft tissues and the elevation of flaps, facilitating subsequent dissection.*

Source: https://www.researchgate.net/figure/Showed-I-shaped-incision-on-the-body-of-the-deceased-in-the-supine-position-The-figure_fig2_365065214 [accessed 8 Jul, 2024].

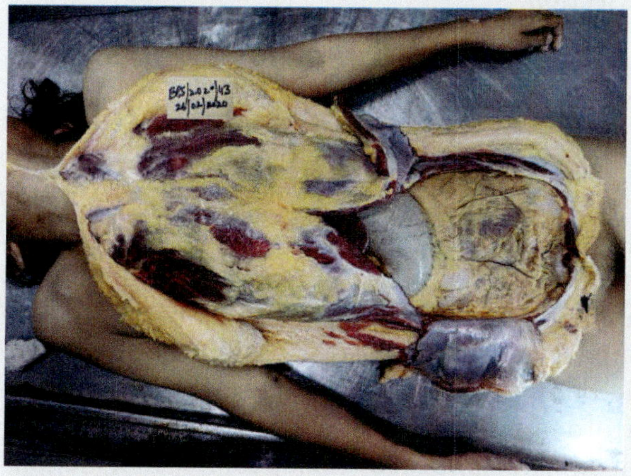

Figure 6.3. *Observed a vertical incision in the shape of the letter "I" on the body of the deceased while lying face up. The diagram depicted an I-shaped cut that began at the suprasternal notch of the manubrium and extended to the symphysis pubis. This incision was made to lift the flaps of skin on both sides of the abdomen. The abdominal cavity was then opened along the midline, below the subcostal margins. The muscular flaps of the abdomen were then pulled aside to allow for the internal dissection of the abdominal organs.*

Source: *https://www.researchgate.net/figure/Showed-I-shaped-incision-on-the-body-of-the-deceased-in-the-supine-position-The-figure_fig2_365065214 [accessed 8 Jul, 2024].*

6.11.2. Y-Shaped Incision

This incision is commonly used to access the abdominal and thoracic cavity. The Y-shaped incision begins below the mastoid process on both sides, forming two limbs of a Y. It then descends in an anterior-inferior direction and meets at the midline, specifically at the level of the suprasternal notch. From there, it continues downward until it reaches the pubic symphysis, curving around the umbilicus laterally, resembling an I-shaped skin incision. This incision technique is employed in forensic autopsies to systematically dissect the layers of the neck, revealing any neck injuries and ligature marks, such as those caused by hanging or strangulation. It is particularly useful for examining the large superficial neck veins in cases of asphyxia resulting from neck compression. There is a possibility of artifactual air embolism, as shown in Figures 6.4–6.6.

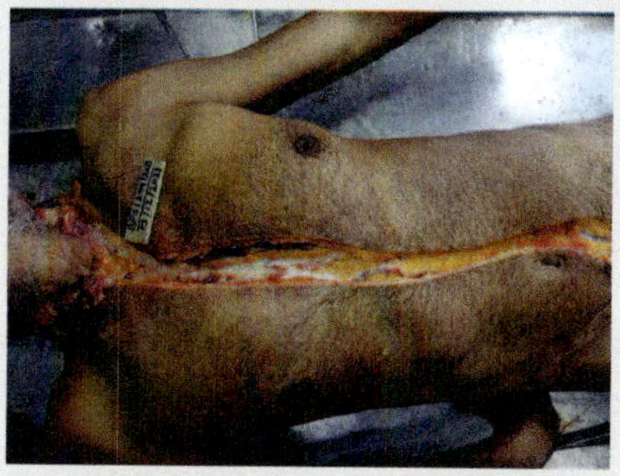

Figure 6.4. *Displayed a Y-shaped cut on the deceased individual's body while lying face up. The Y-shaped incision begins just below the*

mastoid process on both sides, forming two limbs of the Y. It then descends in an anterior-inferior direction and meets at the midline, specifically at the level of the suprasternal notch. From there, it continues downward until reaching the pubic symphysis, curving around the umbilicus laterally, resembling an I-shaped skin incision.

Source: Goyal, N., & Garg, A. (2022). Creative commons license.

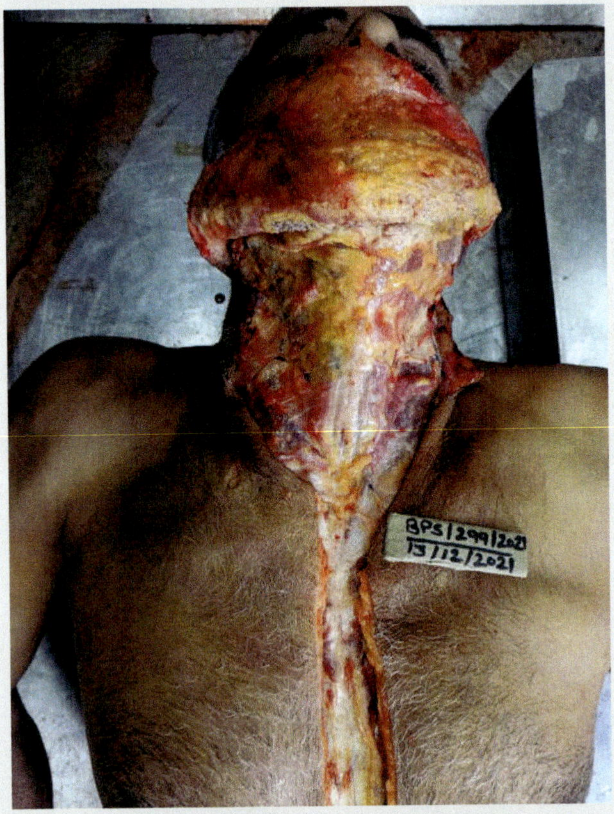

Figure 6.5. *Displayed a Y-shaped cut on the neck and chest of the deceased while lying face up. The skin flap is pulled back upwards to the level of the chin and the lower border of the mandible in a V-shaped pattern. This will provide an unobstructed area for careful examination of the neck.*

Source: Goyal, N., & Garg, A. (2022). Creative commons license.

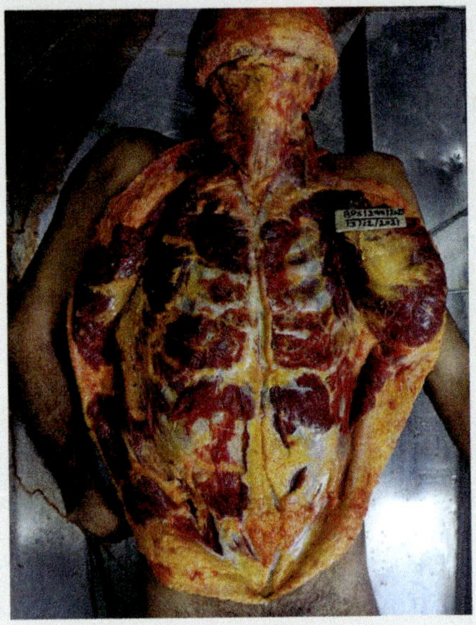

Figure 6.6. *Displayed a Y-shaped laceration on the cadaver's body while lying face up. The diagram depicted a Y-shaped incision originating from each mastoid process and converging at the midline, specifically at the level of the suprasternal notch of the manubrium. From there, the incision continued downwards, curving along the umbilicus and involving the dissection of soft tissues to create flaps on the anterior surfaces of the chest, abdomen, and neck for subsequent dissection.*

Source: Goyal, N., & Garg, A. (2022). Creative commons license.

6.11.3. Modified Y-Shaped Incision

This incision is the third most frequently used method for accessing the abdominal and thoracic cavity. Typically, it is administered to females and individuals of high status, when the body is to be preserved for public viewing in order to prevent disfigurement and public anger. The modified Y-shaped incision begins at the acromion on both sides of the shoulder and then curves downward, following the outer shoulder joint anteriorly. It continues to descend, curving below both breasts and meeting at the midline at the level of the xiphisternum. From there, it proceeds downward to the pubic symphysis, curving around the umbilicus laterally. Please refer to Figures 6.7–6.10 for visual representation.

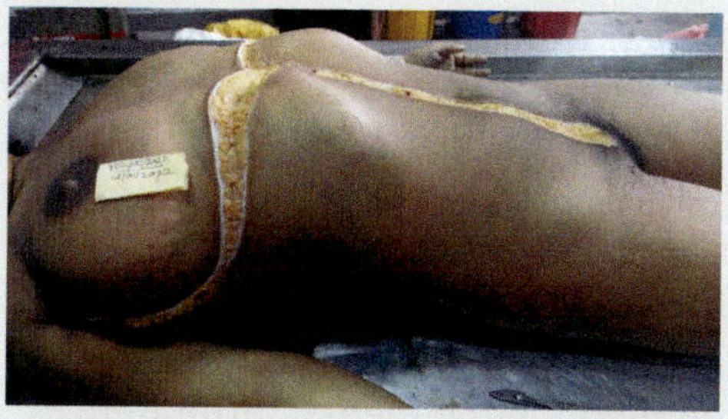

Figure 6.7. *Displayed an altered Y-shaped cut on the body of the deceased female. The modified Y-shaped incision begins at the acromion, descends in a curved path along the outer side of the shoulder, reaches the anterior axillary folds, and curves below both breasts. It then meets at the midline at the level of the xiphisternum and continues downward to the pubic symphysis, curving around the umbilicus laterally.*

Source: Goyal, N., & Garg, A. (2022). Creative commons license.

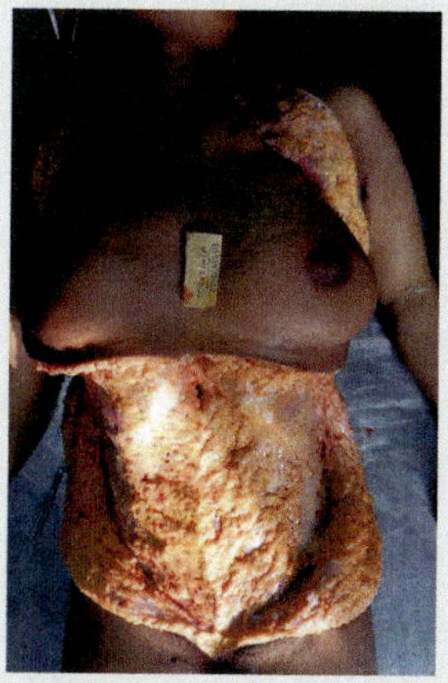

Figure 6.8. *Demonstrated an altered Y-shaped cut in the skin, along with dissection of the underlying soft tissues, on the body of the deceased female. A Y-shaped incision is made and the soft tissues underneath are dissected to raise the abdominal flaps and mammary flaps.*

Source: Goyal, N., & Garg, A. (2022). Creative commons license.

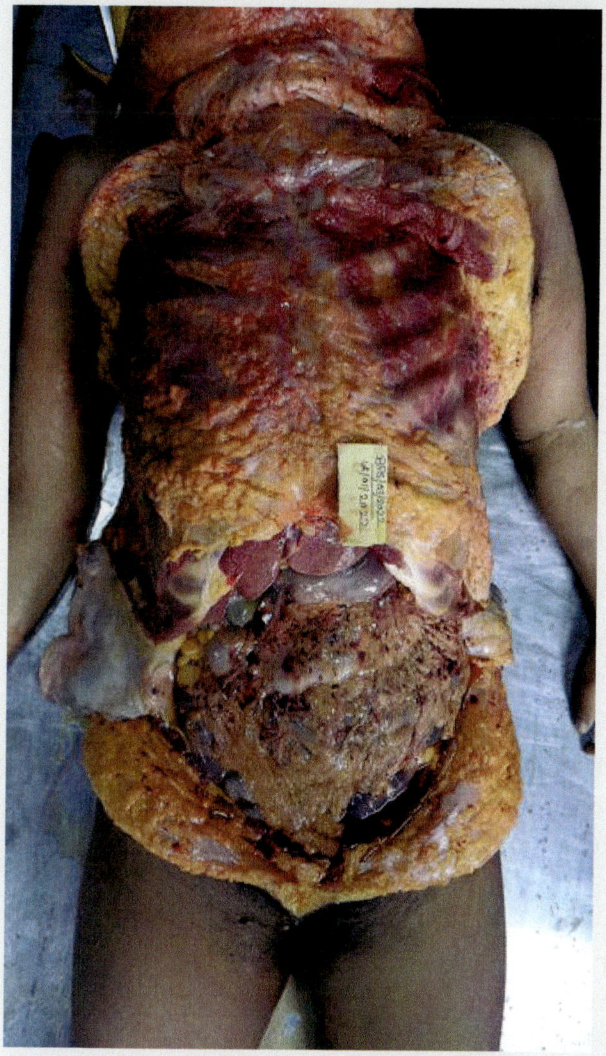

Figure 6.9. *Displayed a revised Y-shaped cut, revealing the underlying soft tissue and dissection of the abdominal wall on the deceased female's body. A revised Y-shaped incision is made, followed by careful dissection of the underlying soft tissues, to elevate both the abdominal flaps and mammary flaps. The midline of the abdominal wall is incised, extending below the sub-costal cartilage, to elevate the flaps of the abdominal wall on both sides of the abdomen and expose the abdominal cavity.*

Source: Goyal, N., & Garg, A. (2022). Creative commons license.

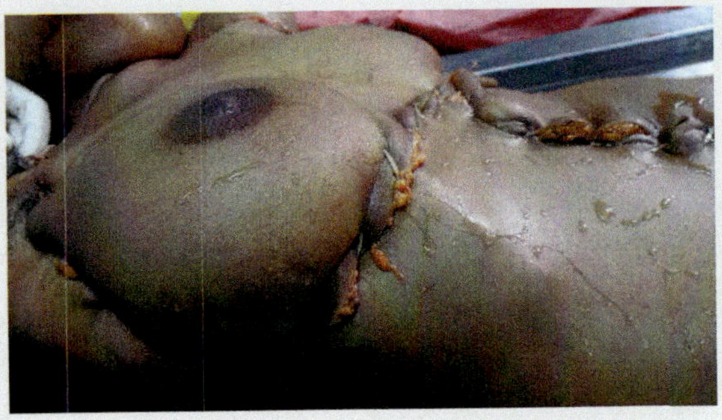

Figure 6.10. *Displayed sutured altered Y-shaped cuts on the corpse of the deceased female. The modified Y-shaped incision is sutured to preserve the anatomical integrity of the deceased's body. The neck and face are aesthetically conserved through the dissection of the underlying tissue after lifting the flaps.*

Source: Goyal, N., & Garg, A. (2022). Creative commons license.

There are few more incisions, other than these three conventional incisions which are used by different autopsy surgeons as per convenience.

6.11.4. Fourth Incision

The aforementioned conventional incisions are located anteriorly on the neck, chest, and abdomen. Consequently, it posed challenges in assessing injuries on the posterior aspect of these regions. In India, it is customary to replace all dissected organs in the abdominal and thoracic cavities through a single incision, as previously mentioned. There is a possibility of blood leakage from this one incision. To address this issue, the author recommended making an additional cut known as the fourth incision. The surgical cut is also aesthetically more pleasing to the immediate legal beneficiaries before the final ceremonies. In the anterior approach, the body is positioned supine with a block placed under the shoulder to extend the neck. The surgical cut is initiated from one edge of the mastoid process to the opposite edge, traversing through the highest point in the coronal plane. The scalp is elevated to the occipital protuberance at the back and the frontal eminence at the front, thereby exposing the cranial bone for subsequent dissection. The incisions on both sides of the mastoid process are extended downwards to the acromion process. They continue in front of the chest, outside the shoulder joint, to the midaxillary line below the axilla. From there, they are further extended to the anterior superior iliac spine. Then, they turn towards the middle along with the inguinal ligaments, ultimately meeting each other in the midline. Currently, the flap is elevated through a shallow dissection, extending to the base of the neck and continuing up to the lower edge of the mandible. Next, the abdominal cavity is accessed by making a vertical incision along the midline. The dissection is performed in the usual manner, followed by suturing the body along the midline. Next, the skin incision is sutured, beginning from the inguinal region on both sides and extending laterally. To perform dissection on the back side of the body, it is positioned in a prone posture with a support placed beneath the chest to elevate it and bend the neck. The incision is extended bilaterally from the right acromion posteriorly, following the outer contour of the shoulder, until it reaches the midaxillary line. It is then further extended to the anterior superior iliac spine on both sides. Now, the scalp flap that has been lifted up to the occipital protuberance is being extended further through the neck, the posterior part of the chest, and the lower back, and is being raised downwards. Now, the fundamental analysis was completed. The suturing on the back is performed following the superior replacement of the flap with an anteriorly replaced scalp flap. Subsequently, the process of stitching the sidewall is carried out.

Some authors have suggested using a fifth or alternative incision to decrease the amount of time required for suturing and to minimize disfigurement of the deceased's body. The body is positioned in a supine posture, with a block placed beneath the posterior aspect of the chest to elongate the neck. The incision originates from the right mastoid process and extends towards the left mastoid process in the coronal plane on the scalp. The incision begins at the right mastoid process and proceeds along the front of the neck to reach the left incision at the left mastoid process, positioned just two fingerbreadths below the lower border of the chin. The cut starting from the right mastoid process extends along the outer side of the neck until it reaches the right acromion process. Starting from the right acromion process, the incision curves in front of the medial end of the right shoulder until it reaches the level of the mid-axillary line of the fourth rib. From there, it descends towards the right anterior superior iliac spine, then continues towards the left side on the front of the abdomen near the inguinal ligament, and finally reaches the left anterior superior iliac spine.

The dissection of the underlying tissues is performed horizontally to elevate the flap of skin on the anterior surface of the chest and abdomen. To access the abdominal cavity, a muscular incision is made above the right anterior superior iliac spine. The incision extends towards the left anterior superior iliac spine along the inguinal canals, then continues upwards to the level of the tenth rib costal cartilage. Finally, it extends towards the right side until reaching the right costal margin near the midaxillary line. Following this surgical cut, the muscular abdominal wall is lifted towards the right side. Following the dissection, the flap is repositioned without suturing, and then the body is stitched, beginning from the skin incision adjacent to the left anterior superior iliac spine and extending to the right mastoid process.

If dissection is necessary on the posterior aspect of the body, the body is positioned in a prone posture, with a support placed beneath the chest to facilitate neck flexion. Beginning from the initial cut made in the front of the body, the incision is continued towards the back on the outer side of the right shoulder, starting from the right acromion process and extending up to the right mid-axillary line, where it meets the previously made incision in the front. The incision must be extended from the anterior superior iliac spine along the upper curved edges of the buttocks, starting from the right and continuing to the left anterosuperior spine.

The dissection is performed tangentially, and the flap on the posterior side of the chest and lower back is lifted on the left side, separating the underlying muscles and body attachments. After dissecting the back, the skin is stitched from the left anterosuperior spine to the right acromion process. The length of this incision is shorter than the fourth incision mentioned earlier, but longer than the conventional I, Y, and Modified Y-shaped incisions. Therefore, suturing can be performed earlier compared to the fourth incision. Nevertheless, like the fourth Incision, it possesses an aesthetically pleasing appearance and prevents the leakage of contents that commonly occurs with traditional skin incisions.

6.12. Methods of Removal of Organs During an Autopsy

There are four conventional methods known to remove organs from the body of the deceased during autopsy.

6.12.1. Rokitansky's Technique or Method of Removal of Organs

This technique was created by a German pathologist named Carl Rakitansky (1804–78), as indicated by its name. This technique involves conducting an autopsy dissection in its original location. Advantages: Can be easily performed in individuals with infections as well as in pediatric patients. Drawback: Executing this technique in adults is challenging.

6.12.2. Virchow's Technique or Method of Removal of Organs

This technique was conducted by Rudolph Virchow, a German pathologist, as indicated by its name. This technique involves the sequential extraction and analysis of individual organs. Advantages: Facilitates the examination of individual organs. Drawback: The interconnection between organs is severed. Consequently, significant data may be forfeited.

6.12.3. Letulle's Technique or Method of Removal of Organs

This technique was conducted by a French pathologist named Maurice Letulle (1853–1929), as indicated by its name. This technique involves the simultaneous removal of multiple organs, from the tongue to the prostate, as a single mass.

- **Benefits:** This technique effectively ensures the preservation of interpersonal relationships. The connections to blood vessels, lymphatic vessels, and nerves are intact and undamaged.
- **Drawback:** This technique is laborious and managing all organs is challenging.

6.12.4. Ghon's Technique or Method of Removal of Organs

This technique was conducted by an Austrian pathologist named Anton Ghon (1866–1936), as indicated by its name. This technique involves the extraction of organs in three distinct segments. This technique combines both Virchow's and Letulle's techniques into a single setting. This technique is alternatively referred to as the Enbloc Method.

- **Benefits:** Organs are extracted in three distinct blocks. The interdependence among the organs within each unit is effectively preserved. Manipulating organs is simpler in comparison to Letulle's technique, which involves removing organs.
- **Drawbacks:** Analyzing interrelationships becomes challenging when the disease spreads across multiple blocs.

6.13. Viscera/Samples to be Collected with Preservatives Used for Medicolegal Cases

In medicolegal cases, various samples are collected depending on the case to case.

6.13.1. Stomach

An incision is made at the greater curvature of the stomach, allowing the contents to be poured into a jar. It is preferable to use a glass jar with a tight lid. The entire stomach is secured above and below the stomach opening. The stomach wall is everted, and the mucosa is inspected for signs of congestion, ulceration, and adhesive substance. The contents of the stomach are additionally analyzed for their texture, smell, and hue. The stomach and its entire contents are conserved in a concentrated solution of sodium chloride to identify toxins in suspected cases of poisoning. Rectified spirit is utilized as a preservative in cases of acid poisoning, except for carbolic acid.

6.13.2. Small Intestine and Large Intestine

The small intestine and large intestine are preserved, along with the stomach, in a jar (ideally a glass jar with a secure lid) to detect poisons.

6.13.3. Spleen, Kidneys, and Liver

The spleen, half of each kidney in the coronal plane, and part of the liver from each lobe or suspected area are also stored in a jar (preferably a glass jar with a tight lid) to detect poisons. In order to conduct a Microbiological examination, swabs of blood are collected from the spleen. The spleen is positioned in a straight manner on the autopsy table. The broad-based, sterilized knife is retrieved and subsequently applied to the spleen on two occasions. This procedure will externally sterilize the spleen. Now, a cross-shaped cut is made on the sterilized surface of the spleen. Microbiological examination is conducted on blood swabs obtained from the cuts on the spleen.

6.13.4. Gallbladder

The entirety of the gallbladder is conserved and submitted for chemical analysis, along with a portion of the livers as previously stated. This is used for the toxins that are eliminated through the Biliary System. Bile can be extracted by making an incision in the gallbladder wall and collecting the bile in a container by inserting a syringe needle and aspirating the bile, or by squeezing the gallbladder through the cystic duct to collect the bile.

6.13.5. Blood

Following the extraction of internal organs, it is recommended to collect a quantity of 10–20 ml of blood. The femoral vein is the most favored location for blood collection, followed by the iliac vein and subclavian vein. Avoid extracting bloody fluid directly from the heart or scooping it from the thoracic or abdominal cavities. Preservatives must not be utilized when sending blood samples for the identification of common toxins. A blood culture vial is utilized to preserve the blood for Microbiological examination. To conduct Dengue serology and other serological tests, it is necessary to preserve the blood in a Red Vacutainer. In order to estimate alcohol levels, it is necessary to preserve blood samples in a solution containing sodium fluoride and potassium oxalate. Alternatively, phenyl mercuric chloride or sodium azide can also be used. To perform blood grouping or DNA/RNA analysis, small amounts of blood are preserved on an FTA Card.

6.13.6. Anal Swabs

These images are captured when there is suspicion of anal intercourse. Two aseptic swabs are placed in glass test tubes labeled A and B. A swab is collected from the rectum. B-Swab is collected from the exterior of the anal canal for control purposes. After collecting the swabs, they are placed on slides and then transferred into their corresponding test tubes. The swabs are then set aside to dry in the air. Before being packaged and sealed for further transportation, they are properly labeled.

6.13.7. Vaginal Swabs

These are captured when there is suspicion of sexual intercourse. A pair of sterilized swabs are collected and placed in glass test tubes, which are labeled as A and B. A swab is collected from the posterior fornix, which is located deep inside the vagina. B-Slide is a method of contraception that is inserted into the vagina to prevent pregnancy. After collecting the swabs, they are placed on individual slides. The swabs are then placed in their respective test tubes and set aside to dry in the air. Before being packaged and sealed for further transportation, the slides and test tubes are labeled. Both anal and vaginal swabs are collected and stored to detect the presence of spermatozoa.

6.13.8. Saliva/Bite Marks

In medicolegal cases, if we come across bite marks then we suspect dried saliva. A cotton swab moistened with saline solution is taken and rotated on the bite mark then the swab is kept aside for drying and then kept back in a glass test tube. Saliva is useful in the detection of the blood group (if secretors) and DNA analysis from mucosal cells in saliva.

6.13.9. Urine

It is usually preserved when we suspect that poison is excreted through urine. The preservative used for Urine is Thymol or Sodium benzoate solution.

6.13.10. DNA Analysis

Long bones are preserved free from skin and muscle tissue preferably in dry ice for DNA Analysis.

6.13.11. Diatom Test

The sternum is preserved to detect diatoms in the bone marrow in suspected cases of drowning.

6.13.12. Feces

For detection of protozoal and helminthic infestation, 5 to 10 g of feces is collected. In Autopsy cases, it is rarely collected these days.

6.13.13. CSF

CSF is collected by using a needle and syringe from cisterna magna.

6.13.14. Vitreous Humor

A volume of 1 to 5 ml of Vitreous Humor is extracted from each eye. It is utilized to ascertain the postmortem interval by analyzing the potassium and other substances' concentration in the vitreous humor and aqueous humor.

The suspected pathological sections of the lungs, brain, kidney, spleen, liver, and skin tissue are collected and sent for histopathological examination. These items should be conserved in a solution of 10% Formalin. The fragments ought to be diminutive. Formalin can rapidly penetrate tissues and reach a wider range of areas. Therefore, the issue of autolysis caused by the absence of tissue preservation is limited.

6.14. The Future

A European survey revealed that various countries have established national guidelines for conducting autopsies. The predominant protocols primarily address cases involving violent or sudden deaths, mass disasters, and medical negligence.

In the future, cutting-edge robotic and advanced microscopy systems and techniques will be employed in the medico-legal field to enhance and standardize autopsy procedures, leading to more accurate identification of natural and traumatic diseases.

To enhance precision and effectiveness, the forensic autopsy will be conducted using a robotic system, employing various techniques such as photogrammetry, optical surface scanning, and image-guided sampling of tissue or liquid.

Atomic force microscopy, a high-resolution scanning probe microscopy technique capable of producing three-dimensional images, can be used to study biological macromolecules and evaluate PMI.

The utilization of MALDI-IMS and SALDI for direct tissue analysis enables the identification, analysis, spatial profiling, and quantification of drugs, heavy metals, proteins, peptides, and metabolites. This application has the potential to enhance diagnostic capabilities and decrease analysis time in forensic cases.

Moreover, MSI will allow for the identification of tissue types based on chemical composition rather than structure. This will reveal the spatial distribution of macromolecules, such as proteins, peptides, nucleic acids, metabolites, and xenobiotics within a specific sample. The SALDI technique enables the detection of small molecules, while MSI offers more advanced applications in forensics, such as determining the cause of death and identifying the PMI. This is achieved by studying the decay of metabolites in cells and analyzing the presence and distribution of xenobiotics in tissues (Patowary, 2010; Smith et al., 2018; Norberti et al., 2019; Herath and Herath, 2021).

A Closer Look

Forensic Lung Pathology

Forensic lung pathology plays a critical role in the field of forensic medicine by examining and diagnosing lung diseases and conditions that contribute to or result from an individual's death. This branch of forensic science focuses on understanding the pathological changes in lung tissues that may offer insights into the cause of death, especially in cases where external factors such as trauma, toxins, or chronic diseases are suspected. The study of forensic lung pathology involves a detailed examination of lung tissues obtained during autopsies to identify pathological changes, such as inflammation, infection, and malignancy, which could have led to or contributed to death.

A key aspect of forensic lung pathology is the identification of diseases that may be overlooked in clinical settings. Chronic conditions such as chronic obstructive pulmonary disease (COPD), asthma, and interstitial lung diseases can be critical in forensic investigations. These conditions may cause significant lung damage, potentially leading to respiratory failure or complications that can be fatal. Forensic pathologists examine lung tissues to identify signs of these chronic conditions, which might explain sudden deaths or deaths that occur under unusual circumstances.

In addition to chronic diseases, forensic lung pathology is crucial in cases of acute lung injury or disease. Forensic pathologists often encounter cases of acute respiratory distress syndrome (ARDS), pneumonia, and pulmonary embolism. Each of these conditions has distinct pathological features that can be identified through histological examination. For instance, ARDS is characterized by diffuse alveolar damage and edema, while pneumonia may show evidence of suppurative inflammation. Accurate diagnosis of these conditions can provide vital information regarding the timing and nature of the lung injury, contributing to a better understanding of the cause of death.

Toxicological investigations are another important component of forensic lung pathology. The lungs are often exposed to environmental toxins, drugs, and pollutants, which can cause significant pathological changes. Forensic pathologists assess the presence of these substances in lung tissues, correlating their effects with the overall pathological findings. For example, exposure to toxic fumes or chemicals can lead to chemical pneumonitis or acute lung injury, which can be crucial in determining whether exposure contributed to the individual's death.

In forensic investigations involving suspected trauma, forensic lung pathology can also play a significant role. Trauma to the chest or lungs may lead to pneumothorax, hemothorax, or contusions. Identifying these injuries and correlating them with the external evidence of trauma is essential for understanding the sequence of events leading to death. Forensic pathologists meticulously examine lung tissues for signs of contusions, hemorrhages, and other injuries that may not be immediately visible on the surface but can reveal important information about the nature of the trauma.

Summary

- The advancement of technology in the field of medico-legal sciences, which started in the late 20th century and continues into the present day, has necessitated an interdisciplinary approach to conducting necroscopic investigations. By employing medico-legal sciences, it becomes possible to identify and describe injuries that may be challenging to quantify objectively. Additionally, these sciences can address specific forensic issues, such as determining the time since death, assessing the vitality of wounds, reconstructing the sequence of injuries, and establishing the timing of natural diseases. The participation and integration of various experts, including forensic pathologists, geneticists, toxicologists, radiologists, anthropologists, microbiologists, and entomologists, have become crucial.
- The conventional autopsy is currently and likely to continue being a crucial method for investigating death, despite significant technological advancements and the potential future use of robotic or virtual autopsies, facilitated by micro- and nanotechnologies.
- Thus, it remains valid to this day. In 1965, L.S. King stated that assuming autopsies alone can advance medical science is a mistake. The progress in the medical field depends not on the number of autopsies performed but on the skills and qualities of the person conducting them. The data obtained from autopsies must be effectively utilized by individuals who possess imagination, originality, tenacity, and mental acuity. However, the most important factor is their adequate and profound scientific preparation. Without this, the observed data from autopsies are entirely useless.
- It is essential for both the Forensic Pathology Services and all the specialists involved in the necroscopic ascertainment, including the forensic pathologist, radiologist, toxicologist, and geneticist, to be certified and accredited. This will guarantee the provision of high-quality services in the forensic field.
- The primary challenge that significantly impacts post-mortem forensic evaluation is primarily the dearth of empirical evidence in scientific understanding.
- The advancement of forensic research will be enhanced by the integration of omics, bio-analytical, and imaging sciences. By developing specific algorithms, the improved accuracy of different forensic disciplines can be used to evaluate the value of evidence provided to the justice system as truth and proof.
- The adage "Justice delayed is justice denied" is widely acknowledged. Medico-Legal Autopsy is a procedure conducted to assist law enforcement agencies in determining the cause of death and providing justice to the deceased and their loved ones. It is imperative that we consistently enhance our knowledge and understanding to assist our law enforcement agencies in promptly delivering justice.

References

1. Bolliger, S. A., & Thali, M. J. (2015). Imaging and virtual autopsy: Looking back and forward. *Philosophical Transactions of the Royal Society B: Biological Sciences*, *370*(1666), 20140253. https://doi.org/10.1098/rstb.2014.0253.

2. Burton, J. L., & Kitsanta, P. (2020). Daily application of post-mortem computed tomography digital autopsy in a public mortuary. *Diagnostik and Histopathology, 26*(9), 358–367. https://doi.org/10.1016/j.diahist.2020.07.006.

3. Herath, J. C., & Herath, S. O. (2021). Is it time for targeted and minimally invasive post-mortem examination using total body computed tomography in a medicolegal autopsy? *Forensic Science, Medicine and Pathology, 17*(2), 175–176. https://doi.org/10.1007/s12024-021-00304-w.

4. Lewis, C., Latif, Z., Hill, M., Riddington, M., Lakhanpaul, M., Arthurs, O. J., Hutchinson, J. C., Chitty, L. S., & Sebire, N. J. (2018). "We might get a lot more families who will agree": Muslim and Jewish perspectives on less invasive perinatal and paediatric autopsy. *PLoS ONE, 13*(9), e0202023. https://doi.org/10.1371/journal.pone.0202023.

5. Moskała, A., Woźniak, K., Kluza, P., Romaszko, K., & Lopatin, O. (2016). The importance of post-mortem computed tomography (PMCT) in confrontation with conventional forensic autopsy of victims of motorcycle accidents. *Legal Medicine, 18*(1), 25–30. https://doi.org/10.1016/j.legalmed.2016.02.001.

6. Norberti, N., Tonelli, P., Giaconi, C., Nardi, C., Focardi, M., Nesi, G., Miele, V., & Colagrande, S. (2019). State of the art in post-mortem computed tomography: A review of current literature. *Virchows Archiv, 475*(2), 139–150. https://doi.org/10.1007/s00428-019-02643-6.

7. Patowary, A. (2010). The fourth incision: A cosmetic autopsy incision technique. *American Journal of Forensic Medicine and Pathology, 31*(1), 37–41. https://doi.org/10.1097/PAF.0b013e3181cf3b2a.

8. Rutty, G. N., & Rutty, J. E. (2011). Perceptions of near virtual autopsies. *Journal of Forensic and Legal Medicine, 18*(6), 306–309. https://doi.org/10.1016/j.jflm.2011.03.002.

9. Smith, A. P. T., Traill, Z. C., & Roberts, I. S. D. (2018). Post-mortem imaging in adults. *Diagnostik and Histopathology, 24*(7), 365–371. https://doi.org/10.1016/j.diahist.2018.03.001.

10. Suvarna, S. K., Kitsanta, P., & Burton, J. L. (2017). The effects of postmortem CT scanning all cases entering a UK public mortuary: A 3-month pilot. *Journal of Clinical Pathology, 70*(10), 903–905. https://doi.org/10.1136/jclinpath-2017-204661.

11. Ukpo, O., & Boger, D. (2018). Chapter 4—The role of virtual autopsy and use of a CT scanner in medico-legal death investigations. In L. Sathyavagiswaran & C. B. Rogers (Eds.), *Multidisciplinary Medico-Legal Death Investigation: Role of Consultants* (pp. 69–73). Academic Press. https://doi.org/10.1016/B978-0-12-812749-0.00004-6.

12. Wagensveld, I. M., Weustink, A. C., Kors, J. A., Blokker, B. M., Hunink, M. G. M., & Oosterhuis, J. W. (2020). Effect of minimally invasive autopsy and ethnic background on acceptance of clinical postmortem investigation in adults. *PLoS ONE, 15*(7), e0232944. https://doi.org/10.1371/journal.pone.0232944.

Chapter 7

VIRTUAL AUTOPSY

Contents

Introduction

In the field of forensic science, an autopsy is a postmortem examination that involves a comprehensive examination of a corpse to determine the cause and manner of death using invasive methods. The term "Virtopsy" refers to a virtual autopsy technique that utilizes imaging methods such as computed tomography (CT) and magnetic resonance imaging (MRI). This technology has demonstrated its benefits in the field of forensic science. It entails the non-invasive scanning of deceased bodies. The alternative to the traditional autopsy offers a comprehensive and systematic examination of the entire body in a shorter time period. This method has advantages in diagnosis and also respects religious beliefs. The method is highly specific, sensitive, and precise, allowing for accurate detection of soft tissue injuries, organ damage, wound severity, and fractures. This method provides compelling and reliable evidence for forensic identification in court. This chapter will discuss the significance of "Virtopsy" in the field of forensic science and its potential for future applications in forensic crime investigations.

Orientation and Directional Terms

Term	Definition	Illustration
Magnetic Resonance Imaging (MRI)	A medical imaging technique that uses strong magnetic fields and radio waves to generate detailed images of organs and tissues inside the body.	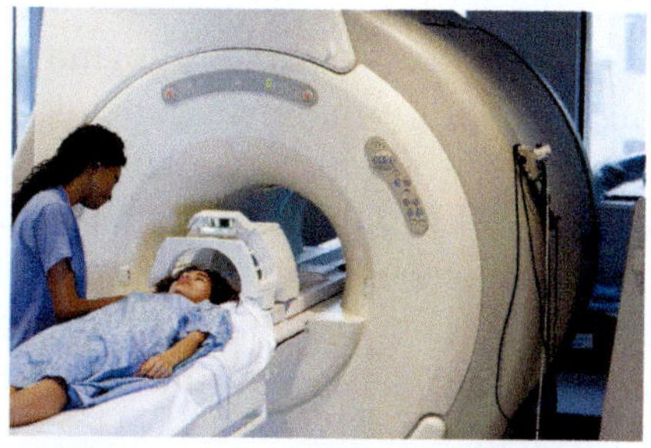
Computed Tomography (CT)	A diagnostic imaging method that uses X-rays and computer processing to create cross-sectional images of the body, providing detailed views of internal structures.	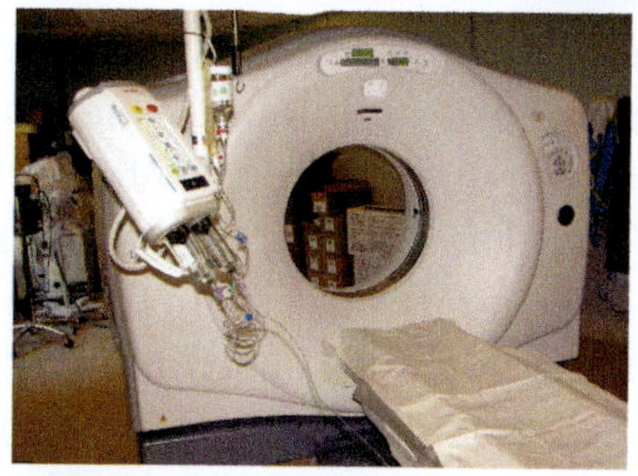
Multi-Slice Computed Tomography (MSCT)	An advanced form of CT imaging that uses multiple detectors to acquire several slices of images simultaneously, allowing for faster scanning and higher resolution.	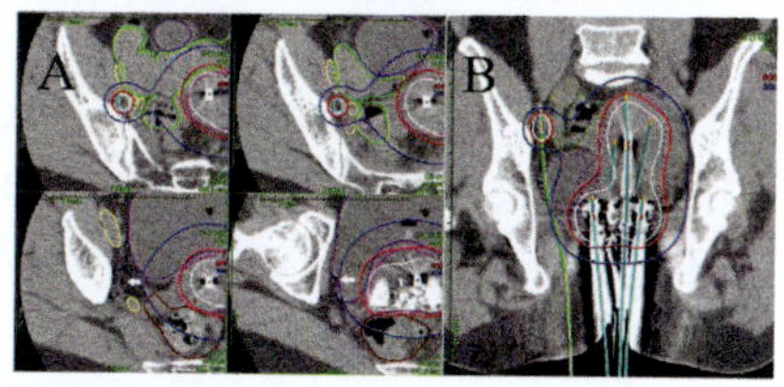
Forensic Odontology	The application of dental science to criminal investigations, including the identification of individuals through dental records and the analysis of bite marks.	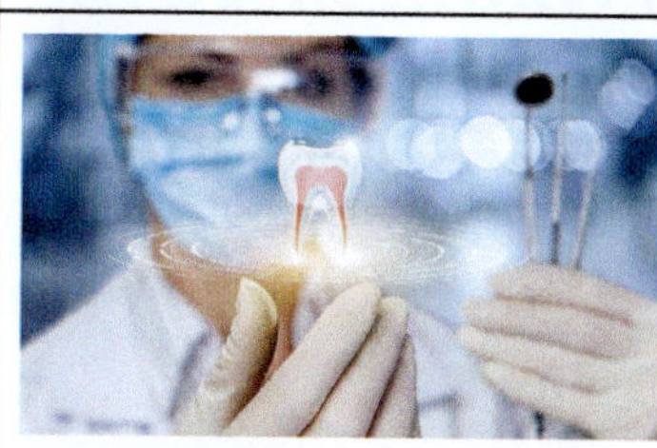
Post-Mortem Computed Tomography (PMCT)	A specialized CT imaging technique used to examine the body after death, aiding in the detection of trauma, disease, and other factors relevant to forensic investigations.	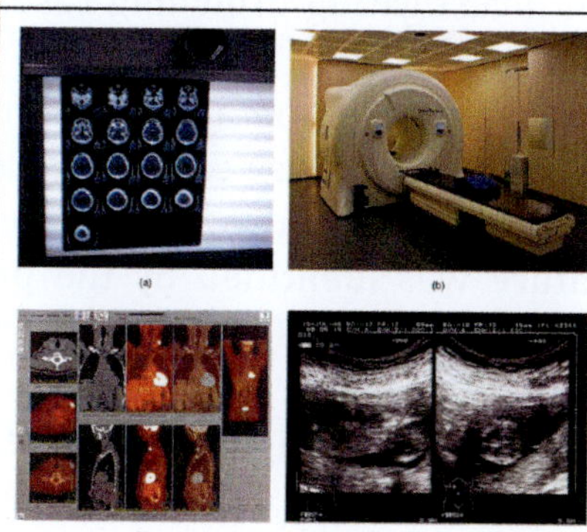

7.1. Virtual Autopsy: A new Approach

The traditional autopsy is a classical method used to investigate and determine the cause and manner of death. This scientific procedure, known as autopsy, involves thoroughly examining the entire surface and internal cavities of a deceased body. The purpose is to document the findings, which can provide valuable information in determining the cause and circumstances of death, and assist law enforcement agencies. Simultaneously, obtaining consent for the forensic autopsy is influenced by the emotions and religious beliefs of the deceased's relatives. In addition, certain religious and cultural beliefs, such as those in Judaism, prohibit the practice of autopsy. The various factors mentioned highlight the necessity for an improved autopsy technique that can overcome these obstacles and demonstrate equal importance to the conventional autopsy method. "Virtual Autopsy" or Virtopsy is an innovative technique that represents a significant advancement in the field of forensic science.

Virtopsy is a contemporary approach that utilizes advanced imaging and measuring technology to perform autopsies without the need for a scalpel. The term was originated by Richard Dirnhofer, the former Director of Forensic Medicine at the Institute of Forensic Medicine, University of Berne in Switzerland. The virtopsy procedure involves a comprehensive combination of advanced imaging techniques, including Three-dimensional (3D) surface scanning using 3D/computer-aided design photogrammetry, multi-slice computed tomography (MSCT), Magnetic resonance imaging (MRI), and MRI spectroscopy. It offers a comprehensive three-dimensional perspective of both the internal and external aspects of the body. The crucial data, including the location, size, and severity of injuries, as well as other pathological conditions, can be collected in a digitized format, thereby enabling a more efficient evaluation of the body's state. This tool is highly promising as it combines advanced scanning and radiographic technology with the computational power and resolution of modern computing. It is particularly useful for investigators, forensic pathologists, and doctors.

7.2. Application of Virtopsy in Forensic Sciences

Virtopsy has demonstrated its extensive range of applications in the forensic field, encompassing various aspects such as investigations into causes of death, firearm injuries, estimation of age and fractures, identification of decomposed bodies, forensic odontology, mass disaster cases, anthropological examinations, drowning cases, analysis of skin lesions, and identification of charred bodies.

When investigating drowning cases, forensic experts must determine whether the drowning occurred before or after death, as well as the precise cause of death. Computed tomography (CT) data provides information about the volume, density, and size of liquid in the lungs, which aids in determining the precise cause of death. In 2007, Levy et al. conducted post-mortem computed tomography (PMCT) on drowning cases and were the first to document the imaging results. The PMCT feature was identified by the presence of foam-covered airway fluid or high-attenuation deposit in the airways of cadavers. Furthermore, the presence of fluid was observed in the paranasal cavity, mastoid air cells, gastric distends, and contents, confirming the cause of death as drowning in 2010. This highlights the effectiveness of post-mortem computed tomography (PMCT) in determining the cause of death in the case of a middle-aged male who passed away after falling into a sewage pool. PMCT imaging revealed blood accumulation in the right external auditory canal, a fracture in the right humerus, small hemorrhages in the subarachnoid space, brain contusion injuries in the left temporal lobe, and scratch and bruise injuries on the right side of the occipital scalp. The combination of these injuries may have resulted in unconsciousness, leading to a coma and rendering the individual unable to save themselves from the pool. Additional observations, such as the detection of fluid in the respiratory tract, paranasal sinuses, and expansion of the stomach and duodenum, suggest that the individual was able to breathe and swallow while submerged in water. Additionally, the evidence that water has infiltrated the respiratory and circulatory systems was confirmed based on the PMCT results, which revealed opacity in both the lungs (Figure 7.1). Jian et al. conducted a study using a rabbit model of drowning.

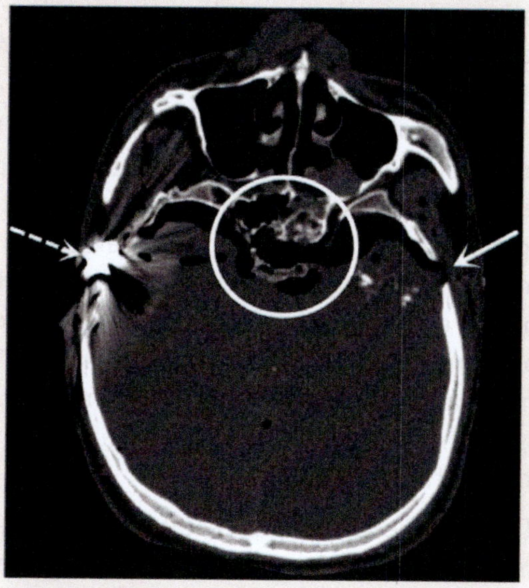

Figure 7.1. *PMCT revealed the bullet's entrance (white arrow), the skull fracture caused by the bullet (white circle), and the bullet and the exit (dotted arrow).*

Source: Ahuja, P., & Ansari, N. (2022). Creative commons license.

The researchers conducted a comparison between animal models of hemorrhagic shock and mechanical asphyxia. The CT values demonstrated a statistically significant increase in lung volumes ($P < 0.05$), suggesting that the virtopsy characteristics can accurately represent key aspects in cases of antemortem drowning.

The Multislice spiral CT can provide a detailed analysis of the permanent damage caused by a bullet, including the bullet's entry and exit points, as well as any diversion caused by anatomical structures, in cases of firearms injury. Gibb showcased the application of CT in actual cases and animal models and delineated the distinct attributes of injuries resulting from various firearms and ammunition types (Figure 7.2). Harcke et al. employed low-intensity CT scans to generate 3D projections and reconstruct the volume of the entire bodies of cadavers with gunshot wounds. The bone damaged, projectile trajectory, and bone fragments in the body were analyzed. The technology demonstrated great significance in accurately detecting the perforation and penetration caused by firearms. In addition, Karger et al. conducted a study on tissue disruption resulting from gunshot wounds to the head, utilizing MRI and PMCT imaging techniques. The researchers noted that the area of permanent tissue damage was clearly delineated, and the bone fragments were readily identifiable within it, a distinction that would not have been possible with a standard autopsy. In China, a police officer took his own life as a result of depression, and a post-mortem examination was conducted. The data unambiguously revealed the location of the bullet's entry and exit points, the presence of a skull fracture, the path taken by the bullet, and other injuries. Additionally, the data provided insights into the manner in which the individual died, as depicted in Figure 7.3.

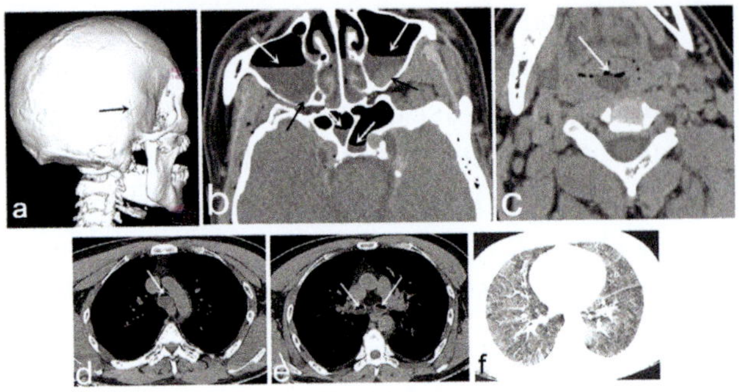

Figure 7.2. *(a) SSD reconstruct revealed the fracture of the right temporal bone (black arrow). (b) Fluid in the paranasal sinuses (white arrows), and dense sediment (black arrows). (c) Fluid in the throat (white arrow). (d) and (e) Fluid in the trachea (white arrows). (f) The diffuse ground-glass opacities in both lungs.*

Source: Ahuja, P., & Ansari, N. (2022). Creative commons license.

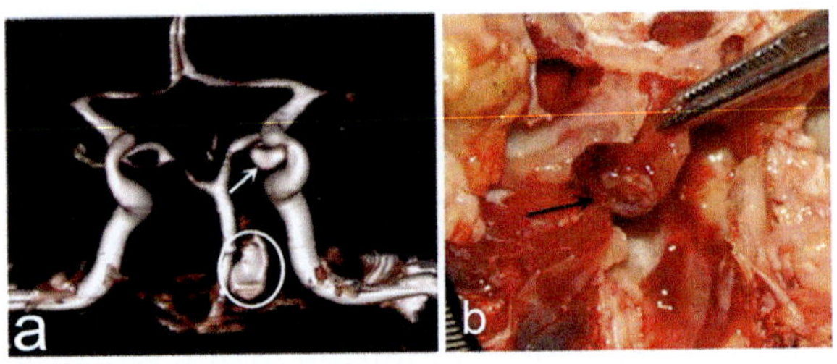

Figure 7.3. *(a) PMCTA results showed a leakage of the contrast agent from the C3 segment of the left internal carotid artery (white arrow) into the adjacent left sphenoidsinus (white circle), suggesting an aneurysm. (b)An aneurysm inside the left sphenoid sinus (black arrow) was confirmed by autopsy, consistent with the PMCTA results.*

Source: Ahuja, P., & Ansari, N. (2022). Creative commons license.

The application of Virtopsy technology in forensic odontology has been demonstrated to be extensive. Human identification and age estimation can be accomplished by analyzing the structure of the teeth, which includes various characteristics of multiple teeth. Dental identification involves the examination and comparison of pre-death and post-death evidence, as well as the analysis of the dental profiles of the deceased individual and the examination of dental DNA. When access to postmortem data of the dentition or oral cavity is obstructed due to factors such as rigor mortis, the utilization of virtopsy can provide an accurate and efficient means of preserving the information. Oesterhelweg et al. reported a case in which a foreign object (food bolus) became lodged in the respiratory tract. Traditional autopsies do not provide information about the depth of these materials, but the use of CT and MRI scans can overcome this limitation. Personal identification was accomplished by overlaying and comparing the data from pre-death orthopantomograms and post-death reconstructed panoramic images obtained from cranial CT scans. Dentistry plays a role in determining the age of charred bodies. CT scans have been shown to be effective in this process, as described by Dedouit et al. Age estimation techniques using CT scans were used to achieve personal identification of the Australian bushfire victims. Scientists have successfully showcased the application of Virtual Autopsy in situations involving large-scale fires by accurately simulating the entire scenario. Jackowski et al. examined the effects of various restoration materials, including composites, ceramics, and temporary fillings, when exposed to high temperatures. They then analyzed the CT scans of these materials.

Cerebral hemorrhages resulting in death are commonly observed in forensic investigations. In 2017, Qian et al. conducted a study on a case involving an individual who died as a result of the rupture of cerebrovascular distortion. The PMCT scan revealed a significant hemorrhage extending to the ventricular system in the right frontal region of the brain. The histological examination confirmed the findings of PMCT angiography, indicating that the cause of death was an arteriovenous distortion (Figure 7.4).

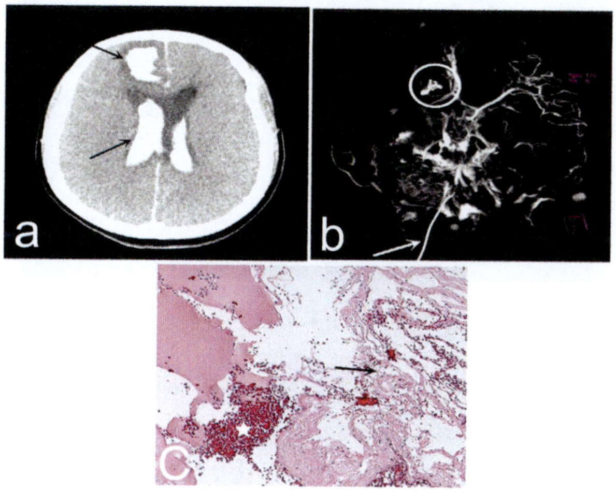

Figure 7.4. *(a) Massive hemorrhage in the brain's right frontal region, extending into the ventricular system (white arrow); (b)a mass of irregular, tortuous vessels in areas of hemorrhage in the right frontal lobe of the brain (white circle); a contrast agent was injected into the basilar artery (white arrow); (c) Lumps of abnormal blood vessels within the region of hematoma (star); small blood vessels were dilated and tortuous, and the thickness of the vessel wall varied (black arrow).*

Source: Ahuja, P., & Ansari, N. (2022). Creative commons license.

In 2017, Shao et al. performed postmortem computed tomography angiography (PMCTA) on a deceased individual who experienced a head injury as a result of a traffic accident. The patients exhibited fractures in the left frontal and sphenoid bones. The PMCT angiography revealed the rupture of an aneurysm in the internal carotid artery. Therefore, the virtopsy, autopsy, and histo-pathological examination all confirmed that the injury observed was a pseudo aneurysm in the sinusoidal vascular system, which was caused by the traffic accident. Virtopsy can be utilized in cases where the investigator is unaware of the actual cause of the damage (Figure 7.5).

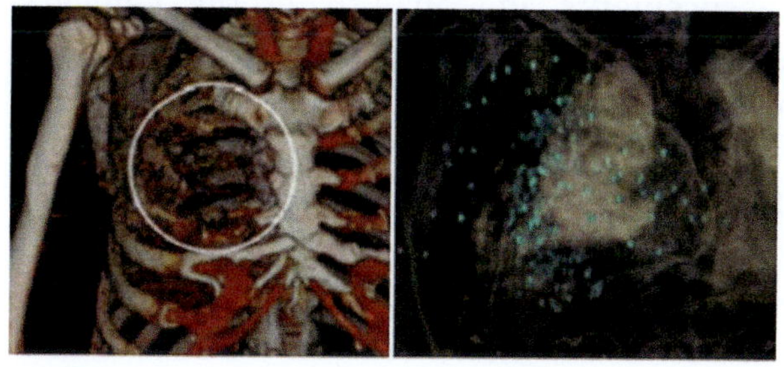

Figure 7.5. *Left: computed tomography threedimensional reconstruction shows fractures in right ribs 2–4 (white circles); Right: computed tomography threedimensional reconstruction shows scattered bullets (bluegreen).*

Source: Ahuja, P., & Ansari, N. (2022). Creative commons license.

7.3. Reconstruction

Michael J. Thali et al. pioneered the utilization of three-dimensional data based on geometric methodology. It utilizes radiological CT/MRI, scanning photogrammetry, and optical surface techniques to analyze the surface features and internal injuries of both living and deceased bodies in a non-invasive and non-destructive manner. These results can be highly consequential for the reconstruction in crime scene cases. Data fusion and animation techniques can be employed to answer reconstructive questions regarding patterned injuries and their connection to the suspect or the instrument that caused the injury. The documentation pertaining to forensic aspects was constrained to the conventional methods of 2D photography, radiographs, sketches, and witness accounts. This recent advancement in 3D imaging has introduced a novel method for conducting forensic examination and reconstruction. Thali et al. utilized these technologies in cases involving the reconstruction of automobile accidents. They generated three-dimensional (3D) data of the injuries and connected it to the animation-generated data that depicts the bodily injuries and damage to the vehicle. The comprehensive measurements and analysis of the vehicle's damages not only facilitated the identification of the points of impact, but also aided in determining the forces involved and the speed of the vehicle. Utilizing 3D real data documentation allows for a novel approach to analyzing forensic evidence, reconstructing events, and generating animated representations of the incidents involved in a case investigation, as depicted in Figures 7.6 and 7.7. In 2007, Buck et al. utilized high-resolution surface scanning and multi-slice CT/MRI scanning to create three-dimensional models of human injuries and vehicles involved in traffic accidents. The scanning yielded valuable data for assessing the locations of vehicles. Several authors have demonstrated the application of 3D scanning in analyzing injuries, determining cause of death, and assessing vehicle damage in vehicular accidents. The researchers determined that combining post-mortem computed tomography (PMCT) with autopsy is the most effective method for determining the cause and manner of death in traffic accidents.

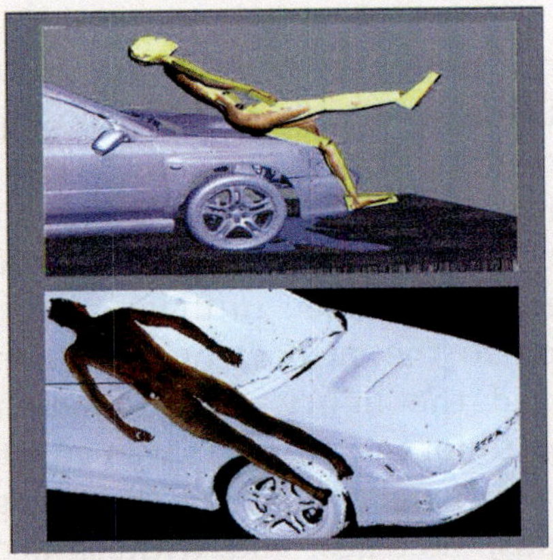

Figure 7.6. *It is feasible to use 3D geometric data for forensic analysis and reconstructive animation. Analyzing investigative opinions can aid in the formation of an expert opinion.*

Source: Ahuja, P., & Ansari, N. (2022). Creative commons license.

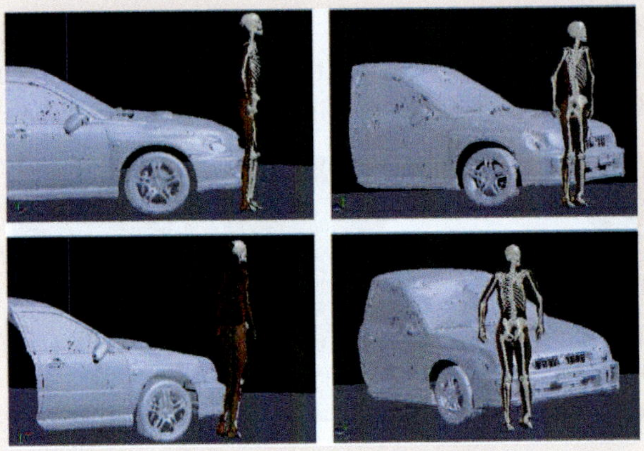

Figure 7.7. *Integrating the skeletal and joint information into the car's dataset enables accurate and personalized simulation of body movements using real data.*

Source: Ahuja, P., & Ansari, N. (2022). Creative commons license.

7.4. Advantages

An essential benefit of this technique is that it is a non-destructive method of examination, meaning it does not require the use of a scalpel. It is a morally satisfying outcome of the technology that makes body examinations more acceptable without causing emotional distress to the family and also preserves the body's structure. The process is more efficient and the data produced in the form of images can be easily transferred and reused for future research. It is the most efficient method for examining injuries and determining the connection with the likely weapon used in the commission of a crime. The 3D scanning also adds to the weightage of the forensic report and make the work easy for the experts in describing the reconstructions or animations of the case investigations. The examination can be performed with ease without causing any damage to the authenticity in a non-destructive manner in both living and non-living individuals. Forensic documentation can be accomplished by storing the data in image format acquired through photogrammetric and 3D optical scanning. A virtual autopsy also reduces the chances of infections, radionuclides, toxic substances or other biohazards. The imaging system has proven to be a reliable tool in contemporary forensic analysis, with diverse applications in various fields.

7.5. Disadvantages

While the technique offers numerous benefits, it also has some inherent drawbacks. Some pathological conditions, such as the extent of infection in the cadaver, and alterations in physical characteristics such as color, odor, and minor tissue damage, may be difficult to define or may be overlooked. The system lacks a database that would be beneficial for comparison. Distinguishing between ante-mortem and post mortem injuries can be challenging. The accuracy of data can be called into question when merging data from multiple technologies, which can also lead to a complete reliance on the imagery system.

A Closer Look

Virtual Post-Mortem Computed Tomography

Post-Mortem Computed Tomography (PMCT) is an advanced imaging technique that has increasingly been utilized in forensic pathology to enhance the investigation of cause and manner of death. Unlike traditional autopsy methods, PMCT offers a non-invasive approach, making it valuable for cases where conventional autopsy is not possible or desired. This technology employs computed tomography (CT) to capture detailed cross-sectional images of the body, providing a comprehensive view of internal structures and potentially revealing information that might be missed through external examination alone.

One of the primary advantages of PMCT is its ability to quickly and accurately visualize internal injuries and anomalies without the need for physical dissection. This is particularly useful in scenarios where the cause of death is uncertain or when examining bodies that have been extensively decomposed or subjected to environmental factors that obscure physical evidence. PMCT can identify fractures, foreign objects, and signs of internal hemorrhage, which can be critical in determining the cause of death and aiding in the reconstruction of events leading up to it.

The process of PMCT involves a high-resolution CT scanner that captures multiple images of the body from various angles. These images are then reconstructed into detailed 3D models, allowing forensic pathologists to examine the body in various planes and perspectives. The technology is capable of differentiating between different types of tissues and materials, making it effective for detecting subtle internal injuries and anomalies. Additionally, PMCT can be complemented with other imaging techniques, such as digital radiography or MRI, to provide a more comprehensive assessment of the body. One of the significant benefits of PMCT is its ability to preserve the integrity of the body, which is important for cultural, legal, or religious reasons. In cases where families or communities prefer not to have a traditional autopsy performed, PMCT provides a non-invasive alternative that still yields valuable diagnostic information. Furthermore, PMCT can be employed as a preliminary diagnostic tool before deciding whether a full autopsy is necessary, thereby potentially reducing the number of invasive procedures performed.

Despite its advantages, PMCT has limitations. The technique is less effective in detecting certain types of injuries, such as those caused by soft tissue trauma or those that do not produce significant radiological changes. Additionally, PMCT cannot provide information about the biochemical or histological changes that might be present in cases of disease or poisoning. As a result, while PMCT is a powerful tool, it is often used in conjunction with traditional autopsy methods to provide a more comprehensive evaluation.

Summary

- This chapter introduces a revolutionary approach to traditional autopsies by utilizing advanced imaging techniques such as CT and MRI scans. This method, termed "virtual autopsy" or "virtopsy," allows for a non-invasive examination of the deceased, preserving the body and enabling detailed analysis without the need for dissection. Virtual autopsy provides numerous advantages, including the ability to visualize and assess internal injuries and pathologies in three dimensions, which enhances the accuracy and comprehensiveness of forensic investigations. Additionally, it offers a permanent digital record that can be re-examined and shared among experts, improving collaborative efforts and educational opportunities. The adoption of virtual autopsy is seen as a significant advancement in forensic medicine, promising to augment the capabilities of medico-legal autopsies while addressing ethical and cultural concerns associated with traditional autopsy procedures.

References

1. Augestad, L. B., & Levander, S. (1992). Personality, health and job stress among employees in a Norwegian penitentiary and in a maximum-security hospital. *Work & Stress*, *6*(1), 65–79. https://doi.org/10.1080/02678379208256829.
2. Barilan, Y. M. (2017). The role of doctors in hunger strikes. *Kennedy Institute of Ethics Journal*, *27*(4), 341–369. https://doi.org/10.1353/ken.2017.0019.
3. Beauchamp, T. L., & Childress, J. F. (2001). *Principles of Biomedical Ethics* (5th ed.). Oxford University Press.
4. Curcă, G. C. (2013). *Elemente de etică medicală. Norme de etică în practica medicală. Despre principiile bioeticii*. Casa Cărţii de Ştiinţă.
5. Elger, B. S., Handtke, V., & Wangmo, T. (2015). Informing patients about limits to confidentiality: A qualitative study in prisons. *International Journal of Law and Psychiatry*, *41*, 50–57. https://doi.org/10.1016/j.ijlp.2015.04.003.
6. Elger, B. S., Handtke, V., & Wangmo, T. (2015). Paternalistic breaches of confidentiality in prison: Mental health professionals' attitudes and justifications. *Journal of Medical Ethics*, *41*(6), 496–500. https://doi.org/10.1136/medethics-2014-102408.
7. García-Guerrero, J. (2013). La huelga de hambre en el ámbito penitenciario: Aspectos éticos, deontológicos y legales. *Revista Española de Sanidad Penitenciaria*, *15*(1), 8–15. https://doi.org/10.4321/S1575-06202013000100002.
8. Garland, B., & Wilson, G. (2012). Prison inmates' views of whether reporting rape is the same as snitching: An exploratory study and research agenda. *Journal of Interpersonal Violence*, *28*(7), 1201–1222. https://doi.org/10.1177/0886260512453820.
9. Herman, J. L. (1992). Complex PTSD: A syndrome in survivors of prolonged and repeated trauma. *Journal of Trauma & Stress*, *5*(3), 377–391. https://doi.org/10.1002/jts.2490050305.
10. Hostiuc, S. (2021). *Tratat de bioetică medicală şi stomatologică*. C.H. Beck.
11. Moskop, J. C., Marco, C. A., Larkin, G. L., Geiderman, J. M., & Derse, A. R. (2005). From Hippocrates to HIPAA: Privacy and confidentiality in emergency medicine–Part I: Conceptual,

moral, and legal foundations. *Annals of Emergency Medicine, 45*(1), 53–59. https://doi.org/10.1016/j.annemergmed.2004.08.007.

12. Pont, J., Stöver, H., & Wolff, H. (2012). Dual loyalty in prison health care. *American Journal of Public Health, 102*(3), 475–480. https://doi.org/10.2105/AJPH.2011.300389.
13. Reich, W. T. (1995). *Oath of Hippocrates.* Macmillan.
14. Ross, M. W., Liebling, A., & Tait, S. (2011). The relationships of prison climate to health service in correctional environments: Inmate health care measurement, satisfaction, and access in prisons. *Howard Journal of Criminal Justice, 50*(3), 262–274. https://doi.org/10.1111/j.1468-2311.2011.00271.x.
15. Wolff, N., Blitz, C. L., Shi, J., Bachman, R., & Siegel, J. A. (2006). Sexual violence inside prisons: Rates of victimization. *Journal of Urban Health, 83*(5), 835–848. https://doi.org/10.1007/s11524-006-9060-1.

Chapter

SEXUAL ASSAULT: FORENSIC EXAMINATION

8

Contents

Introduction

The forensic examination of a person who is suspected of having been sexually assaulted may encapsulate the scope of forensic medicine more completely than any other situation that occurs in the practice of forensic medicine. The detection of injury and biological material to support or exclude sexual activity requires a careful and methodical approach to ensure robust evidentiary value. Additionally, an understanding of genito-anal anatomy and sexual physiology is required to interpret the significance of an injury or biological material for the courts. This is true whether the individual in question is alive or deceased. Rather than being an exhaustive guideline, the purpose of this chapter is to provide a general overview of the key components of forensic sexual assault examination. It will focus on the common and different aspects that are present in both living and deceased individuals.

Orientation and Directional Terms

Term	Definition	Illustration
Sexual Assault	An act involving non-consensual sexual contact or behavior, including rape, attempted rape, and other forms of sexual violence or coercion.	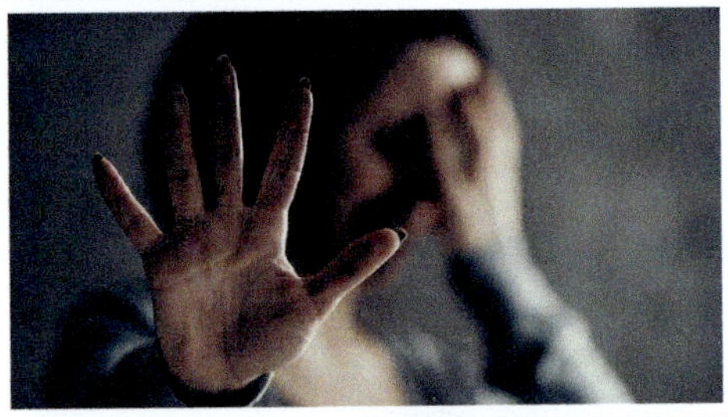
Colposcopy	A medical procedure that uses a colposcope, a special magnifying instrument, to examine the cervix, vagina, and vulva for signs of disease or abnormality.	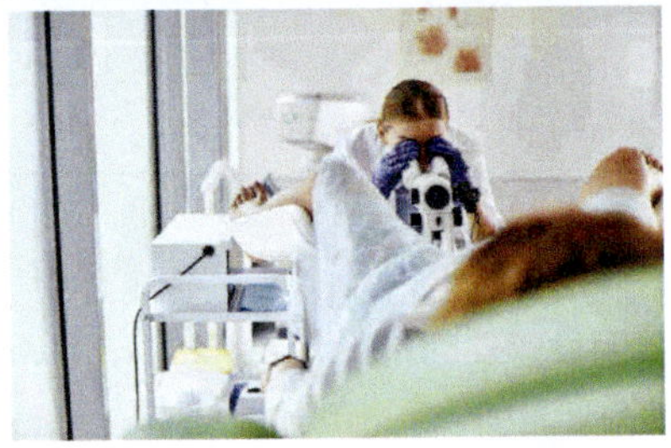
Genito-anal Injuries	Injuries that affect both the genital and anal regions, often resulting from trauma or abuse.	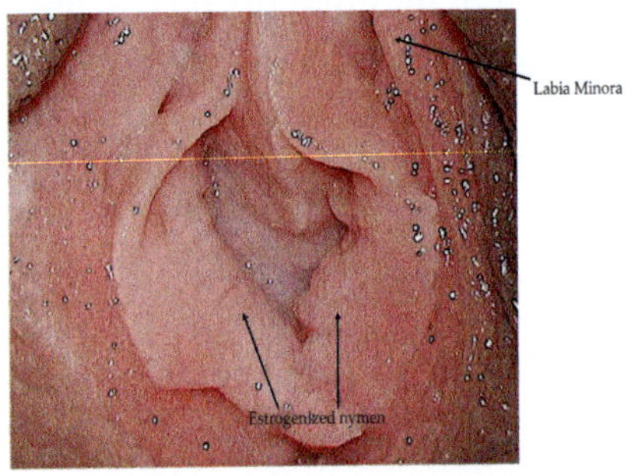
Spermatozoa	The male reproductive cells or sperm, which are responsible for fertilizing the female egg in sexual reproduction.	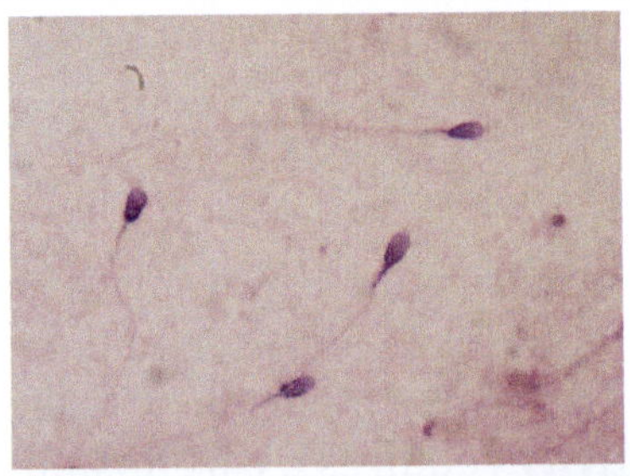
DNA Markers	Specific sequences of DNA used in genetic analysis to identify individuals, track inheritance, or detect genetic conditions.	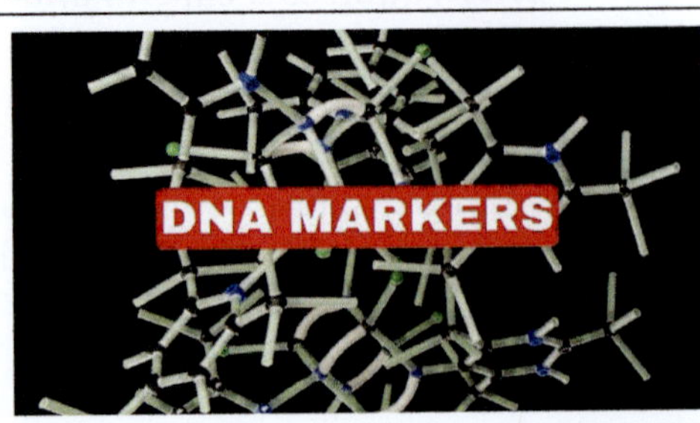

8.1. Sexual Assault: An Overview

As with all other areas of medicine, the literature that is currently available on the forensic medical aspects of sexual assault is written from the point of view of the various authors' experiences. As a result, the literature varies greatly depending on whether it originates from an environment that focuses on primary care, emergency medicine, trauma, surgical, or pathology. Clinicians who work in rape crisis centers will see injuries that are different from those that their colleagues who work in forensic pathology will see. Additionally, the persistence and ability to retrieve biological material will vary depending on the circumstances. The field of sexual assault medicine has reaped significant benefits from the interaction and collaboration between forensic clinicians and pathologists, whether it be at the bedside of a patient in the hospital, in the mortuary, or in the courtroom. In the field of forensic pathology, the jurisdictions that are responsible for conducting both autopsies and clinical forensic examinations are the ones that are responsible for conducting important research.

Even though sexual offense laws, clinical and laboratory practices, and service resources vary from jurisdiction to jurisdiction, the development of standardized protocols for forensic examination and evidence collection kits has made it easier to investigate sexual offenses and has increased the likelihood that medical evidence will be relied upon. Although injuries can serve as evidence of penetration, they are not capable of establishing consent. This is since injuries can be the result of sexually consenting sexual encounters. There is a possibility that biological material, such as sperm, saliva, or sperm, can provide evidence of sexual penetration or contact, such as sperm or saliva on the genitalia or sperm in the vagina or anus. Lawyers who are involved in cases involving sexual assault will vary their reliance on the probative value of injury and biological evidence depending on the characteristics of the case. This includes proving sexual contact or corroborating a physical struggle. It is the responsibility of the forensic medical examiner to conduct a comprehensive examination and collect all evidence that may be of potential value. This is since a forensic examination is typically carried out at an early stage in the investigation process, frequently before witness interviews and scene processing have taken place. As a result, the likely issues of a case are still unclear.

One of the most common obstacles that arises in the process of prosecuting sexual assault cases is the presence of forensic medical evidence that is either of poor quality or insufficient quantity. The presence of injury has been found to influence decisions at all stages of the legal process, including investigation, prosecution, conviction, and sentencing; minor injury may be of significance depending on the nature of a case. Although sexual assault does not always result in injury, it has been found that the presence of injury influences decisions at all stages of the legal process. Furthermore, because criminal investigation teams are comprised of members from a variety of disciplines, the manner in which forensic medical evidence is utilized in cases involving sexual assault is significantly impacted by the quality of communication that exists between law enforcement, medical examiners, personnel working in laboratories, attorneys, and judges.

8.2. Role of Information in Directing an Examination

Although the complainant's account of events will, to some extent, direct the forensic sexual assault examination that takes place in a clinical setting, it is possible that such information may not always be available due to the effects of recent trauma, altered consciousness, or intoxication. They might not be aware of minor injuries that are relevant to forensics, and they might not be able to determine whether ejaculation or penetration took place, or whether a condom was present. It is possible to collect all possible evidence by employing a standardized protocol for the examination and collection of samples. This is true even in situations where there is a limited amount of information available. When dealing with a deceased individual, the lack of a personal account of the events brings about an increase in the significance of the standardized approach. Nevertheless, it is important to recognize that the diverse nature of sexual assault scenarios may necessitate the use of examiner discretion to maximize evidence collection. For instance, the examiner may be required to collect additional swabs or use a different examination technique.

8.2.1. Identifying General Bodily Injury

In the clinical setting, the detection of injuries on the body is used to either confirm or disprove the account of events provided by a complainant. On the other hand, these injuries may be the only indication of what occurred at or around the time of death when they are examined during an autopsy. Minor injuries could prove to be life-threatening in either scenario. Finger pad bruising on the limbs or neck, suction-type bites, circumferential bruising to wrists or ankles, bruising to the inner lips or behind the ear pinna, petechiae in the eyes or on the palate, brush abrasions on the knees or bony prominences of the back, and bruising to the inner lips or behind the ear pinna are all examples of injuries that can shed light on the events that led up to the death. These injuries should be meticulously documented through written descriptions, diagrams, and photographs. In a similar vein, the absence of any instances of bodily injury can be informative and allow for the elimination of certain scenarios.

If it is necessary, dissection and histology can accurately identify the nature of the findings in a deceased person, whereas in a clinical setting, it may not be possible to say with absolute certainty whether the findings are the result of traumatic experiences or not. In a similar manner, non-visible traumatic bruising on the surface of the body can be located through the process of dissection.

8.2.2. Identifying Oral, Genital, and Anal Injury

The use of transparent plastic speculae and anoscopes is necessary for the detection of injuries in the mouth, vagina, or anus. In the case of vaginal and anal forensic examination, it is also necessary to have adequate lighting in order to avoid obscuring the sites of potential injuries (Figure 8.1). It is possible that increasing the use of a swab or a Foley balloon catheter to display hymenal edges will improve injury detection. Sexually transmitted injuries to the vaginal walls and cervix are not frequently observed in clinical settings. This may be since it is difficult to visualize the vaginal fornices using a speculum and the entire mucosal surface due to the presence of rugae. During the autopsy, dissection will make it possible to conduct a thorough examination of all mucosal surfaces for signs of injury.

Figure 8.1. *The placement of a vaginal speculum.*

Image Credit: Diana Kryski. Creative commons license.

Abrasions, bruises, and petechiae are some of the most common types of oral injuries that can be caused by penile penetration. These injuries can occur on the frenula, palate, gums, and buccal surface of cheeks, tongue, and lips. Penile penetration can be either consensual or nonconsensual.

In the absence of other recent nonsexual penetrative events, such as the use of a tampon or a speculum examination, as well as injuries that occurred during the forensic examination itself, the presence of a recent injury in the vagina or Ano-rectum will provide evidence that penetration occurred. This is because legal definitions of the vagina and the anus support the idea that penetration occurred. The lack of injury, on the other hand, will not rule out the possibility.

The appearance of the genitalia and the Ano-rectum can vary greatly, and it is essential to be familiar with the normal, non-injured genitalia and the Ano-rectum in order to prevent the false identification of injuries in these areas of the body. After both vaginal and anal penetration, it is possible to observe injuries such as lacerations, abrasions, and bruises. When engaging in vaginal sex, the posterior fourchette, fossa navicularis (Images 8.2 and 8.3), labia minora, and hymen/hymenal remnant are the areas of the genital region that are most likely to sustain injuries. As a result of the fact that the posterior wall and the posterior fornix are more firmly connected to the pelvic musculature and, as a result, less flexible, the posterior wall and posterior fornix laceration is the most commonly described of the more severe vaginal injuries that are associated with sexual activity. While sexual penetration of the female genitalia can result in a variety of blunt force injuries, the following table describes these injuries.

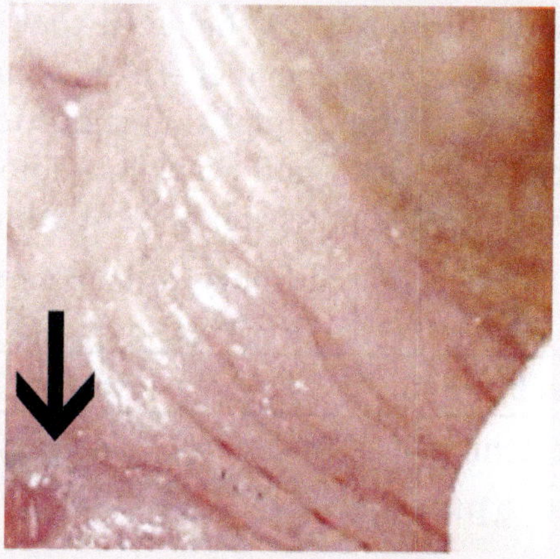

Figure 8.2. *Fossa navicularis lacerations.*

Source: Girardin BW, Faugno DK, Seneski PC, et al. (1997c). Color atlas of sexual assault St. Louis: Mosby; Creative Commons license.

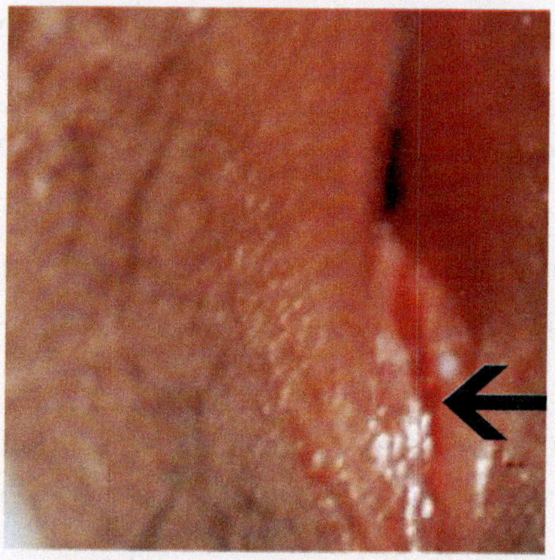

Figure 8.3. *Posterior fourchette lacerations seen with separation.*

Source: Girardin BW, Faugno DK, Seneski PC, et al. Color atlas of sexual assault St. Louis: Mosby; c1997. Creative Commons license.

Examination enhancement techniques such as magnification (colposcopy), staining with toluidine blue, or the use of ultraviolet light will increase the likelihood of detection of sex-related genital injuries, which are typically small and superficial. Female genitalia, with its many creases and rugae, can be difficult to detect because of the numerous creases and rugae that are present. Although it is believed that toluidine blue does not compromise biological evidence, false negatives can occur if there is a barrier that covers the lesions. Additionally, false positives may occur in certain genital skin conditions, such as vulvitis and herpes (indicated in Figure 8.3). In particular, it was found that ultraviolet light was particularly helpful for detecting submucosal hemorrhage and scar tissue, both of which are difficult to see in normal light illumination.

Table 8.1. Blunt Force Injury to Female Genitalia

Mechanism	**Injury Type**	**Site**
Stretching of genital tissue due to penetration	"Split-type" lacerations, radially orientated	Hymenal tissue Labia minora Posterior fourchette Fossa navicularis
	Bruising, circumferential or interrupted	Hymenal tissue
Direct impact	Bruising Abrasions Lacerations	Any site
Frictional force	Abrasions, circumferential or interrupted	Any site
Compression of tissue against bony pelvis	Bruising "Crush-type" lacerations	Labia Hymenal tissue Vaginal wall
Shearing/tearing of fixed or "tethered" tissue (e.g., perineal body)	Bruising Lacerations	Posterior fourchette Perineum
Adhesion of non-lubricated surface followed by movement	Bruising	Free edge of labia or hymen
	Lacerations	Between labia major and minor (inter-labial)

Source: Lincoln CA, 2019.

Vaginal penetrative sex, regardless of whether it is conscientious, has the potential to result in genital injury. On the other hand, it is observed more frequently because of sexual activity that is not consented to than it is because of sexual activity that is consented to. Depending on the type of examination that was performed (for example, macroscopic, colposcopic, staining, or combinations of these), the prevalence rates can range anywhere from 0% to 73% for consensual groups and from 4% to 89% for non-consensual groups.

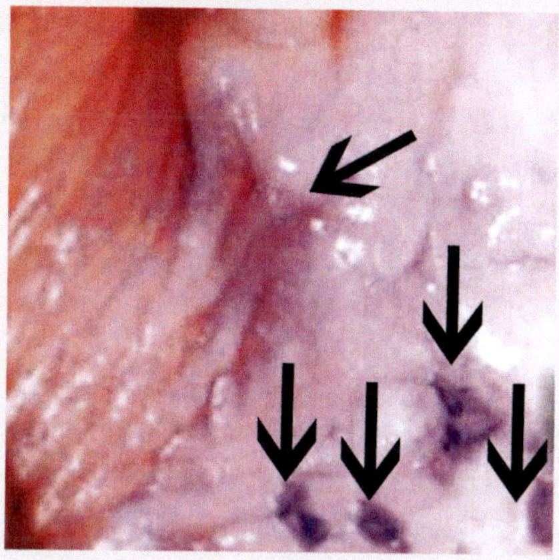

Figure 8.4. *Lacerations shown in Figure 8.2 highlighted with toluidine blue dye uptake.*

Source: Girardin BW, Faugno DK, Seneski PC, et al. Color atlas of sexual assault St. Louis: Mosby; c1997. Creative Commons license.

This was demonstrated by a review of the most important studies that were conducted in this field. The existence of serious genital injuries was not taken into consideration in these studies, which were conducted primarily in primary care settings. Macroscopically detected consensual group injury rates ranged from 10–34%, while nonconsensual group injury rates were found to be higher than 55% in more recent prospective primary care research studies. These studies tried to reduce the number of confounding variables. While there have been attempts to identify patterns of injury that differentiate sex-related genital injury that occurs in a consensual setting from injury that occurs in a nonconsensual setting, there have not been any results that can be considered definitive. On the other hand, single lacerations at the posterior aspect of the vaginal opening have been consistently identified as the most common injury that occurs as a result of consensual vaginal penetration (20). On the other hand, nonconsensual vaginal penetration is more likely to result in more than one injury, more than one type of injury, and more than one site of injury.

Less information is available regarding injuries that are the result of anal penetration, and published research almost exclusively focuses on nonconsensual study groups. In a recent study, 27% of 174 women who reported nonconsensual completed anal penetration sustained injury, the most common type of which was perianal lacerations. As a result of anal penetration, perianal lacerations are typically radial, do not confine themselves to the midline, and frequently extend into the anus (Figure 8.4).

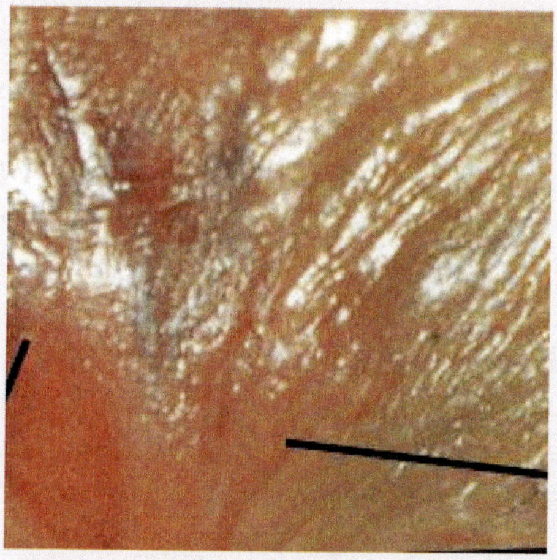

Figure 8.5. *Perianal lacerations and redness.*

Source: Girardin BW, Faugno DK, Seneski PC, et al. Color atlas of sexual assault St. Louis: Mosby; c1997. Creative Commons license.

There is little information available with respect to sex-related male genital injury in consensual or nonconsensual settings or in sex offenders.

8.2.3. Documenting Injury

Recording injuries in a comprehensive manner, including descriptive, diagrammatic, and photographic documentation, maximizes the value of the evidence and the interpretation of the evidence. The inclusion of specific diagram templates for documentation of internal oral, vaginal, and Ano-rectal mucosal surface findings in forensic examination protocols, as well as the utilization of "clock-face" position references, enables the forensic examiner to record injuries as they are observed and eliminates the possibility of ambiguity.

8.2.4. Genito-Anal Pain

It is not possible to provide a response to the question of consent using medical evidence. The variance in individual responses to pain, as well as the existence of sexual practices that involve the intentional infliction of painful injury on participants, both contribute to a reduction in the weight of injury evidence concerning consent. While a deceased person is unable to describe any pain that they experienced during a sexual act, a complainant in a clinical setting is able to describe any pain that they experienced during a sexual act. In order to provide advice regarding the likelihood that an injury was painful or to explain why a woman may have been unaware of a serious vaginal injury or retained foreign body, it is helpful to have an understanding of the female genito-anal sensorineural supply, as well as the degree of sensation and the extent of sensitive clitoral tissue in various parts of the genitalia. It is not widely known that the upper portion of the vaginal canal is not sensitive to touch or pressure and that it possesses a significantly lower number of free nerve endings in comparison to the lower vagina and the external genitalia.

8.2.5. Severity of Injury

Does the sexual assault contribute directly to death, as in the case of severe hemorrhage from a vaginal laceration? Did it occur as part of an assault that led to death without the sexual act being the cause of death, as in the case of fatal blunt trauma or strangulation? Or is there evidence of sexual activity that is unrelated to the circumstances of death, having occurred at some time before or after death? in the case of the deceased, sexual assault is considered in the context of the cause of death. The forensic sexual assault examination that takes place in the mortuary can involve the full spectrum of general and genito-anal injury severity, in contrast to the clinical setting, where the majority of injuries, if uncovered, will be minor.

In terms of general body injuries, a recent large primary care study discovered that 29% of women who reported an acute sexual assault did not sustain any visible injuries, while 52% only sustained mild injuries. In primary care settings, most of the research on genito-anal injuries related to sexual activity is carried out. This research describes the prevalence and typology of these injuries, but it does not address the issue of severity. To differentiate between injuries sustained during consensual and nonconsensual sexual encounters, several researchers have investigated the validity of a genital injury severity scale. However, to acknowledge the full spectrum of sexually related injuries that are seen in primary care, surgical gynecology, and autopsy, then it is necessary to address the significant practical challenges that are currently being faced.

8.2.6. Biological Evidence

The contamination of biological evidence led to the wrongful conviction and imprisonment of an Australian man for the crime of rape in the year 2009. The United Kingdom conducted a review of 20 mortuaries in the late 1990s and discovered that 50% of them had quantifiable DNA on instruments and surfaces of the mortuary. As a result of the serious implications of environmental DNA contamination and contamination during the collection of biological material, it is necessary to pay meticulous attention to the protocols for cleaning before and after the examination, to collect examination surface control swabs to assist in determining the potential locations of contamination, and to use single-use equipment whenever it is feasible to do so. At all times during the sampling process and when handling specimens, it is imperative to wear double gloves that are not sterile.

The detection of spermatozoa or semen can be extremely significant depending on the circumstances of an investigation. It can provide a means of identifying the perpetrator, evidence of sexual activity and sexual contact between a complainant and the perpetrator, and it also has the potential to provide evidence of sexual penetration. Nevertheless, the absence of sperm or sperm does not rule out the possibility of sexual activity or penetration having occurred.

Laboratory practices that involve the use of sperm microscopy, the detection of seminal biomarkers, and DNA/RNA markers will vary from one jurisdiction to another. In most cases, the guidelines for collection will be determined by local protocols and persistence data. The detection of male DNA through the use of Y-short tandem repeat techniques has resulted in improved outcomes and improved detection times. While recommendations for time scales for sample collection in clinical settings are based on maximum times in published persistence data, it is necessary to exercise discretion on an individual basis for each individual case. There has been a significant amount of research conducted on oral or anal samples, and even less research has been published on the postmortem recovery of sperm and semen in cases of rape-homicide. This is in contrast to the large amount of information that has been published regarding the persistence of sperm on vaginal samples taken from sexual assault kits. Concerning the detection of sperm in males, one study discovered that the use of postmortem prostate specific antigen (PSA) and acid phosphatase (AP) screening was not very useful. Sperm appear to survive for longer periods of time after death; the cessation of biological processes that expel sperm and sperm from the body, as well as the supine position of deceased individuals, are likely factors that contribute to the ability to detect sperm and sperm for longer intervals.

Speculum examination is required to gain access to the posterior fornix, which is where the best sperm recovery occurred in a study that investigated the persistence of sperm following consensual vaginal sex. Furthermore, sperm were consistently discovered on the external genitalia when they were detected in the posterior fornix, even though they were present in considerably lower quantities. When it comes to sperm recovery, other studies have demonstrated that the posterior fornix is superior to external genital and cervical samples; however, the combination of these sample sites yields the best results.

It is important to exercise caution when interpreting the results of semen-positive anal swabs during genital examinations. Sperm or sperm from vaginal sex may drain to perianal and anal sites when the patient is in the supine position. This is the reason why it is recommended to take a sample from the Ano-rectal region before performing an internal vaginal examination. The optimal sequence for Geni-to-anal examination and sampling is as follows: first, the external genital region, then the peri-anal, anal, and rectal regions using an anoscope, and finally, the internal vaginal region using a speculum. The order in which swabs are taken ought to be reflected in their labels. When only anal penetration is reported, it is recommended that the full sequence of genital sampling be performed in the clinical setting in addition to Ano-rectal swabs. This is done to identify semen transfer between sites, and it is recommended that two swabs be taken from each site.

It is important to conduct forensic sampling as soon as it is feasible to do so; in a clinical setting, the probability of obtaining negative genital swab results following sexual activity increases by approximately 3 percent for every hour. International recommendations for routine sampling from the vagina and cervix range from three to 10 days after vaginal intercourse; from the mouth (including oral rinse and peri-oral swab) up to 48 hours after oral penetration; and from the Ano-rectum up to 72 hours after anal penetration, depending on the resources available in the laboratory (for example, the ability to analyze fluid samples and the availability of Y-STR testing).

If it is determined that male genital swabs are necessary, they should be taken from the penile shaft and external foreskin, if it is present; the coronal sulcus and internal foreskin; and the penile glans. It is recommended that sampling be done up to 72 hours after sexual activity.

Table 8.2. Potential Biological Material Transfer in Different Sexual Contact Scenarios

Penile to genito-anal	Semen/sperm Epithelial cells Blood Hairs Feces Saliva, if used as lubricant
Hand/fingers to genito-anal	Epithelial cells Semen/sperm (if prior masturbation) Blood Feces Saliva, if used as lubricant
Mouth to genito-anal, breasts,	Saliva other

Source: https://www.ncbi.nlm.nih.gov/pmc/articles/PMC6491537/table/table2-1925362118821490/.

Dry swabs can be used to sample moist skin or mucosa, and swabs that have been moistened with sterile water can be used to sample dry skin. Researchers have demonstrated that the "double-swab" technique, which involves using a wet swab first and then a dry swab, is more effective at retrieving material. It is preferable to roll the swab onto the skin rather than rub it in order to ensure that all of its parts come into contact with the skin. Even after taking a shower, it is beneficial to perform a saliva test on the skin in areas where the perpetrator's mouth has come into contact with the victim's areas of skin. It is possible to concentrate sampling efforts on bite marks when they are visible; however, the process is essentially "blind" in all other respects. Current research in this field is investigating methods for directing surface sampling (for example, the utilization of alternative light sources) or sampling large areas of the body (for example, the utilization of vacuum devices or tapelifts). The retrieval and careful labeling of any foreign hairs or other material discovered during the course of an examination is a necessary step. Fingernail scrapings or clippings are only considered to be of value when they have been in contact with body fluids (for example, the fingers of a perpetrator after digital penetration), as opposed to when they have been reported to have been scratched. This is because background DNA determines the value of these samples. In a variety of sexual contact scenarios, it is important to consider the possibility of the transfer of a wide variety of biological material (see Table 8.2). Collection of clothing worn at the time of or since the incident, in particular, underpants into which semen may have drained, should be separately bagged in the paper. A recent study using alternative light source, acid phosphatase testing, and sperm microscopy demonstrated that sperm persisted on some fabric (cotton and terry towel) after six wash cycles.

A Closer Look

Colposcopy in Forensic Medicine

Colposcopy in forensic medicine is a specialized procedure used to enhance the examination of the cervix, vagina, and vulva, particularly in cases involving sexual assault, trauma, or suspected abuse. This diagnostic tool is integral for forensic investigations, offering detailed visualization of the epithelial surface and enabling the identification of abnormalities that may not be visible with the naked eye. Colposcopy involves the use of a colposcope, a binocular microscope equipped with a light source, which magnifies and illuminates the areas of interest, providing a high-resolution view of the mucosal surfaces.

The procedure begins with a thorough examination of the patient's medical and sexual history, followed by a physical examination. During the colposcopic examination, the patient is positioned in a gynecological chair, and a speculum is inserted to visualize the vaginal walls and cervix. The colposcope is then positioned at the vaginal opening, and the examiner uses it to closely observe the cervix and vaginal walls, often applying various solutions, such as acetic acid or iodine, to highlight abnormal cells or lesions. Acetic acid, for instance, causes abnormal cells to appear white, enhancing the contrast and making it easier to identify potentially malignant or precancerous lesions.

In forensic cases, colposcopy plays a crucial role in documenting injuries, identifying signs of trauma, and collecting evidence of sexual assault or abuse. The detailed images obtained can reveal bruising, abrasions, or other trauma that might be indicative of forced or non-consensual acts. Moreover, it helps in detecting sexually transmitted infections (STIs) that could corroborate allegations of sexual violence. Forensic colposcopy is performed with meticulous care to ensure the collection of accurate and reliable evidence. Samples from abnormal areas may be biopsied for histological examination, which can provide further insights into the nature of the abnormalities.

The findings from a colposcopic examination are meticulously documented and can be used in legal proceedings as part of the forensic evidence. The documentation typically includes detailed descriptions of the observed lesions or injuries, photographs of the colposcopic images, and, if applicable, biopsy results. This comprehensive documentation is crucial for supporting the legal process, providing objective evidence that can help in the prosecution or defense in cases of sexual assault or abuse.

Colposcopy in forensic medicine not only aids in the immediate assessment and documentation of injuries but also contributes to the broader understanding of patterns and types of injuries associated with sexual violence. The procedure underscores the importance of specialized medical examinations in forensic investigations, ensuring that survivors receive appropriate care and that evidence is collected and preserved in a manner that upholds the integrity of the legal process.

Summary

- In the case of sexual assault, forensic examination reflects many of the fundamental principles of forensic medicine, including Locard's principle and the interpretation of injuries. The interpretation of medical evidence, on the other hand, is dependent on practical experience and the knowledge gained from a wide variety of medical specialties, such as gynecology, dermatology, gynecology, and surgery, among others.
- When primary care clinicians, hospital professionals, and forensic pathologists interact with one another, whether they do so within or outside of the mortuary, there is a significant possibility that this interaction will improve understanding of the full spectrum of HIV medicine. With the combined knowledge and experience of everyone involved in this field, as well as the collaboration to maximize the quality of patient care, medical evidentiary value, and medicolegal death investigation, there is the potential to improve understanding of the forensic aspects of sexual assault, which would be to everyone's benefit.

References

1. Avrahami, R. (1995). Laparoscopic vs. conventional autopsy: A promising perspective. *Archives of Surgery, 130*(4), 407. https://doi.org/10.1001/archsurg.1995.01430280031006.
2. Avrahami, R. (1995). Thoracoscopy vs. conventional autopsy of the thorax: A promising perspective. *Archives of Surgery, 130*(9), 956. https://doi.org/10.1001/archsurg.1995.01430290038007.
3. Avrahami, R., Watemberg, S., Daniels-Philips, E., Kahana, T., & Hiss, J. (1995). Endoscopic autopsy. *American Journal of Forensic Medicine and Pathology, 16*(2), 147–150. https://doi.org/10.1097/00000433-199506000-00008.
4. Ayoub, T., & Chow, J. (2008). The conventional autopsy in modern medicine. *Journal of the Royal Society of Medicine, 101*(4), 177–181. https://doi.org/10.1258/jrsm.2008.070568.
5. Blokker, B. M., Wagensveld, I. M., Weustink, A. C., Oosterhuis, J. W., & Hunink, M. G. M. (2016). Non-invasive or minimally invasive autopsy compared to conventional autopsy of suspected natural deaths in adults: A systematic review. *European Radiology, 26*(4), 1159–1179. https://doi.org/10.1007/s00330-015-3961-1.
6. Buja, L. M., Barth, R. F., Krueger, G. R., Brodsky, S. V., & Hunter, R. L. (2019). The importance of the autopsy in medicine: Perspectives of pathology colleagues. *Academic Pathology, 6.* https://doi.org/10.1177/2374289519851486.
7. Cacchione, R. N., Sayad, P., Pecoraro, A. M., & Ferzli, G. S. (2001). Laparoscopic autopsies. *Surgical Endoscopy, 15*(6), 619–622. https://doi.org/10.1007/s004640010161.
8. Fan, J. K., Tong, D. K., Poon, J. T., Lo, O. S., Beh, P. S., Patil, N. G., & Law, W. L. (2010). Multimodality minimally invasive autopsy—A feasible and accurate approach to post-mortem examination. *Forensic Science International, 195*(2–3), 93–98. https://doi.org/10.1016/j.forsciint.2009.12.016.
9. Friberg, N., Ljungberg, O., Berglund, E., Berglund, D., Ljungberg, R., Alafuzoff, I., & Englund, E. (2019). Cause of death and significant disease found at autopsy. *Virchows Archiv, 475*(6), 781–788. https://doi.org/10.1007/s00428-019-02648-2.

10. Kunz, S., Bergsdóttir, Þ., & Jónasson, J. (2020). Autopsy rates in Iceland. *Scandinavian Journal of Public Health, 48*(5), 486–490. https://doi.org/10.1177/1403494819896850.

11. Latten, B. G. H., Overbeek, L. I. H., Kubat, B., Zur Hausen, A., & Schouten, L. J. (2019). A quarter century of decline of autopsies in the Netherlands. *European Journal of Epidemiology, 34*(11), 1171–1174. https://doi.org/10.1007/s10654-019-00575-2.

12. Rentschler, L., Märkl, B., Schaller, T., Hirschbühl, K., Kleinlein, I., Dintner, S., & Vlasenko, D. (2023). All-body-cavity (ABC)-scopy—An approach for a feasible method of minimally invasive autopsy to allow for postmortem tissue sampling in cases where a conventional autopsy is denied. *Pathology - Research and Practice, 241*, 154263. https://doi.org/10.1016/j.prp.2023.154263.

13. Rosendahl, A., Mjörnheim, B., & Eriksson, L. C. (2021). Autopsies and quality of cause of death diagnoses. *SAGE Open Medicine, 9*. https://doi.org/10.1177/20503121211022872.

14. Skowronek, R., & Chowaniec, C. (2010). Ewolucja techniki sekcyjnej–od Virchowa do Virtopsy®. *Archiwum Medycyny Sądowej i Kryminologii, 60*(1), 48–54. https://doi.org/10.5114/amsik.2010.17104.

15. Świderski, P., Rzepczyk, S., Bożek, B., & Żaba, C. (2023). Minimally invasive autopsy—Endoscopic approach to post-mortem diagnostics. *Videosurgery and Other Miniinvasive Techniques, 18*(2), 122–128. https://doi.org/10.5114/wiitm.2023.118553.

16. van der Linden, A., Blokker, B. M., Kap, M., Weustink, A. C., Riegman, P. H. J., & Oosterhuis, J. W. (2014). Post-mortem tissue biopsies obtained at minimally invasive autopsy: An RNA-quality analysis. *PLoS ONE, 9*(8), e115675. https://doi.org/10.1371/journal.pone.0115675.

17. Wagensveld, I. M., Hunink, M. M., Wielopolski, P. A., van Kemenade, F. J., Krestin, G. P., Blokker, B. M., & Weustink, A. C. (2019). Hospital implementation of minimally invasive autopsy: A prospective cohort study of clinical performance and costs. *PLoS ONE, 14*(4), e0219291. https://doi.org/10.1371/journal.pone.0219291.

18. Wang, Z., Ma, K., Zou, D., Liu, N., Li, Z., Shao, Y., & Chen, Y. (2020). Diagnosis of drowning using postmortem computed tomography combined with endoscopic autopsy: A case report. *Medicine, 99*(43), e19182. https://doi.org/10.1097/MD.0000000000019182.

Chapter 9

INFECTIOUS DISEASES: THE ROLE OF THE FORENSIC PHYSICIAN

Contents

Introduction

Since ancient times, infections have been a source of difficulty for medical professionals, both in terms of diagnosing the specific diseases that they cause and in terms of identifying and then treating the agents that cause them. As new organisms come into existence, some of the organisms that already exist develop resistance to the drugs or vaccines that are currently available, and there are shifts in epidemiology and prevalence, there is an ongoing demand for information. In the 21st century, the importance of acquiring this information has never been higher than it is nowadays. Because of population migration and the relatively low cost of flying, people can bring infectious diseases that are not familiar to industrialized countries. An example of this would be the outbreak of severe acute respiratory syndrome (SARS), which was identified for the first time in the year 2003. It took several months to identify the agent, develop a diagnostic test, and devise a plan for disease reporting and isolation, despite the fact that modern technology and a significant amount of money were also involved in the process.

Orientation and Directional Terms

Term	Definition	**Illustration**
Swine Influenza	A respiratory disease of pigs caused by influenza A viruses, which can occasionally infect humans, causing flu-like symptoms.	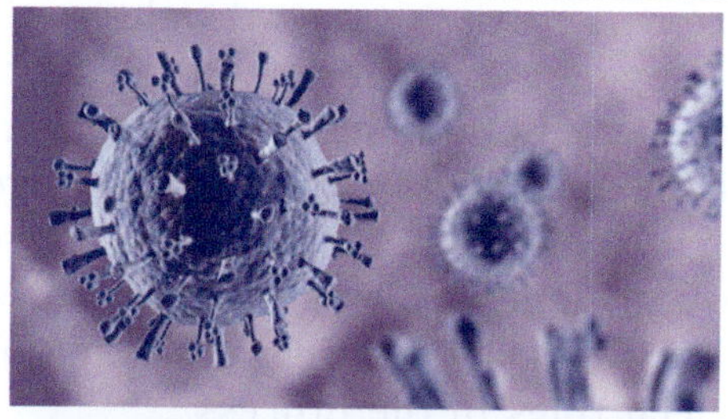
Human Immunodeficiency Virus (HIV)	A virus that attacks the immune system, specifically CD4 cells, leading to progressive immunodeficiency and potentially AIDS if untreated.	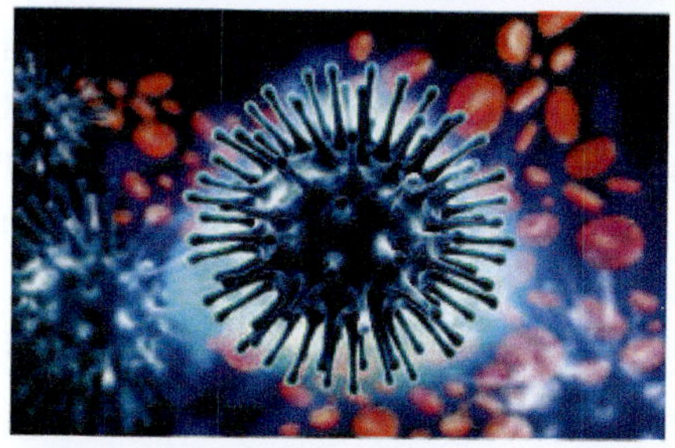
Hepatitis B Virus (HBV)	A virus that infects the liver, causing inflammation and potentially leading to chronic liver disease, cirrhosis, or liver cancer.	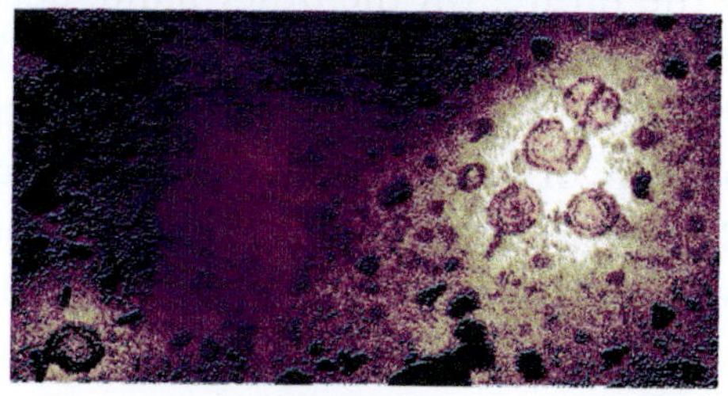
Hepatitis C Virus (HCV)	A virus that primarily infects the liver, often leading to chronic liver inflammation, which can result in cirrhosis or liver cancer over time.	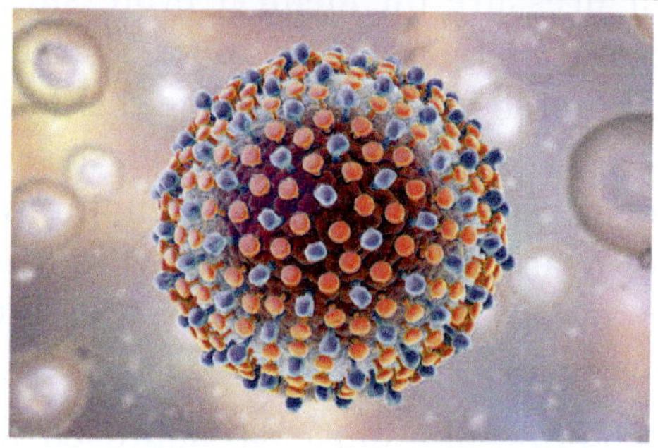

9.1. Spreading of Infections

Throughout history, infections have posed challenges for healthcare professionals, both in diagnosing specific diseases they cause and in identifying and treating the agents responsible. As new organisms emerge, existing ones develop resistance to available drugs or vaccines, leading to shifts in epidemiology and prevalence, creating a continuous need for information. In the 21st century, the importance of obtaining this information has never been greater. Due to population migration and affordable air travel, individuals can introduce unfamiliar infectious diseases to industrialized nations. An instance of this is the emergence of severe acute respiratory syndrome (SARS) in 2003. It took several months to identify the causative agent, develop a diagnostic test, and establish protocols for disease reporting and isolation, with modern technology and substantial funding playing crucial roles in the process.

The appearance of swine influenza A (H1N1) is yet another illustration of how population migration can take place, which can lead to the spread of disease. Mexico was the location where the first case was reported in March of 2009. By June of that same year, over 22,000 cases had been reported in 70 different countries, which meant that the pandemic had been established. After that, there were difficulties in making decisions regarding treatment, and then there were difficulties in distributing and administering specific vaccines.

There is no question that additional fascinating diseases that are brand new will continue to emerge in the future. On the other hand, dealing with infections presents two primary challenges for the forensic physician. In the first place, the management of detainees or police personnel who have contracted a disease and may be infectious or ill, and in the second place, the management of complainants of assault, including police officers, who may have been exposed to an infectious disease. The latter can be upsetting for those who are involved, and another factor that can contribute to this is the inconsistency of management guidelines if such guidelines do in fact exist.

As a result of the introduction of human rights legislation, authorities are exerting an increasing amount of pressure on medical professionals with regard to the detainee's consent and the confidentiality of their information. Therefore, it is prudent to preempt such situations before the consultation begins by obtaining the detainee's consent, either verbally or in writing, to allow certain pieces of information to be disclosed. This can be done to avoid any potential problems. The doctor is responsible for determining whether or not withholding pertinent details will put the lives or health of those working within custody or other individuals with whom they may have had close contact (whether or not it was intentional) in jeopardy. If they do not agree, then the doctor must make the decision.

The adoption of a universal approach with all detainees will bring about a reduction in the risk of the staff acquiring such diseases, as well as a reduction in the needless overreaction and the unjustified disclosure of sensitive information. An approach that is more open-minded is required for those who have been victims of sexual or violent assault. It is possible to make an informed assessment of the risk of certain diseases by determining the lifestyle of the individuals who are responsible for the attack if the perpetrator is known. If, on the other hand, the perpetrator of the attack is unknown, then it is prudent to assume the worst. The purpose of this chapter is to provide an overview of the infections that are most frequently encountered by forensic physicians. The objective is to debunk the "urban myths" that have been prevalent and to present a rational strategy for achieving efficient management.

9.2. Universal Precautions

The adoption of measures that are considered to be good practice in the United Kingdom, the United States of America, and Australia can help reduce the risk of exposure to infections, particularly blood-borne viruses (BBVs).

Those who work in the medical field, including forensic physicians and other professionals, should wash their hands both before and after coming into contact with prisoners or victims. It should be a requirement for law enforcement personnel to wash their hands after coming into contact with bodily fluids or excreta. When it is likely that they will come into contact with body fluids, mucous membranes, or skin that is not intact, all employees should wear gloves. Additionally, gloves should be worn whenever one is cleaning up body fluids or handling clinical waste, including contaminated laundry among other things. Only gloves designed for a single use should be worn, and they must be under the requirements of European Standard 455 or an equivalent standard. In addition, those who are allergic to latex should have access to a synthetic alternative that is in accordance with the same standards!

Every member of the staff is responsible for applying a waterproof dressing to any open skin lesions, fresh wounds (those that are less than 24 hours old), or breaks in exposed skin. Gloves are not able to prevent percutaneous injuries; however, they can reduce the likelihood of contracting a blood-borne viral infection by limiting the amount of blood that is transmitted through the bloodstream. The only time gloves should be worn is when blood is being drawn, provided that doing so does not reduce manual dexterity and consequently raises the risk of accidental percutaneous injury.

Within the best case scenario, a designated individual should be assigned the responsibility of ensuring that the clinical room is kept clean and that sharps containers and clinical waste bags are removed consistently. The disposal of clinical waste is required to take place in "hazard bags," which must not be filled to the brim. Following their use, they should be placed in two separate bags and then sealed with "hazard tape." Placement of the bags in a designated waste disposal area (preferably outside the building) and removal of the bags by a professional company are both recommended.

If cells have been contaminated with bodily fluids, it is imperative to contact a professional cleaning company as soon as possible to provide assistance. Since that time has not yet arrived, the cell ought to be considered "out of action."

9.2.1. Sharps Awareness

Under the Environmental Protection Act (1990) and the Control of Substances Hazardous to Health Regulations 1994 (COSHH), it is a legal requirement in the United Kingdom to dispose of sharps in a container that has been approved. At the Centers for Disease Control and Prevention (CDC) website in the United States of America, the Division of Healthcare Quality Promotion (DHQP) offers comparable guidance. When sharps containers are transported off-site from the custody facility, they are required to be of a type that has been approved.

The Carriage of Dangerous Goods (Classification, Packaging and Labeling) and Use of Transportable Pressure Receptacles Regulations 1996 in the United Kingdom include a provision that stipulates the necessity of such a requirement. Taking these precautions helps to reduce the likelihood of suffering an injury by accident. To take additional precautions, it is important to always wear gloves when handling sharp objects and to avoid bending, breaking, or resheathing needles before their disposal. There should never be an excessive amount of sharps in the bins, nor should they be left on the floor or positioned above the eye level of the smallest member of the staff.

9.2.2. Contaminated Bedding

Any bedding that is visibly stained with body fluids should be handled with gloves. There are only three acceptable ways of dealing with contaminated bedding:

1. Laundering with a detergent at a minimum temperature of 71°C (160°F) or at a lower temperature (22–50°C) with water containing detergent and 50–150 ppm of chlorine bleach.
2. Dry cleaning at elevated temperatures/dry cleaning cold followed by steam pressing.
3. Incineration.

It is not considered acceptable practice to share bedding between detainees.

9.2.3. Other Measures

As the risk of infection is low in the custodial setting, staff members don't need to wear masks or protective eyewear in order to prevent infection.

On the other hand, in the event that an individual is accidentally exposed to eyewash, it ought to be available in the clinical room or contained within other first aid kits that are situated within the police station location. Before washing one's eyes, it is important to remove any contact lenses.

9.3. Formulation of Guidelines

An example of good practice can be found in a document that was published in 1998 by the United Kingdom's Department of Health. This document states that "it is the responsibility of Health Authorities, Health Boards, and NHS Trusts to create their own local guidelines to prevent the spread of BBVs in the health care setting." There may be no such guidelines in place at other places of employment. The formulation of these should take place as quickly as possible if this is the case. When working for the Royal Military Police in the United Kingdom, forensic physicians can consult the "Good Practice Guidelines." The pre-arrangement of a referral system with the nearest hospital that has access to a specialist, a genito-urinary department, and an accident and emergency department is another best practice that should be considered. It is possible that the latter represents a consultant in the fields of virology, microbiology, infectious diseases, or genito-urinary medicine. "The Guideline for Infection Control in Health Care Personnel" is a document that provides guidance that is comparable in the United States of America.

Even though accidents can occur regardless of how much care is taken, the majority of exposures to staff members are typically the result of a failure to maintain accepted practice. In the custody system, all forensic physicians and other healthcare professionals must have a comprehensive understanding of what constitutes a risk. The first step in this process is to compile a comprehensive account of the incident, which should include the nature of the exposure, the bodily fluids that were involved, and the occurrence date.

From the very beginning, this information has the potential to alleviate any unnecessary anxiety that may have been present, and it will also guarantee that the individual who has been exposed to the substance is referred, if necessary, to the designated hospital at the earliest possible opportunity. While it is not necessary to have knowledge of specific treatment protocols, it is beneficial to be able to explain to the recipient what they can anticipate from the treatment. A voluntary baseline blood sample will be collected for storage, and depending on the nature of the exposure, a number of follow-up samples will be collected for testing. For instance, the individual will be asked to provide a baseline blood sample. The human immunodeficiency virus (HIV), hepatitis B (HBV), and hepatitis C (HCV) are three viruses that are particularly pertinent to this discussion. In most cases, this will be finished within a period of 12 weeks; however, there are some instances in which testing may be extended to a period of six months after the incident.

The best course of action would be to refer victims of sexual assault to specialized centers if such facilities are available. Since the atmosphere is frequently hostile and there is no ready access to the necessary treatment and ongoing management, a police station should only be used as a last resort.

9.4. Routes of Transmission

It's possible for organisms to choose more than one path. To make the infections that are discussed in this chapter more easily understandable, they have been categorized according to their primary route of transmission. These primary routes include transmission through blood and body fluids, transmission through contact with lesions or organisms, transmission through the respiratory route, and transmission through the fecal-oral route.

9.5. Transmission Through Blood and Body Fluids

Blood-borne viruses (BBVs) that are associated with persistent viral replication and viremia are the ones that pose the greatest risk of cross-infection to staff members or victims. Hepatitis B (HBV), hepatitis C (HCV), hepatitis D (HDV), and human immunodeficiency virus (HIV) are some of the viruses that fall into this category.

The potential for exposure to blood or other bodily fluids is the primary factor that contributes to the transmission of blood-borne viruses (BBVs). In accordance with the sections that are pertinent to the topic at hand, the level of risk varies depending on the virus in question. A percutaneous injury, mucocutaneous exposure, or exposure through contamination of fresh cuts or breaks in the skin are all represented in Figure 9.1, which illustrates the immediate management that should be administered thereafter.

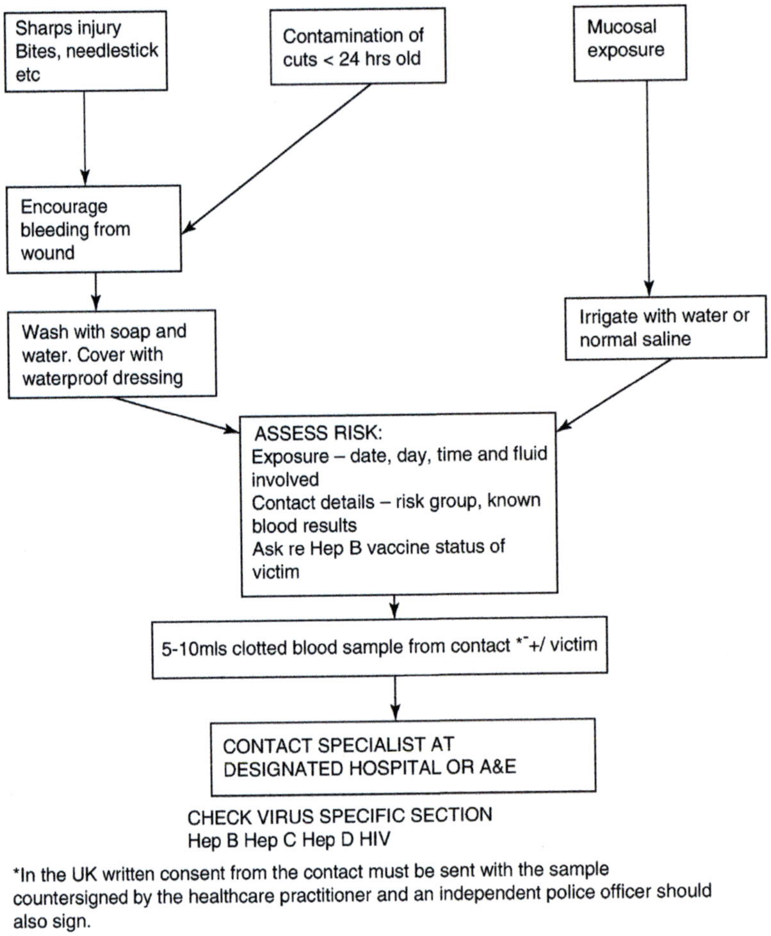

Figure 9.1. *Immediate management following occupational exposure to blood-borne viruses (BBVs).*

Source: Nicholson F. (2011). Infectious diseases: The role of the forensic physician. Clinical Forensic Medicine, 95–340.

9.5.1. Hepatitis B

9.5.1.1. Epidemiology and Prevalence

Although the prevalence of HBV varies from population to population, the virus is considered to be endemic everywhere in the world. Over 350 million people have a chronic infection with HBV, which accounts for approximately 2,000 million people who have been infected with the virus. HBV is responsible for the deaths of approximately 1 million people annually across the globe. The World Health Organization (WHO) recommended that the HBV vaccine should be incorporated into national immunization programs by the year 1995 in those countries with a chronic infection rate of 8% or higher, and by the year 1997, it should be included in all countries. This recommendation was made in 1982, when a vaccine that was both safe and effective was developed. 135 countries had accomplished this objective by the end of the year 2001; however, the poorest countries, which frequently have the highest prevalence, have been unable to afford it. China, the Indian Subcontinent, and Sub-Saharan Africa are three examples of these region's particular significance.

The ability to transmit infection is present in individuals who are either in the early stages of infection or who have chronic carrier status, which is defined as the presence of a hepatitis B surface antigen for more than six months. There is an overall prevalence of chronic HBV in the United Kingdom that is somewhere between 0.2 and 0.3%. Table 9.1 provides a comprehensive breakdown of the items.

Table 9.1. Prevalence of Chronic Hepatitis B (HBV)

Blood-donning population – <1%
Intravenous drug users – 10–15%
Homosexual/bisexuals – 10–15%
Institutionalized patients – no data available
People from high-risk endemic areas, e.g., China and the Far East, up to 30% of the population are carriers and 75% have evidence of past infection. In Africa, 5–10% are carriers

Source: Nicholson F. (2011). Infectious diseases: The role of the forensic physician. Clinical Forensic Medicine, 295–340.

9.5.1.2. Symptoms and Complications

The incubation period lasts somewhere between six weeks and six months on average. This virus primarily affects the liver, as the name of the virus suggests. Malaise, anorexia, nausea, mild fever, and abdominal discomfort are some of the typical symptoms that one may experience before the gradual onset of jaundice. These symptoms can last anywhere from two days to three weeks. The formation of immune complexes can also result in the development of skin rashes and pain in the joints. Most of the time, infections in newborns do not present any symptoms.

In the majority of cases, patients who have acute HBV can make a full recovery and develop immunity. After an acute infection, approximately one in every 300 patients will develop liver failure, which can ultimately lead to death.

Around 90% of newborns, 50% of children, and 5 to 10% of adults acquire a chronic infection at some point in their lives. In most cases, newborns and children do not exhibit any symptoms. Adults may only experience mild symptoms, or they may not experience any symptoms at all. Cirrhosis is a condition that can develop in approximately 15–25% of chronically infected individuals throughout a number of years, depending on the age at which the infection came about. There is also the possibility that this will lead to liver failure or other serious complications, such as hepatocellular carcinoma, although the latter is extremely uncommon. Less than 5 percent is the estimated mortality rate associated with HBV in the general population.

9.5.1.3. Period of Infectivity

The presence of HBsAg in the blood of a person is considered to be infectious. It is possible for this to last for as long as six months during the acute phase of the illness. A person is considered to be a carrier of the HBsAg virus if the virus continues to be present after this period. It is common for carriers to transmit the disease for life. Many factors, including the stage of the disease and the markers listed in Table 9.2, influence the degree of infectiousness.

Table 9.2. Significance of Markers

Name	Infectivity	Immunity	Risk Following Needle Stick (%)
HBsAg	Yes	No	Only marker = 10–20
HBeAg	Yes	No	With HBsAg = 30–40
HBeA	Yes	Yes	With HBsAg = <10
HBCA	No	Yes	0
HBSA	No	Yes	0

Source: Nicholson F. (2011). Infectious diseases: The role of the forensic physician. Clinical Forensic Medicine, 295–340.

HBsAg Hepatitis B surface antigen; *HbeAg* hepatitis B e antigen; *HBeA* hepatitis B e antibody; *HBCA* hepatitis B core antibody; *HBSA* hepatitis B surface antibody

9.5.1.4. Routes of Transmission

The primary transmission routes include parenteral (such as needlestick injuries, bites, unscreened blood transfusions, tattooing, acupuncture, and dental procedures with insufficient sterilization of equipment); exposure of mucous membranes (including the mouth, eyes, and genital mucous membranes); and contamination of recently broken skin (particularly within 24 hours).

9.5.1.5. At-Risk Groups

Hepatitis B virus (HBV) poses a risk to individuals who may encounter blood or body fluids contaminated with blood through the mentioned pathways. HBV can be transmitted solely through saliva. Studies have demonstrated that the saliva of individuals infected with HBV may contain HBV-DNA concentrations that are 1/1,000 to 1/10,000 of the concentration found in their blood serum. This is particularly applicable to deep puncture wounds. Infection resulting from contact with other bodily fluids, such as bile, urine, feces, and cerebrospinal fluid (CSF), has never been proven unless these fluids are tainted with blood.

Individuals who engage in intravenous drug use and engage in the practice of sharing needles or other paraphernalia are also susceptible to potential harm. HBV can also be transmitted through unprotected sexual contact, regardless of sexual orientation. The risk is heightened when blood is present. Sexual assault survivors should be encompassed within this category.

Empirical data has demonstrated that the virus can be transmitted within a family through intimate household contact. Transmission is believed to occur through activities such as kissing, sharing toothbrushes, razors, bath towels, and so on. This mode of transmission likely pertains to patients who are in institutional care, although there is currently no data available to support this.

Research conducted on incarcerated individuals in western countries has revealed a greater occurrence of antibodies to Hepatitis B virus (HBV) and other blood-borne viruses (BBVs) compared to the general population. The primary risk factor frequently reported in these studies is the use of intravenous drugs. Nevertheless, the actual rate of transmission of blood-borne viruses (BBVs) in British prisons remains uncertain due to the challenges associated with gathering accurate data. Hepatitis B virus (HBV) can be transmitted from mother to baby during the perinatal period. Approximately 80% of infants born to mothers with either acute or chronic HBV are infected, and the majority of them will develop chronic HBV. The administration of the HBV vaccine to the neonate has restricted this. All pregnant women in developed nations undergo screening for HBV. The vaccine is administered to the neonate ideally within the first 12 hours after birth, and at least two additional doses are given at specified intervals. The World Health Organization (WHO) advises that this should be done routinely for all women in countries with a high prevalence. Nevertheless, the logistical challenges of distributing a vaccine that requires precise temperature control and the limited availability of medical services result in a substantial decline in the number of people receiving and responding to the vaccine.

9.5.1.6. Disease Prevention

In industrialized countries, HBV vaccination is recommended for those deemed at risk of acquiring the disease

1. Through occupational exposure
2. Homosexual/bisexual men
3. Intravenous drug users
4. Sexual partners of people with acute or chronic HBV
5. Family members of people with acute or chronic HBV
6. Newborn babies whose mothers are infected with HBV. If the mother is HBeAg positive, then HBV-specific immunoglobulin (HBSIG) should be given at the same time as the first dose of the vaccine
7. Institutionalized patients and prisoners

Preferably, the HBV vaccine should be given before any potential exposure. The routine schedule (RS) involves administering three doses of vaccine at intervals of 0, 1, and 6 months. It is recommended to assess the levels of antibodies between 4 and 16 weeks following the administration of the final dose. An adequate response has been achieved if the titers exceed 10 miU/ml. In the UK, this is regarded as offering protection for a period of 5 to 10 years, after which an additional dose would be administered. In the United States, if an initial sufficient response has been attained, additional doses of vaccine are deemed unnecessary.

The administration of vaccines following exposure varies depending on the timing of the incident, the level of risk, and the individual's vaccination status. A shortened timetable (AS) is employed to prevent perinatal transmission by administering the third dose 2 months after the initial dose, followed by a booster shot one year later. If there are high levels of risk, it may be necessary to implement a rapid schedule (RDS). The doses are administered at 0, 7, and 21–28 days following the initial presentation, with an additional booster dose given at 6–12 months. The current licensing for this schedule is exclusively with Engerix B.

HBIG can be administered either independently or in combination with a vaccine. The precise dosage administered is contingent upon the individual's age, but it must be delivered via a deep intramuscular injection at a distinct location from the vaccine. In adults, the injection is typically administered into the gluteus muscle.

HBIG is administered concurrently with the initial vaccine dose to individuals considered to be at a high risk of contracting the disease, and this is done within 72 hours of the occurrence. It is also utilized for newborns born to mothers who test positive for HBeAg.

Approximately 5 to 10% of adults do not exhibit a response to the standard vaccination regimen. It is advisable to administer an additional complete course of vaccine before classifying them as "non-responders." Individuals who have been exposed to a high-risk situation should receive two doses of HBIG, with each dose administered one month apart. Optimally, the initial dosage should be administered within 48 hours following exposure and should not exceed a period of 2 weeks after exposure.

Additional measures involve reducing the likelihood of being exposed to risks by implementing the safe working practices described in the "Universal Precautions" section. It is important to address any possible exposures promptly. HBV screening is a routine practice in industrialized nations for blood, blood products, and organs.

It is advisable to promote vaccination among intravenous drug users and to discourage them from sharing needles or any other drug-related equipment.

9.5.1.7. Management in Custody

It is prudent to establish a protocol for prompt handling and risk assessment for both staff members and individuals who come into contact with the disease. Figure 9.1 illustrates an example. Although forensic physicians are not required to provide medical treatment, it is often beneficial to inform individuals about what they can anticipate. Tables 9.3 and 9.4 provide a comprehensive overview of the treatment protocols utilized in the United Kingdom.

Table 9.3. Management Following High-Risk Exposure

Vaccination Status	Hepatitis B-Specific Immunoglobulin (HBSIG)	Hepatitis B Vaccine	Follow Up	Notes
Not vaccinated	Yes if <3 days after exposure	Yes	AS via GP	
	No if >3 days	Yes	Rapid schedule (RDS) via GP	Advise GP of timing
Vaccinated: non-responder	Yes if within 3 days	No	Repeat HBSIG at 1 month	Consider trying newer vaccines at later stage

Course completed. Levels >10 miU/ml	No	Yes if primary course >3 years ago	No	
Course completed within 3 years. Levels not checked	No	Yes	GP to check results of baseline blood test	If baseline antibodies <10 miU/ml advise RDS
If >3 years see below				
Incomplete course (one or two doses)	Yes if within 3 days	Yes	GP to check results of baseline blood test	>10 miU/ml – RS
	No if >3 days	Yes		<10 miU/ml – RDS

Source: Nicholson F. (2011). Infectious diseases: The role of the forensic physician. Clinical Forensic Medicine, 295–340.

Contact in a high-risk group or HBsAg positive and person has had a high-risk exposure

Table 9.4. Management Following Low-Risk Exposure

Vaccination Status	HBSIG	Vaccine	Follow up	Notes
Not vaccinated	No	Yes	RS via GP	
Vaccinated non-responder	No	No		Consider using newer vaccines
Course completed	No	Yes if not checked or >3 years since 1° course		
Incomplete course	No	Yes	GP to check results of baseline test	<10 miU/ml complete RS

Source: Nicholson F. (2011). Infectious diseases: The role of the forensic physician. Clinical Forensic Medicine, 295–340.

The individual is either in the low-risk group or has been confirmed to be negative for HBsAg. Additionally, they have experienced an exposure that is low-risk.

Detainees who have a disease can typically be effectively handled while in custody. Once the detainee has left, if there is any bleeding, the cell should be considered unusable until it can be cleaned by a professional. The appropriate course of action for handling contaminated bedding is outlined in the section titled "Contaminated Bedding." If the individual in custody has a persistent Hepatitis B Virus (HBV) infection and is currently taking an antiviral medication such as Lamivudine, it is recommended to maintain the ongoing treatment regimen, if feasible.

9.5.2. Hepatitis C

9.5.2.1. Epidemiology and Prevalence

HCV is prevalent in the majority of regions worldwide. Hepatitis C virus (HCV) infects around 3% (200 million) of the global population. Prevalence data is not available for many countries.

Studies on seroprevalence conducted among blood donors have revealed that Egypt has the highest prevalence rate, ranging from 17% to 26%. The cause of this can be attributed to the use of contaminated needles during the treatment of schistosomiasis, which occurred from the 1950s to the 1980s.

Eastern Europe, the Mediterranean, the Middle East, the Indian Sub-continent, and parts of Africa and Asia have an intermediate prevalence of 1–5%. The prevalence of this condition is low (0.2–0.5%) in Western Europe, most of Central America, Australia, and certain regions in Africa, including South Africa.

In the past, America was categorized as having a low occurrence of HCV. However, a report published in 2003 revealed that nearly 4 million Americans, which is equivalent to 1.8% of the population, have antibodies to HCV. This indicates that they either currently have or have had an HCV infection in the past. Additionally, it is indicated that HCV is responsible for approximately 15% of cases of acute viral hepatitis in the United States.

The United Kingdom and Scandinavia have the lowest prevalence rates, ranging from 0.01% to 0.1%. However, certain demographic groups within a country are more likely to be carriers of HCV. In the United Kingdom, these figures are presented in Table 9.5.

Table 9.5. Prevalence of Hepatitis C (HCV)

General blood-donning population	0.06%
Organ donors	0.72%
Hemophiliacs	100%[a]
Intravenous drug users	28–57%
Homosexual/bisexuals	<5%

[a]Statistics apply to all who received blood products before the mid-1980s.

Source: Nicholson F. (2011). Infectious diseases: The role of the forensic physician. Clinical Forensic Medicine, 295–340.

9.5.2.2. Symptoms and Complications

The acute phase of the disease typically lasts for about 2 to 3 years following an incubation period of 6 to 8 weeks. Unlike hepatitis A (HAV) or HBV, patients with this disease typically do not show any symptoms. As a result, the disease often goes unnoticed unless the individual has reported a specific exposure and is under observation. Additional instances may be discovered incidentally when elevated liver enzymes are detected during a routine blood examination.

After the acute phase, a period known as the "silent phase" occurs, during which the virus remains inactive and the levels of liver enzymes typically return to normal. This time frame has a duration of approximately 10–15 years. Subsequent reactivation may ensue. Following viral replication, the hepatocytes are harmed, resulting in an increase in liver enzymes to either moderate or high levels.

Regardless of their liver enzyme levels, 80% of individuals who test positive for HCV antibodies are capable of transmitting the infection. Roughly 80% of individuals experience long-term infection, with one out of every five individuals advancing to cirrhosis. Hepatocellular carcinoma is significantly more strongly associated with HBV. Approximately 1.25–2.5% of individuals diagnosed with cirrhosis caused by hepatitis C virus (HCV) are at risk of developing liver cancer. Spontaneous resolution occurs in less than 2% of chronic cases.

9.5.2.3. Routes of Transmission

Approximately 75% of cases are transmitted through parenteral routes, such as needlestick injuries. Sexual transmission of HCV is rare and only becomes significant when there is repeated contact with one or more individuals who are infected with the virus. Vertical transmission from mother to baby is considered to be infrequent, but cases have been documented. In theory, household transmission can occur when individuals share toothbrushes or razors that are contaminated.

Since the disease is often silent, there is a need to raise awareness among the general population on how to avoid infection and to encourage high-risk groups to be tested. Healthcare professionals should receive proper education to prevent acquiring infections in the workplace. An exemplification of exemplary methodology can be found in the document titled 'Hepatitis C strategy for England,' which was published by the Department of Health in 2002.

9.5.2.4. Risks from Exposure to HCV RNA-Positive Person

For a risk to occur, there must be the presence of blood or body fluids that are stained with blood. Saliva alone is not considered to be a significant threat. The probability of contracting an infection from a single needlestick incident is 1.8%, with a range of 0–7%. The estimated rate of infection through contact with a contaminated cut is 1%. There is a lack of data regarding penetrating bite injuries, but it is only considered risky if blood is present. Transmission through mucous membrane exposure requires the involvement of blood or body fluids that are stained with blood. This could explain the lower-than-anticipated occurrence among the homosexual community.

9.5.2.5. Management in Custody

9.5.2.5.1. Staff/Victims in Contact with Disease

Adhere to the prompt management flow chart, ensuring that all accessible information is acquired. Notify the specified medical facility and/or expert promptly. If the individual in question is identified and believed to have a weakened immune system, and if they have permitted to provide a blood sample, it is crucial to inform the specialist. This is because their antibody tests may yield falsely negative results. In this case, it is advisable to employ an alternative test known as polymerase chain reaction, which is capable of detecting viral RNA.

The staff member/victim will be requested to provide an initial blood sample, followed by additional samples at 4–6 weeks and 12 weeks. If the test results are negative after 12 weeks, but the initial risk is considered to be high, then the follow-up period may be extended for a maximum of 24 weeks. If any of the subsequent samples yield positive results, the initial baseline sample will undergo testing to determine if the infection was acquired as a result of the specific exposure.

Treating chronic HCV may involve a combination of pegylated or non-pegylated interferons and ribavirin. The success of treatment relies on various factors, such as the stage of the disease and the viral genotype. Early intervention is highly effective in treating infections during the initial stages, irrespective of the genotype. Therefore, timely detection is crucial.

Detainees who have a disease can be kept in custody unless their condition is extremely severe. Special precautions are necessary solely in the event of bleeding.

If there is a possibility of coming into contact with blood, custody staff should wear gloves. Proper handling of contaminated bedding and professional cleaning of the cell should be conducted after use.

9.5.3. Hepatitis D (Delta Agent)

This faulty transmissible virus, which was found in 1977, relies on HBV for its replication. It is globally distributed in connection with HBV, affecting around 15 million individuals. HDV is more common in southern Italy, the Middle East, and certain regions of Africa and South America. It affects over 20% of people who have HBV but show no symptoms, and over 60% of those with chronic liver disease related to HBV. Although HBV is highly prevalent in China and South East Asia, the occurrence of HDV in these countries is infrequent.

HDV is linked to both acute (co-infection) and chronic hepatitis (superinfection) and can worsen existing liver damage caused by HBV. The transmission routes and groups at risk are identical to those of HBV. Individuals who have potentially been exposed to a disease and those who are infected should be treated in the same manner as those with Hepatitis B virus (HBV). Interferon-alpha, such as Roferon, is effective in treating patients with chronic HBV and HDV. However, it is not feasible to continue this treatment in a custodial setting.

9.5.4. Human Immunodeficiency Virus

9.5.4.1. Epidemiology and Prevalence

The identification of HIV occurred in 1983, following reports to the CDC in Atlanta, GA, of a higher occurrence of two uncommon diseases (Kaposi's sarcoma and Pneumocystis carinii pneumonia) among the homosexual community in San Francisco, which had been reported two years earlier. The magnitude of the virus became apparent over time, and by the conclusion of 2002, approximately 42 million individuals worldwide were afflicted with HIV or AIDS. Africa and India are home to more than 80% of the global population. According to a report published by UNAIDS and the WHO in 2002, the prevalence of HIV or AIDS among adults in Lesotho, Malawi, Mozambique, Swaziland, Zambia, and Zimbabwe was estimated to be 20%. China, Papua New Guinea, and other countries in Asia and the Pacific are anticipated to experience a significant increase in HIV cases in the coming years.

By the end of 2002, the cumulative data in the UK indicated that 54,261 individuals had been reported to have HIV or AIDS, including deaths from AIDS. However, it is probable that this figure is lower than the actual number. By the conclusion of 2006, the number of individuals affected by HIV had risen to 78,000, with approximately one-third of them remaining undiagnosed. Men who have sex with men (MSM) remain the most vulnerable group to HIV transmission in the United Kingdom, with a 5.4% infection rate among individuals aged 15–44.

The estimated prevalence of intravenous drug use among drug users is 1 in 73 overall, but in London, it is higher at 1 in 20. During the 1980s, it was reported that as many as 90% of individuals in Edinburgh and Dundee were HIV positive. However, the majority of these individuals have since passed away. In 2006, a total of 78,000 new cases were identified, with approximately half of them occurring in individuals of black African descent. Annually, there is an increasing number of HIV infections being contracted through heterosexual transmission in the United Kingdom.

The prevalence of mother-to-baby transmission has been calculated to be 15% in Europe and approximately 45% in Africa. The transmission rates among African women are believed to be significantly higher due to a combination of factors. These factors include a larger number of women with advanced-stage disease and a higher viral load, as well as concurrent placental infection, which makes it easier for the virus to pass through. Administering anti-retroviral therapy during pregnancy and advising against breastfeeding has been effective in reducing the transmission of HIV from HIV-positive women to their children and to others in the western world. For individuals residing in developing nations, the situation is harsh and uncompromising. Access to medical treatment is restricted and there is no practical alternative to breast milk, which serves as a valuable source of antibodies against other potentially fatal infections. The inclusion of patients who receive blood transfusions, organs, or blood products without routine screening is also necessary.

9.5.4.2. Incubation Period and Phases of Infection

The period of incubation is estimated to range from 2 weeks to 6 months following exposure. The ability of current laboratory tests to detect HIV antibodies or viral antigen partially determines this. Most cases are currently diagnosed within a span of 12 weeks. The sensitivity of viral RNA detection has been enhanced through the advancement of PCR technology.

During the acute phase of the infection, about 50% experience a seroconversion "flu-like" illness. Currently, the person is contagious because the blood contains viral antigen (p24). Once the antibodies begin to develop, the viral antigen vanishes, and the individual transitions into the latent phase. They are non-contagious and remain in good health for a variable duration of time (7–15 years). The emergence of AIDS signifies the final stage of the disease. The viral antigen resurfaces, leading to the individual becoming infectious once more. The initiation of AIDS has been significantly postponed through the implementation of anti-retroviral therapy.

9.5.4.3. Routes of Transmission

Parenteral transmission encompasses the transmission of pathogens through various means, such as needle stick injuries, bites, unscreened blood transfusions, tattooing, acupuncture, and dental procedures where equipment is not adequately sterilized. The risk of transmission is higher in cases of deep penetrating injuries caused by visibly bloodstained hollow bore needles, particularly when the device has been previously used in the source patient's artery or vein. Additional pathways of exposure include contact with mucous membranes, such as the eyes, mouth, and genital mucous membranes, as well as contamination of compromised skin.

As the viral load in the contact increases, the risk of transmission also increases. This is most probable during the final stage of the infection. HIV is primarily transmitted through blood or other body fluids that are visibly contaminated with blood, excluding semen, vaginal fluid, and breast milk. It is highly improbable for saliva to transmit infection on its own. Thus, individuals who have experienced penetrating bite wounds can be assured that they are not in danger, as long as there was no bleeding from the mouth during the contact.

9.5.4.4. Risk of Seroconversion

The likelihood of infection resulting from a single percutaneous exposure through a hollow bore needle is minimal, and the probability of infection from a single mucocutaneous exposure is even lower.

The risk of contracting a sexually transmitted infection (STI) can vary depending on the type of sexual activity. However, it seems that engaging in receptive anal intercourse carries a higher risk compared to engaging in receptive vaginal intercourse.

9.5.4.5. Body Fluids Containing HIV

High-risk fluids include blood, semen, vaginal fluid and breast milk. There is little or no risk from saliva, urine, vomit or feces unless they are visibly bloodstained. Other fluids that constitute a theoretical risk include CSF, peritoneal, pleural, synovial or pericardial fluid.

9.5.4.6. Management in Custody of Staff/Victims in Contact with Disease

The management of staff or victims who have come into contact with a disease involves following the immediate management flow chart (Fig.9.1) and informing the designated hospital or specialist about the details of the exposure. If feasible, acquire a blood specimen from the individual in question. Similar to HBV and HCV, blood samples collected for HIV testing in the United Kingdom must adhere to the requirement of informed consent. The forensic physician does not need to provide an in-depth explanation of the test's significance. However, it is advisable to urge the individual to visit the genito-urinary department (or a similar department) at the designated hospital to discuss the test results. If the contact person declines to provide a blood sample, the specialist may find it helpful to consider information regarding their lifestyle, ethnic background, and health condition to determine whether the recipient should receive post-exposure prophylaxis (PEP). If a bite injury only involves saliva, it is highly justifiable to reassure the person that there is minimal risk of contracting HIV. Nevertheless, it is prudent to seek guidance from an expert.

In the United Kingdom, the current recommended treatment for post-exposure prophylaxis (PEP) is to take one tablet of Truvada (containing 254 mg of tenofovir and 200 mg of emtricitabane) once a day, along with two film-coated tablets of Kaletra (containing 200 mg of lopinavir and 50 mg of ritonavir) twice a day.

The risk of HIV transmission is only present when there has been significant exposure to a high-risk fluid that is visibly bloodstained and when the contact is known or highly likely to be HIV positive. Optimally, initiation of treatment should occur within 60 minutes following exposure, and definitely within a maximum of 72 hours. PEP may be administered after a longer period following exposure if there are exceptional circumstances that are not covered in this chapter. The typical duration of administration is 4 weeks unless the individual is later determined to be HIV-negative or experiences tolerance or toxicity issues. Regular monitoring of the recipient should occur every week during treatment to enhance compliance, assess drug toxicity, and address any other concerns.

Additional pertinent factors that could impact the decision to administer the standard treatment regimen or opt for alternative medications include potential drug interactions with other medications the recipient is currently using, prior history of anti-retroviral therapy, and pregnancy status of the recipient. There is no available data regarding the effectiveness of PEP beyond cases of occupational exposure. PEP is not recommended for individuals who have been exposed to low or no risk fluids through any route, or in cases where the source of exposure is unknown, such as a discarded needle. Although PEP has been used correctly and administered at the appropriate time, there have been instances of its failure.

9.5.4.7. Management in Custody of Detainees with HIV

Unless they are in a critical condition, they can be detained. It is imperative to exert every effort to maintain the continuation of any ongoing treatment they are receiving. Employ universal precautions when handling the detainee and make sure to handle contaminated cells and/or bedding suitably.

9.6. Transmission Through Contact with Lesions or Organisms

9.6.1. Varicella (Chicken Pox)

9.6.1.1. Epidemiology and Prevalence

Instances of this highly contagious illness are present year-round but are more prevalent during the winter and early spring. The occurrence of this seasonal pattern seems to be becoming less distinct due to the effects of global warming. The age group with the highest prevalence in the UK is 4–10 years. Immunity is present in 90% of individuals aged 40 and above. Comparable rates have been documented in other regions of Western Europe and the United States. Varicella primarily affects adults in South East Asia. Consequently, individuals who were born in these countries and have relocated to the UK are at a higher risk of contracting chicken pox.

A significant association exists between a past occurrence of chicken pox and the presence of serologic immunity, with a high percentage (97–99%) of individuals showing this immunity. The majority of adults in industrialized countries with a questionable or unfavorable past of chicken pox are also seropositive, with a prevalence ranging from 70% to 90%. A live-attenuated vaccine was authorized for use in the United States in March 1995, along with the implementation of a policy to vaccinate children and healthcare personnel who are susceptible to the disease.

Varilrix, a live-attenuated vaccine, was launched by GlaxoSmithKline in the UK during the summer of 2002. In December 2003, the Department of Health, based on advice from the Joint Committee on Vaccination and Immunization (JCVI), advised that the vaccine should be administered to healthcare workers who are not immune to chickenpox and are at high risk of coming into direct contact with infected individuals. Healthcare workers without a prior history of chicken pox should undergo screening for immunity. If no antibodies are detected, they should be administered two doses of vaccine, spaced 4–8 weeks apart. Currently, the vaccine is not advised for children and should be avoided during pregnancy.

9.6.1.2. Incubation Period and Symptoms

After a period of 10–21 days of incubation (which may be shorter in individuals with weakened immune systems), there is typically a preliminary illness resembling the flu before the appearance of the rash. The occurrence of this coryzal phase is more common in adults. The lesions usually manifest in clusters, rapidly transitioning from red papules to vesicles and eventually forming open sores that subsequently scab and detach within a span of 10 days. The rash is distributed in a centripetal manner, meaning it is more prevalent on the trunk and face compared to the limbs. This is the opposite of smallpox. In adults, the disease typically presents with more severe symptoms, characterized by the presence of lesions on the scalp and mucous membranes of the oropharynx.

9.6.1.3. Complications

In children, the disease typically manifests as a mild condition, unless they have a weakened immune system, in which case the likelihood of experiencing complications is low. Among individuals aged 15 years or older, the situation is notably distinct. Secondary bacterial infection is frequently encountered but seldom poses a significant threat. There is a higher probability of developing permanent scarring. Hemorrhagic chickenpox usually manifests on the second or third day after the appearance of the rash. Typically, this is restricted to the leakage of blood into the skin, but it is possible for life-threatening conditions such as melaena, epistaxis, or hematuria to occur.

Varicella pneumonia can vary in severity, ranging from localized lung consolidation to more severe pneumonitis. It is estimated to occur in approximately 1 out of every 400 cases of varicella. It may manifest in individuals who were previously in good health, especially adults, but the likelihood is higher in those who smoke. Individuals with compromised immune systems are most susceptible to developing this complication. Varicella-zoster virus infection progresses rapidly and is the most frequent cause of death associated with Varicella.

Survivors may experience fibrosis and develop permanent respiratory impairment. Immediate treatment should be administered to any individual showing signs of lung involvement, and both detainees and staff members should be promptly sent to the hospital. The central nervous system (CNS) can be affected by various conditions, such as meningitis, Guillain–Barre syndrome, and encephalitis. The latter, referring to a specific condition or situation, is more frequently observed in individuals with weakened immune systems and has the potential to result in death.

9.6.1.4. Period of Infectivity

This is taken 3 days before the first lesions appear to the end of new vesicle formation and the last vesicle has crusted over. This typically is 5–7 days after onset, but may last up to 14 days.

9.6.1.5. Routes of Transmission

The primary route is through direct contact with open lesions of chicken pox. However, it is also spread through aerosols or droplets from the respiratory tract. Chicken pox may also be acquired through contact with open lesions of shingles (Varicella zoster), but this is less likely as shingles is less infectious than chicken pox.

9.6.1.6. At-Risk Groups

Individuals who do not have immunity are susceptible to contracting a disease. Roughly 10% of the adult population who were born in the UK and less than 5% of adults in the USA belong to this particular group. Thus, the probability of encountering chicken pox in the custodial setting is higher among individuals born outside the UK, especially in South East Asia, or those who are immunocompromised and have lost immunity. Pregnant women who do not have immunity are susceptible to experiencing complications.

Pneumonia may develop in as many as 10% of pregnant women who contract chicken pox, and its severity seems to be heightened during the later stages of pregnancy. Additionally, they can transmit infection to the fetus. If an individual acquires the infection within the initial 20 weeks, the likelihood of it resulting in congenital Varicella syndrome is less than 3%. Neonatal Varicella can occur if there is an infection during the final trimester of pregnancy unless there is a gap of more than 7 days between the appearance of a rash in the mother and delivery. During this time, antibodies can pass through the placenta, resulting in a mild or unnoticed infection in the newborn. Given this circumstance, it is imperative to promptly administer Varicella immunoglobulin (VZIG) to the infant following delivery.

9.6.1.7. Management in Custody

Employees who have contracted chicken pox should refrain from coming to work until the conclusion of the contagious phase, which typically lasts around 7 to 14 days. Individuals who have not developed immunity to the disease or have no previous history of the disease should get in touch with the assigned occupational health physician. If feasible, individuals who are afflicted with an illness should not be held in detention, particularly pregnant women. If this situation cannot be avoided, then staff members who are not immune or who have compromised immune systems should refrain from entering the cell or having close contact with the detainee.

Individuals who are not immune due to immunocompromisation or pregnancy and have been exposed to chickenpox should consult a medical expert or receive VZIG treatment. Immunocompromised individuals with chicken pox should receive Aciclovir, or a similar antiviral medication, promptly. It is important to take into account individuals who are 15 years old or older, as they have a higher likelihood of experiencing complications.

Individuals who are suspected of experiencing severe complications should be immediately referred to a hospital.

9.6.2. Herpes Zoster (Shingles)

9.6.2.1. Epidemiology

Following a bout of chicken pox, the virus remains inactive in the dorsal root or cranial nerve ganglia but can reactivate and usually affects a single dermatome. The specific location of involvement is determined by the sensory ganglion that is initially affected. Shingles is more prevalent among individuals aged 50 and above unless they have a weakened immune system, in which case it can occur at a younger age. The latter group is also more vulnerable to subsequent attacks and the involvement of multiple dermatomes. Bilateral zoster is an even more uncommon occurrence, but it does not have any correlation with increased mortality rates.

In the United Kingdom, the estimated occurrence rate is between 1.2 and 3.4 per 1,000 person-years.

9.6.2.2. Symptoms

A prodromal period characterized by paranesthesia and burning or shooting pains in the affected segment may occur. Subsequently, a cluster of vesicles typically emerges. Occasionally, the vesicles do not manifest and the individual only experiences pain. This condition is referred to as zoster sine herpete. In immunocompromised individuals, the duration of the disease may be extended and there is a possibility of the disease spreading, although it is uncommon for it to result in death.

The severity of shingles during pregnancy is typically mild. The fetus is only impacted if viremia happens before the maternal antibody being able to pass through the placenta.

9.6.2.3. Complications

The most common complication of shingles is post-herpetic neuralgia occurring in about 10% of cases. It is defined as pain lasting more than 120 days from rash onset. It is more frequent in people over 50 and can lead to depression. It is rare in children including the immunocompromised. Infection of the brain includes encephalitis, involvement of motor neurons leading to ptosis, paralysis of the hand, facial palsy or contralateral hemiparesis. Involvement of the oculomotor division of the trigeminal ganglion can cause serious eye problems including corneal scarring.

9.6.2.4. Period of Infectivity

Shingles is far less infectious than chicken pox and is only considered to be infectious up to 3 days after lesions appear.

9.6.2.5. Routes of Transmission

Shingles is only infectious following prolonged contact with lesions. Unlike chickenpox, airborne transmission is not a risk.

9.6.2.6. At-Risk Groups

Immunocompromised individuals may experience the reactivation of the latent virus and subsequently develop shingles. Individuals who have not previously contracted primary Varicella are susceptible to acquiring chicken pox after prolonged direct exposure to shingles.

Contrary to common belief, it is false that individuals with a healthy immune system who have had chicken pox will develop shingles when exposed to either chicken pox or shingles. Such events are purely coincidental unless there is a decrease in immunity.

9.6.2.7. Management in Custody

Employees who have shingles should refrain from coming to work until the skin lesions have completely healed, unless they are able to adequately cover the affected areas. Staff who have previously contracted chicken pox possess immunity, including pregnant women, and are therefore not susceptible to the disease. If individuals are not immune (typically defined as those without a prior history of chickenpox), they should refrain from prolonged contact with detainees who have shingles. Pregnant women who do not have immunity should completely avoid any form of contact.

Individuals who are being held in custody and have an illness may be detained, and any visible sores or wounds should be covered. There is ample evidence to support the fact that receiving timely treatment lessens the intensity of the illness, shortens the period of viral shedding, speeds up the healing of lesions, and decreases the severity and duration of pain. Additionally, it decreases the probability of developing post-herpetic neuralgia. Immediate administration of Famciclovir (500 mg three times a day for a duration of 7 days, for instance) is recommended if symptoms appear within 3 days. Additionally, it should be taken into account after this period whether the detainee is above the age of 50. Pregnant detainees who have shingles can be assured that the risk to both the mother and the unborn child is minimal. It is advisable to seek expert advice before starting treatment for the mother.

9.6.3. Scabies

9.6.3.1. Epidemiology

The *Sarcoptes scabiei* mite, a minuscule parasitic organism, has been plaguing humans for more than 2,500 years. According to experts, the number of cases worldwide each year is estimated to be over 300 million. The female mite rapidly penetrates the skin, particularly in areas such as the hands, feet, and male genitalia, within approximately 2.5 minutes. Eggs are deposited and subsequently hatch into larvae that migrate to the skin surface as recently formed mites.

9.6.3.2. Symptoms

The mite induces severe pruritus, which is frequently exacerbated during nighttime and intensified by high temperatures and humidity. The irritation extends beyond the initial site of infection as a result of an allergic response to the excrement of mites. The irritation may endure for approximately 2 weeks following treatment but can be relieved by antihistamines.

Crusted scabies is an extremely severe manifestation of the disease. Extensive regions of the body may be affected. The crusts conceal numerous live mites and eggs, rendering them challenging to address. Norwegian scabies, also known as crusted scabies, is more prevalent among older individuals or those with weakened immune systems, particularly individuals with HIV.

9.6.3.3. Incubation Period

Following primary exposure, it takes about 2–6 weeks before the onset of itching. However, further exposures reduce the incubation time to around 1–4 days.

9.6.3.4. Period of Infectivity

Without treatment, this is assumed to be indefinite. With treatment, the person should be considered infectious until the mites and eggs are destroyed – usually 7–10 days. Crusted scabies is highly infectious.

9.6.3.5. Management in Custody

Due to the mode of transmission being direct skin-to-skin contact with an infected individual, it is advisable to wear gloves when interacting with individuals who are suspected of being infested. Typically, extended contact is required for transmission, unless the individual has crusted Scabies, which facilitates easier transmission. The risk of transmission is significantly higher in households where there is a high likelihood of repeated or prolonged contact.

Given that mites can endure in bedding or clothing for a maximum of 24 hours, it is advisable to wear gloves while handling these items. Bedding should be treated using one of the aforementioned methods. Professional cleaning of the cell is necessary only in instances of crusted scabies.

9.6.3.6. Treatment

Permethrin cream (5%) or aqueous Malathion (0.5%) are the recommended treatments for scabies. Both treatments must be applied to the entire body and left on for a minimum of 8 hours for permethrin and 24 hours for Malathion before being washed off. Lindane is no longer the preferred treatment option due to potential pregnancy complications.

While treatment in custody may not be feasible, it should be taken into account when the detainee is suspected to have Norwegian scabies.

9.6.4. Head Lice

1. **General Information:** Like scabies, head lice occur worldwide and are found in the hair close to the scalp. The eggs or nits cling to the hair and are difficult to remove, but are not harmful. If you see nits then you can be sure that lice are also present. The latter is best seen when the hair is wet. The lice bite the scalp and suck blood causing intense irritation and itching.
2. **Route of Transmission:** They can only be passed from direct hair-to-hair contact.
3. **Management in Custody:** Gloves are required solely for the purpose of examining the head. There is no need to clean the cell after use, as the lice reside on or near the skin. Bedding may contain shed skin and

should be handled with gloves and either washed or burned.

If live lice are present, treatment is necessary, either through physical removal using a comb or by applying an insecticide. The latter option may be more feasible in terms of custody arrangements. The application of a 0.5% solution of Malathion in water to dry hair is recommended, followed by rinsing after 12 hours. Subsequently, the hair should be cleansed with shampoo in the usual manner.

9.6.5. Crabs or Body Lice

1. **General Information:** These organisms are typically more prevalent in the hair located in the pubic area, armpits, chest, and legs. Additionally, eyelashes and eyebrows may also be affected. They are linked to individuals who do not engage in regular bathing or changing of clothes. The individual typically experiences severe pruritus or irritation.
2. **Routes of Transmission:** The primary mode of transmission is through direct person-to-person contact, although it is worth noting that eggs can adhere to fibers, necessitating cautious handling of clothing and bedding.
3. **Management in Custody:** Staff should always wear gloves if they are likely to come into contact with any hirsute body part. Clothing or bedding should be handled with gloves and either laundered or incinerated.

Treatment of a detainee in custody is good in theory but probably impractical as the whole body has to be treated.

9.6.6. Fleas

1. **General Information:** Fleas lay eggs on floors, carpets and bedding. In the UK, most fleabites come from cats or dogs. The eggs and larvae fleas can survive for months and are reactivated in response to animal or human activity. Since animal fleas jump off humans after biting, most detainees with fleabites will not have fleas, unless they are human fleas.
2. **Management in Custody:** Treatment is only necessary if fleas are seen. After use, the cell should be vacuumed and cleaned with a proprietary insecticide. Any bedding should be removed wearing gloves, bagged and either laundered or incinerated.

9.6.7. Bedbugs

1. **General Information:** Bedbugs live and lay eggs on walls, floors, furniture and bedding. If you look carefully, fecal tracks may be seen on hard surfaces. If they are present for long enough, then they emit a distinct odor. Bedbugs are rarely found on the person but may be brought in on clothing or other personal effects.
2. **Symptoms:** Bedbugs bite at night and can cause sleep disturbance.
3. **Management in Custody:** The detainee does not need to be treated, but the cell should be deemed out of use until it can be vacuumed and professionally cleaned with an insecticide solution. Any bedding or clothing should be handled with gloves and disposed of as appropriate.

9.6.8. Methicillin-Resistant Staphylococcus aureus

9.6.8.1. Epidemiology

Staphylococcus aureus is frequently present on the skin or in the nasal passages of individuals who are in good health. Around 25–30% of the population is harboring the bacteria, but they remain in good health. Occasionally, the bacteria can result in minor skin infections that typically do not necessitate antibiotic treatment. However, more serious problems can occur, e.g., infection of surgical wounds, drug injection sites, osteomyelitis, pneumonia or septicemia. Over the past five decades, there has been a progressive rise in the resistance of bacteria to penicillin-based antibiotics, and in the last two decades, this resistance has extended to a growing range of alternative antibiotics. Methicillin-resistant S. aureus (MRSA) refers to bacteria that are resistant to multiple antibiotics.

Methicillin-resistant *Staphylococcus aureus* (MRSA) is widely distributed across the globe. Similar to non-resistant staphylococci, it can go unnoticed as a source in individuals who are colonized, but it can also cause clinical illness. It is more prevalent among the elderly, individuals with weakened health or compromised immune systems, or those with open wounds. Since 1981, there have been reports of groups of skin infections caused by MRSA among injecting drug users in America. More recently, similar strains have been discovered in the UK among injecting drug users in the community. This is especially important for forensic physicians when they are treating sores in injecting drug users. Individuals with a fully functioning immune system seldom contract MRSA and should not be regarded as being susceptible to the infection. From April 2003 to December 2008, there were a total of 74 documented instances of community-acquired MRSA among individuals who inject drugs in England and Wales.

9.6.8.2. Route of Transmission

The bacteria are usually spread via the hands of staff after contact with colonized or infected detainees or devices, items (e.g., bedding, towels, soiled dressings) or environmental surfaces that have been contaminated with MRSA-containing body fluids.

9.6.8.3. Management in Custody

Standard precautions should be implemented for both confirmed and suspected cases, including all abscesses/ulcers in injecting drug users being treated as infectious. Personnel must don gloves when coming into contact with mucous membranes, compromised skin, blood or other bodily fluids, or any objects that may be contaminated. Individuals should be actively encouraged to cleanse their hands using an antimicrobial substance, regardless of whether or not they have used gloves. Following use, gloves should be discarded in a yellow "hazard" bag and should not come into contact with any surfaces. It is recommended to exclusively wear masks and gowns during procedures that produce aerosols of blood or other bodily fluids. Given the low probability of this situation occurring in the custodial environment, it is unnecessary to have them. It is advisable to wear gloves when handling bedding or clothing, and all items should be discarded properly. Immediate attention should be given to the covering of any exposed wounds. If there is a possibility of contamination, it is advisable to have the cell cleaned by professionals after use.

9.6.9. Other Bacteria Associated with Abscess Formation in Injecting Drug Users

9.6.9.1. Epidemiology

In the past 10 years, there has been a growing recognition of the bacterial flora that inhabit injection sites, which could potentially cause severe infections that could be fatal. In 1997, there was a sudden rise in needle abscesses caused by a genetically identical strain of Group A Streptococcus among intravenous drug users who were hospitalized in Berne, Switzerland. A recent study conducted in the UK revealed that the most prevalent strain is *S. aureus*, while Streptococcus species account for slightly less than one-fifth of the total (50% being beta-hemolytic streptococci). There have also been reports of both non-sporing and sporing anaerobes (e.g., Bacteroides and Clostridia species including *Clostridium botulinum*). From a numerical standpoint, injecting drug use accounted for 20% of Group A streptococcal infections in the United Kingdom during the 2003–2004 period, making it a significant risk factor. In recent times, there has been a consistent decrease in the number of cases each year.

Specifically, in the year 2000, laboratories in Glasgow were documenting instances of *C. novyi* being found in intravenous drug users (IDUs) who were experiencing a "severe unexplained illness." As of June 12, 2000, there were a total of 42 reported cases, with 18 being definite and 24 being probable. A definitive case was characterized as an intravenous drug user (IDU) exhibiting both severe localized and systemic inflammatory responses. A probable case was defined as an intravenous drug user (IDU) who arrived at the hospital with an abscess or notable inflammation at an injection site. Additionally, the individual exhibited either a severe inflammatory response at or near the injection site or a severe systemic reaction resulting in multiorgan failure and a high white cell count.

In the United Kingdom, the occurrence of *C. botulinum* in infected injection sites is a recently observed phenomenon. Until the conclusion of 1999, the PHLS did not receive any reported cases. Since then, there has been a rise in the number of reported cases in the UK and Eire, with a total of 13 cases being reported since the start of 2002. These cases are believed to be linked to tainted batches of heroin. The concurrent administration of cocaine enhances the risk by promoting anaerobic conditions. Anaerobic flora in wounds may have serious consequences for the detainee but the risk of transmission to staff is virtually non-existent. By the end of 2008, a cumulative total of 132 suspected cases had been reported from the United Kingdom, with 86% of cases occurring in England. A total of four cases were reported exclusively in the year 2008.

In December 2009, two injecting drug users in Scotland died from anthrax-contaminated heroin. Following this, two further deaths occurred in England in February 2010. An alert was issued first by the Department of Health and then, by the National Treatment Agency warning any drug user of the possible risks. Spores from *Bacillus anthracis* can contaminate heroin without any obvious signs. Anthrax can be acquired by injecting, smoking or inhaling heroin. Obvious symptoms include excessive swelling and redness at injection sites, fever, headache or shortness of breath when the heroin is smoked. Users are advised to go straight to the Emergency Department if they are at all worried. Such infections with spore-forming bacteria will always occur from time to time. Healthcare practitioners should be mindful at all times.

9.6.9.2. Management in Custody

Personnel must be instructed to wear gloves when handling detainees who have infected skin sites oozing pus or serum. Additionally, any used dressings discovered in the cell should be properly disposed of in the designated yellow bag labeled as "clinical waste" located in the medical room. Similarly, it is necessary to place any bedding in a bag and clean it through laundering or dispose of it by incineration once it has been used. Once the detainee has left, the cell should be declared unusable and thoroughly sanitized.

It is imperative for the healthcare professional overseeing the detainee to promptly cleanse and bandage any exposed wounds in order to mitigate the risk of infection transmission. If there is abscess formation, signs of cellulitis, or if the detainee is systemically unwell, it may be suitable to initiate a course of antibiotics. Nevertheless, infections frequently manifest as low-grade due to the repeated penetration of the skin, which damages the skin, venous, and lymphatic systems. Common manifestations in such instances encompass lymphedema, enlarged lymph glands, and hyperpigmentation of the skin in the affected region. Fever may or may not be present, but septicemia is rare unless the person has a weakened immune system, such as being HIV positive. Co-Amoxiclav is the preferred treatment due to its broad coverage of staphylococci, streptococci, and anaerobes. The dosage administered depends on the severity of the infection.

Necrotizing fasciitis and septic thrombophlebitis are infrequent yet perilous complications of intravenous drug use. Any individual who is suspected of either of these conditions requires medical attention at a hospital. It is important to provide guidance on harm reduction as well. This entails promoting the use of smoking as a preferable alternative for drug users, as opposed to injecting. Alternatively, it involves advising them to refrain from injecting drugs into their muscles or skin. While many individuals who use drugs by injection are conscious of the dangers associated with sharing needles, they may not be fully aware that sharing any equipment related to drug use can also pose a significant risk. It is advisable to use a minimal quantity of citric acid to dissolve the heroin, as excessive acid can harm the tissue beneath the skin, creating an environment where bacteria can thrive. Drugs should be injected at different sites using fresh works for each injection. It is especially crucial to consider this when "snowballing" because crack cocaine produces an environment without oxygen. Medical help should be requested if any injection site becomes painful and swollen or shows signs of pus collecting under the skin. Since intravenous drug users are at increased risk of acquiring HBV and HAV, they should be informed that vaccination against both diseases is advisable.

Another serious but relatively rare problem is the risk of broken needles in veins. Embolization can take anything from hours to days or even longer if it is not removed. Complications may include endocarditis, pericarditis or pulmonary abscesses. IVDUs should be advised to seek medical help as soon as possible, and should such a case present in custody, then send the detainee straight to the hospital.

9.6.10. Management of Human and Dog Bites

The Forensic Physician May Encounter Bites in Four Circumstances

1. During the examination of victims of assault (both children and adults) where presentation is more likely to be late;
2. Among police officers bitten during the arrest of a detainee;
3. In detainees during the arrest if dogs have been used; and
4. Where detainees have been involved in a fight either around the time of arrest or earlier

With any bite that has penetrated the skin, the goals of therapy are to minimize soft tissue deformity and to prevent or treat an infection.

9.6.10.1. Epidemiology

In the UK and USA, dog bites represent approximately three-quarters of all bites presented to Accident and Emergency departments. A single dog bite can produce up to 220 psi of crush force in addition to the torsional forces as the dog shakes its head. This can result in massive tissue damage. Human bites may cause classical bites or puncture wounds (e.g., impact of fists on teeth) resulting in crush injuries.

9.6.10.2. Rates and Risks of Infection

Approximately 10–30% of dog bites and 9–50% of human bites result in infection. Contrast this with approximately 1–12% of non-bite wounds treated in Accident and Emergency Departments.

Puncture wounds, hand injuries, full-thickness wounds, wounds requiring debridement, and those involving joints, tendons, ligaments or fractures all carry a heightened risk of infection.

Additional medical conditions such as diabetes, asplenia, chronic edema of the area, liver dysfunction, the presence of a prosthetic valve or joint, and an immunocompromised state can also heighten the likelihood of infection.

9.6.10.3. Other Complications of Bites

Infection may spread beyond the initial site, leading to septic arthritis, osteomyelitis, endocarditis, peritonitis, septicemia and meningitis. Inflammation of the tendons or synovial lining of joints may also occur. If enough force is used, bones may be fractured or the wounds may be permanently disfiguring.

9.6.10.4. Initial Management

An evaluation regarding the necessity of hospital treatment should be conducted promptly. Always seek medical attention if the wound is experiencing profuse bleeding or if it does not cease bleeding when pressure is applied. Immediate referral is necessary for penetrating bites that involve arteries, nerves, muscles, tendons, hands or feet, or result in a moderate-to-serious facial wound, as well as crush injuries.

If it is deemed suitable for the management of custody, inquire about the individual's present tetanus vaccine status, HBV vaccination status, and any known allergies to antibiotics.

Wounds that have breached the skin should be irrigated with 0.9% (isotonic) sodium chloride or Ringer's lactate solution in preference to antiseptics, as the latter may delay wound healing.

Observe for any clinical indications of infection, such as redness, swelling, inflammation, pus discharge, or swollen lymph nodes in the surrounding area. Apply a clean, non-sticky dressing to the wound. Wound closure is generally discouraged due to evidence indicating that it may heighten the likelihood of infection. This is especially applicable to wounds that are not on the face, deep puncture wounds, hand bites, wounds that are clinically infected, and wounds that occurred more than 6–12 hours before seeking medical attention. Head and neck wounds in areas that are important for appearance can be stitched if they are less than 12 hours old and show no signs of infection.

9.6.10.5. Pathogens Involved

1. Bacteria
    i. **Dog Bites:** *Pasteurella canis, P. multocida, S. aureus*, other staphylococci, *Streptococcus* species, *Eikenella corrodens, Corynebacterium* species and anaerobes including *Bacteroides fragilis* and *C. tetani*.

   ii. **Human Bites:** *Streptococcus* species, *S. aureus, E. corrodens*, and anaerobes including *Bacteroides* (often penicillin resistant), peptostreptococci species, and *C. tetani*. TB and syphilis may also be transmitted.

2. Viruses
   i. **Dog Bites:** Outside of the UK, Australia and New Zealand, rabies should be considered. In the USA, domestic dogs are mostly vaccinated against rabies, and police dogs have to be vaccinated, so the most common source is from raccoons, skunks and bats.
   ii. **Human Bites:** HBV, HCV, HIV, and herpes simplex.

9.6.10.6. Antibiotic Prophylaxis

Antibiotics are typically unnecessary for wounds that are over 2 days old and show no signs of infection. Additionally, superficial wounds that are not infected and are evaluated early can be left open to heal naturally in individuals who are compliant with their treatment and have no significant underlying health conditions. Antibiotics should be prescribed for high-risk wounds that affect the hands, feet, face, tendons, ligaments, joints, or suspected fractures. They should also be given for any penetrating bite injury in individuals with diabetes, asplenia, cirrhosis, or immunosuppression.

Co-amoxiclav, which consists of amoxicillin and clavulanic acid, is the recommended initial treatment for mild to moderate infections caused by dog or human bites that are being managed in primary care. The recommended dosage for adults is 500/125 mg three times a day, and for children, it is 40 mg per kilogram of body weight three times a day, based on the amoxicillin component. The duration of treatment should be maintained for a period of 10 to 14 days. It is the primary drug used for prevention when the same dosage regimen should be prescribed for a period of 5–7 days. If the person has a confirmed or suspected penicillin allergy, alternative antibiotics such as tetracycline (e.g., doxycycline 100 mg twice daily) and metronidazole (500 mg three times daily), or an aminoglycoside (e.g., erythromycin) and metronidazole can be prescribed. In the United Kingdom, the utilization of doxycycline is limited to individuals who are 12 years of age and older, while in the United States, it is restricted to those who are 8 years of age and older. Pregnant women should seek specialist advice.

Individuals experiencing a severe infection or those who are medically unstable should be directed to a hospital for further evaluation and treatment. The administration of the tetanus vaccine is recommended if the initial series of doses or the most recent booster was administered over a decade ago. Human tetanus immunoglobulin should be administered in cases of tetanus-prone wounds, such as those caused by soil contamination, puncture wounds, signs of devitalized tissue, or wounds that are more than 6 hours old. If an individual has not received any immunization for tetanus or is uncertain about their tetanus status, it is recommended to administer a complete three-dose course, with each dose spaced at least one month apart.

9.7. Infections Transmitted Through the Respiratory Route

9.7.1. General Information

Respiratory tract infections are prevalent and typically have a mild and self-limiting course.

However, they may necessitate symptomatic treatment with paracetamol or a non-steroidal anti-inflammatory drug. The viruses responsible for these illnesses are primarily rhinoviruses (80%) and coronaviruses (20%), which cause the common cold. Other viruses such as adenoviruses, influenza and parainfluenza are also involved. Additionally, enteroviruses are more prevalent during the summer and early autumn. Particular emphasis should be placed on individuals with asthma or compromised immune systems, as infection in these individuals can have more severe consequences, especially if it affects the lower respiratory tract.

The subsequent section comprises respiratory pathogens that are particularly noteworthy due to their potential to endanger both detainees and staff members who have close contact with them.

9.7.2. Meningococcal Meningitis (Neisseria meningitidis)

9.7.2.1. General Information and Epidemiology

Neisseria meningitidis is classified into five serogroups: A, B, C, W135, and Y. The incidence of the various types differs from one country to another. Currently, there is no existing vaccine for type B, however, there are two other vaccines (C and ACWY) that are currently accessible. In general, 10% of the population in the UK are carriers of *N. meningitidis*, with the percentage rising to 25% among individuals aged 15–19.

In the United Kingdom, the majority of meningitis cases are sporadic, with less than 5% occurring as clusters or outbreaks among school children. From 1996 to 2000, the majority of cases (59%) were classified as group B, while group C accounted for 36% of the cases. The remaining 5% of cases were attributed to W135 and A. There is a cyclical fluctuation with a pronounced surge in cases during winter and a decrease during summer. The most vulnerable age group is children under the age of 5, with the highest occurrence of risk observed in infants under 1 year old. There is a second peak that happens in the age group of 15 to 19 years old. In Sub-Saharan Africa, the disease is more common during the dry season, but in many countries, there is a constant presence of the disease throughout the year. The serogroup A is the most common.

In the UK, routine immunization against group C was implemented in November 1999 for individuals up to the age of 18, as well as for all first-year university students. Subsequently, the scope of this has been expanded to encompass individuals who are below the age of 25. Due to the implementation of the vaccination program, there has been a significant decrease of 90% in group C cases among individuals under the age of 18 and an 82% decrease in cases among those under the age of 1.

In 2000, there was an occurrence of meningitis caused by serogroup W135 among the pilgrims participating in the Hajj. Instances were documented in numerous countries, including the UK. In the UK, there is now an official requirement to be vaccinated with the quadrivalent vaccine (ACWY Vax) before going on a pilgrimage (Hajj or Umra), but illegal immigrants may enter the country who have not been vaccinated.

9.7.2.2. Symptoms

After a period of 3–5 days of incubation, the disease may start either gradually with mild initial symptoms or suddenly and intensely. Initial indications consist of general discomfort, elevated body temperature, and the act of expelling stomach contents forcefully. Symptoms such as severe headache, stiffness in the neck, sensitivity to light, feeling sleepy, and the appearance of a rash may occur. The rash may exhibit petechiae or purpura and typically does not fade when pressure is applied. Meningitis in infants tends to have a gradual and subtle onset, and may not exhibit the typical symptoms. Septicemia is the main characteristic in around 15–20% of cases. Despite receiving prompt antibiotic treatment, the mortality rate is 3–5% for meningitis and 15–20% for individuals with septicemia.

9.7.2.3. Period of Infectivity

A person should be considered infectious until the bacteria are no longer present in nasal discharge. With treatment, this is usually approximately 24 h.

9.7.2.4. Routes of Transmission

The disease is spread through infected droplets or direct contact from carriers or those who are clinically ill. It requires prolonged and close contact, so there is a greater risk for people who share accommodation, utensils, and kisses. It must also be remembered that unprotected mouth-to-mouth resuscitation can also transmit disease.

9.7.2.5. Management in Custody

It is impossible to determine whether a detainee is a carrier. However, the likelihood of contracting an infection from an infected and ill individual is minimal unless they have performed mouth-to-mouth resuscitation. Any staff member who believes they have been exposed to a potential danger should promptly notify the Occupational Health Department (or equivalent) or the nearest emergency department to receive a vaccination.

If mouth-to-mouth resuscitation has been performed, it is advisable to administer prophylactic antibiotics before receiving vaccination. Rifampicin, ciprofloxacin, and ceftriaxone are viable treatment options, but ciprofloxacin offers several distinct advantages. A solitary dosage of 500 mg (for adults and children above 12 years old) is sufficient and exhibits fewer adverse effects and contraindications compared to rifampicin. Administration of ceftriaxone necessitates injection, making it less suitable for use in custodial environments.

If a staff member is pregnant, it is advisable to consult with a specialist obstetrician before using ciprofloxacin, as it is not recommended in such cases.

Individuals who frequently interact with undocumented immigrants, particularly those from the Middle East or Sub-Saharan Africa, such as immigration officials, detention center staff, medical professionals, and interpreters, should strongly consider receiving the ACWY Vax vaccination. A solitary injection confers immunity for a duration of 3 years. Individuals who are suspected of having a disease should be immediately transported to a hospital for further evaluation and treatment.

9.7.3. Tuberculosis

9.7.3.1. Prevalence and Epidemiology

Tuberculosis (TB) in humans is a result of being infected with either *Mycobacterium tuberculosis*, *M. bovis*, or *M. africanum*. It is classified as a notifiable disease according to the specific laws of different countries. In the UK, it falls under the jurisdiction of the Public Health (Control of Disease) Act 1984. In 1993, the World Health Organization (WHO) designated tuberculosis (TB) as a worldwide crisis, with approximately 7–8 million new cases and 3 million deaths reported annually. The majority of these cases and deaths were concentrated in Asia and Africa. Nevertheless, these statistics are prone to underestimation as they rely on the precision of reporting, and in economically disadvantaged nations, the surveillance systems are frequently insufficient due to insufficient funding. In the UK, there has been a lack of consistency in reporting, especially when it comes to individuals who have a simultaneous infection with HIV. Until 1997, certain physicians faced a dilemma regarding confidentiality. However, this issue was resolved when the codes of practice were revised to promote reporting with the patient's consent.

Due to the introduction of rapid identification tests and treatment, as well as the implementation of BCG vaccination for prevention, the incidence of tuberculosis decreased in the United Kingdom during the first half of the twentieth century. Nevertheless, starting from the early 1990s, there has been a gradual rise in numbers, with approximately 6,800 cases being reported in 2002. In 1998, 56% of the reported cases were attributed to individuals who were not born in the UK, while 3% were linked to HIV infection.

London has been identified as a region with a substantial issue. The reasons for this can be attributed to several factors, including the population's high mobility, the presence of diverse ethnic groups, a significant prevalence of HIV, and the emergence of drug-resistant strains (1.3% in 1998 – PHLS unpublished data – Mycobnet).

In 1985, a comparable image was first discovered in the United States, coinciding with a reversal of a persistent decline. Nevertheless, during the period from 1986 to 1992, there was a rise in the number of cases from 22,201 to 26,673. In addition, hospitals in New York City and Miami experienced significant occurrences of multi-drug-resistant TB (MDR-TB). Relevant factors contributing to the overall increase included the emergence of HIV, the growing influx of immigrants from countries with a high incidence of tuberculosis, and, potentially more importantly, the discontinuation of specific federal funding for control efforts in 1972. This resulted in the collapse of the public health infrastructure for tuberculosis (TB) control. Since 1992, there has been a reversal in the trend as the CDC allocated a majority of its funds to tuberculosis surveillance and treatment programs in states and major cities. Between 1992 and 2001, there was an average annual decline of 7.3%. However, in the subsequent year, this decline was reduced to 2%, suggesting that there was no reason to be overly confident. The World Health Organization (WHO) has taken proactive measures by reallocating funding to countries that are facing the greatest need. The global partnership Stop TB was established in October 1998 to coordinate all aspects of tuberculosis (TB) control. By 2002, the partnership had garnered membership from more than 150 countries. A goal was established to identify a minimum of 70% of contagious cases by the year 2005.

The acquisition of tuberculosis infection does not inevitably result in disease, as the infection has the potential to heal spontaneously. The disease may not show symptoms for a period of weeks or months, or the infection may remain inactive for years before becoming active again later in life, particularly if the person's health deteriorates or their immune system is weakened. Contrary to commonly held beliefs, most cases of tuberculosis in individuals with a healthy immune system go unnoticed. Out of the cases that have been reported, 75% primarily affect the lungs. However, non-respiratory involvement (such as in the bones, heart, kidneys, or brain) or dissemination of the disease (known as miliary TB) are more frequently observed in immigrant ethnic groups and individuals with weakened immune systems. Additionally, they have a higher probability of developing strains that are resistant. Within the overall population, there is a projected 10% chance that a tuberculosis infection will develop into a disease throughout a person's lifetime.

There has been a rise in the incidence of tuberculosis cases linked to HIV, either as a result of new infection or reactivation. HIV-positive individuals with a lifetime risk exceeding 50% are more prone to the progression of tuberculosis infection into active TB. Tuberculosis can also exacerbate HIV infection by causing an elevation in viral load. Hence, early detection is crucial, although it can be challenging due to the possibility of pulmonary TB displaying nonspecific characteristics, such as bilateral, unilateral, or lower lobe shadowing.

9.7.3.2. Symptoms of Pulmonary TB

After an incubation of 4–12 weeks, symptoms may develop (see Table 9.6).

Table 9.6. Symptoms of TB

Cough lasting >3 weeks
Fatigue
Anorexia and weight loss
Fever and night sweats
Mild hemoptysis (rusty colored)
Cough with phlegm
Swollen lymph glands

Source: Nicholson F. (2011). Infectious diseases: The role of the forensic physician. Clinical Forensic Medicine, 295–340.

9.7.3.3. Routes of Transmission

The main route is airborne through infected droplets, but prolonged or close contact is needed. Non-respiratory disease is not considered a risk unless the *Mycobacterium* is aerosolized under exceptional circumstances (e.g., during surgery) or there are open abscesses.

9.7.3.4. Period of Infectivity

A person is considered infectious as long as viable bacilli are found in induced sputum. Untreated or incompletely treated people may be intermittently sputum-positive for years.

Following 2 weeks of appropriate treatment, the individual is usually considered as non-infectious. This period is often extended for treatment of MDR-TB or for those with concomitant HIV. Patient compliance also plays an important factor.

9.7.3.5. At-Risk Groups

The risk of infection is directly proportional to the degree of exposure. More severe disease occurs in the malnourished, or the immunocompromised (e.g., HIV, etc.) and substance misusers.

Immunocompromised people are at special risk of MDR-TB or *Mycobacterium avium-intracellulare* (MAI).

9.7.3.6. Management in Custody

Employees who are infected with a disease should refrain from coming to work until they have completed their treatment and their consecutive sputum samples no longer contain bacilli. Staff members who have been vaccinated with BCG and have come into contact with the disease have a reduced likelihood of acquiring the disease. However, it is advisable for them to minimize the duration of time spent in the cell. Individuals who have not been administered the Bacillus Calmette-Guérin (BCG) vaccine or those with weakened immune systems should make an effort to minimize any form of interaction with the detainee. Detainees with MAI do not pose a threat to a staff member unless the staff member has a weakened immune system. Pregnant staff members, irrespective of their BCG status or type of tuberculosis, should completely refrain from any form of contact.

Individuals who engage in mouth-to-mouth resuscitation with someone who has untreated or suspected pulmonary tuberculosis should be considered as household contacts. They should promptly inform Occupational Health or their general practitioner if no other means of communication is available. They should also receive education regarding the symptoms of tuberculosis. Individuals who are expected to have frequent interactions with people who are at risk of tuberculosis should receive the BCG vaccine, regardless of their age, even though there is evidence indicating that the effectiveness of BCG decreases when administered in adulthood. This exemption does not pertain to individuals with weakened immune systems or women who are currently pregnant. If the situation is the latter, it is advisable to postpone vaccination until after giving birth.

Detainees who have a disease, whether suspected or diagnozed, and have not received treatment or have incomplete treatment, should be held in custody for the shortest possible duration. Typically, individuals with weakened immune systems who have tuberculosis (TB) are too sick to be held in detention. However, if they are detained, it is important to recognize that they are more likely to spread the disease to staff members. Detainees who have a disease should be advised to consistently cover their mouth and nose when coughing and sneezing.

Personnel must don gloves when coming into contact with the detainee and when handling garments and bedding. After using any bedding, it should be placed in a bag and either washed or burned. The cell should be considered inoperable until it has been properly ventilated and decontaminated by professionals, despite the lack of concrete evidence to support the possibility of transmission through this pathway.

9.7.4. Severe Acute Respiratory Syndrome

9.7.4.1. General Information

On March 14, 2003, the World Health Organization (WHO) issued a worldwide alert to health authorities regarding a novel form of pneumonia known as Severe Acute Respiratory Syndrome (SARS). The initial case is thought to have originated in the Guandong province of China on 16 November 2002. The etiological agent was identified as a novel coronavirus – SARS-CoV. As of June 2003, a total of 8,422 cases had been reported from 31 countries, resulting in 916 deaths. China, including Hong Kong, Taiwan, and Macao, accounted for around 92% of the reported cases. The mortality rate ranged from less than 1% in individuals under 24 years old, to 6% in those aged 25–44, 15% in the 44–64 age group, and over 50% in individuals 65 years or older. On July 5, 2003, the World Health Organization (WHO) announced that the final instance of SARS transmission among humans had been halted, leading to the removal of the ban on all countries. Nevertheless, they cautioned that everyone needed to stay watchful, as there was still a chance of a resurgence of SARS. This prediction was indeed confirmed, with reports continuing until May 2004. Subsequently, there have been no additional documented instances. Our understanding of the epidemiology and ecology of SARS-CoV and the disease it causes is still limited. However, the knowledge gained from the previous outbreak has allowed us to quickly control the spread of the disease, which is evident from the low number of cases reported since December. As of now, no targeted treatment or preventive vaccine has been developed.

9.7.4.2. Incubation Period and Symptoms

The incubation period of SARS is brief, typically lasting 3–6 days (with a maximum of 10 days). Despite the excessive media attention during the initial outbreak, SARS is less contagious than influenza. A clinical case definition for SARS has been formulated specifically for public health purposes.

A person with a history of:

- Fever (at least 38°C)

- one of more symptoms of lower respiratory tract illness (cough, difficulty in breathing, dyspnea)
- radiographic evidence of lung infiltrates consistent with pneumonia or Respiratory Distress Syndrome, or post mortem findings of the above with no identifiable cause
- no alternative diagnosis can fully explain the illness

Laboratory tests have been developed which include detection of viral RNA by PCR from nasopharyngeal secretions or stool samples, detection of antibodies by ELISA or IFA in the blood, and viral culture from clinical specimens.

9.7.4.3. Route of Transmission

The currently available data indicates that the greatest risk of contracting the disease comes from close contact with an infected person through aerosol or infected droplets. The majority of cases occurred among hospital workers who were providing care for either an initial case or their immediate family members.

9.7.4.4. Management in Custody

Although SARS has resurfaced, the chances of encountering a case in the custodial setting at present are extremely low. Nevertheless, forensic physicians must maintain vigilance for the symptoms of SARS and stay informed about recent outbreaks. One can access daily information from the World Health Organization (WHO) through their website. If there is suspicion of SARS, it is necessary for medical personnel to wear gloves and a surgical mask while examining a suspected case. However, masks are typically not accessible in custody. Individuals who are suspected of having SARS should be promptly transported to a hospital, and personnel who have had extended and close interaction with them should be informed about the possible symptoms.

9.8. Infections Transmitted Through the Fecal-Oral Route

9.8.1. General Considerations

Diarrhea is the primary characteristic of diseases that are transmitted through the fecal-oral route, as indicated in Table 9.7. Pathogens encompass bacteria, viruses, and protozoa. Due to the multitude of causes, this chapter cannot comprehensively address all of them. It is safest to treat all diarrhea as infectious unless the detainee has a proven non-infectious cause (e.g., Crohn's disease, ulcerative colitis).

Table 9.7. Common Causes of Infective Diarrhea

Cause	Symptoms	Incubation	Infectivity	Notes
Campylobacter	C, F, N, V, BD	1–10 Days	Untreated – 7 weeks	Requires antibiotics
				Seek advice
				Acute phase exclude from custody

E. coli O157:H7	BD (or WD), F unusual	3–8 Days	Up to 7 days	Person to person spread
				Can be serious with TTP, HUS, dehydration
				Seek advice
Norwalk virus	N, V, D, AP, mild F	24–48 h	Up to 48 h after diarrhea stops	Mild to moderate. Self-limiting
Rotavirus	F, V, WD	24–72 h	Up to 8 days	Symptomatic treatment
			Up to 30 days in immuno-compromised	Persists in environment
Salmonella	H, AP, D, N, F, ±V	6–72 h	Days to weeks	Persistent carriage can occur
				Requires antibiotics
				Seek advice
Shigella	DY/WD, F, N, (C, V)	12–96 h	Up to 4 weeks	Usually mild in U.K
				Can be severe in IC
				Requires antibiotics in custody
				Take advice
				Person to person spread

AP Abdominal pain; H headache; BD bloody diarrhea; HUS hemolytic-uraemic syndrome; C cramps; IC immunocompromised; D diarrhea; N nausea; DY dysentery (blood and mucus); TTP thrombotic thrombocytopaenic purpura; F fever; V vomiting; WD watery diarrhea.

Source: Nicholson F. (2011). Infectious diseases: The role of the forensic physician. Clinical Forensic Medicine, 295–340.

All staff should wear gloves when in contact with the detainee or handling clothing, bedding etc., and contaminated articles should be laundered or incinerated. The cell should be professionally cleaned after use paying particular attention to the toilet area.

9.8.2. Hepatitis A

9.8.2.1. Epidemiology and Prevalence

Viral hepatitis is a global disease that has varying levels of occurrence. The prevalence is greatest in countries with low hygiene standards and where infection is persistent throughout the year. The highest occurrence of this phenomenon is observed during the autumn and winter seasons in regions with temperate climates. However, this pattern is gradually becoming less prominent.

Individuals of all age brackets are vulnerable if they lack immunity or have not received vaccination. The disease typically manifests in early childhood in developing countries, whereas the opposite is observed in countries with a higher standard of living.

From 1990 to 2000, there was a gradual decline in the number of reported cases in the UK. This can be attributed partially to enhanced quality of life and the implementation of a highly efficient vaccine. The highest prevalence is observed in the age group of individuals between 15 and 34 years old. Roughly 25% of individuals aged 40 and above possess inherent immunity, while the remaining population is vulnerable to infection.

Occasionally, there are instances of small clusters that arise due to a deterioration in hygiene. Additionally, there is a growing prevalence of HAV in homosexual or bisexual males and their respective partners. A study conducted in London in 1996, which has not been published, revealed that 23% of gay men tested positive for antibodies in their blood (Young Y et al., unpublished).

9.8.2.2. Symptoms

The clinical presentation varies from no symptoms to severe hepatitis. Unlike Hepatitis B Virus (HBV) and Hepatitis C Virus (HCV), Hepatitis A Virus (HAV) does not endure or advance to long-lasting liver harm. Childhood infections typically manifest as mild or asymptomatic, whereas infections in adults tend to be more severe.

The symptomatic infection begins suddenly with the onset of jaundice, occurring anywhere from 2 days to 3 weeks after the anicteric phase. This occurs after an incubation period of 15–50 days, with an average of 28 days. It has a similar duration and is frequently accompanied by a sudden onset of fever.

Infection with HAV can result in hospitalization across all age groups, but the likelihood of this outcome increases with age, as well as the length of hospital stay.

According to the CDC Fact sheet, the overall mortality rate is below 1%. However, approximately 15% of individuals will experience a prolonged or relapsing illness lasting 6–9 months. Fulminant hepatitis has a prevalence of less than 1%, but it is more common among individuals who are over the age of 65 or have pre-existing liver disease. The case fatality rate in hospitalized patients varies from 2% in individuals aged 50–59 to almost 13% in those aged over 70 years.

9.8.2.3. Period of Infectivity

The individual is most infectious in the 2 weeks before the onset of jaundice when they are asymptomatic. This can make control of infection difficult since the disease is not recognized.

9.8.2.4. Routes of Transmission

The main route is fecal-oral through the ingestion of contaminated water and food. It can also be transmitted by close personal contact including homosexuals practicing anal intercourse and fellatio. There is a very slight risk from blood transfusions if the donor is in the acute phase of infection. It should not be considered a risk from needlestick injuries unless clinical suspicion of HAV is high.

9.8.2.5. Risk Groups

Risk groups include the homeless, homosexuals, IVDUs, travelers abroad who have not been vaccinated, patients with chronic liver disease and chronic infection with HBV and HCV, employees and residents in day-care centers and hostels, sewage workers, laboratory technicians and those handling non-human primates.

Several large outbreaks have occurred among injecting drug users – some with an epidemiological link to prisons. Transmission occurs during the viremic phase of the illness through sharing injecting equipment and via fecal-oral routes because of poor living conditions. There have also been reports of HAV being transmitted through drugs that have been carried in the rectum. A study in Vancouver showed that 40% of injecting drug users had past infection of HAV and they also showed an increased prevalence among men who have sex with men.

9.8.2.6. Management in Custody

Employees who are ill should notify Occupational Health and refrain from working until the infectious period has ended. Individuals who have been exposed to a disease, either through contact with an infected person at home or with an infected detainee, should promptly receive preventive treatment (refer to the information below).

In order to mitigate the potential for disease transmission in custody, it is imperative for staff members to don gloves while interacting with detainees and subsequently cleanse their hands meticulously. Dispose of gloves exclusively in clinical waste bags.

Detainees who are afflicted with an illness should be held in custody for the shortest duration feasible. Patients should only be referred to the hospital if there is a strong suspicion of fulminant hepatitis. Following its use, it is imperative to isolate the cell and ensure that it undergoes thorough decontamination by trained professionals. It is necessary to use gloves when handling any bedding or clothing, and these items should be either washed or burned in accordance with local regulations. Detainees who have reported contact with a disease should receive prophylactic treatment promptly.

9.8.2.7. Prophylaxis and Treatment

Contacts of HAV should receive HAV vaccine (e.g., Havrix Monodose or Avaxim) if they have not been previously immunized or had disease. Human normal immunoglobulin (HNIG) 500 mg deep in gluteal muscle should be used in the following circumstances:

- The contact is over 50.
- Has cirrhosis or pre-existing HBV, HCV, or HDV.
- Contact has occurred >8 days but <28 days from exposure.

Staff at higher risk of coming in contact with HAV should consider being vaccinated prior to exposure. Two doses of vaccine given 6–12 months apart give at least 10 years of protection.

There is no specific treatment for HAV except supportive measures and symptomatic treatment.

9.9. Exotica

While the probability of encountering a tropical disease while in custody is low, it is important to keep in mind. For a forensic physician, it is not imperative to make a specific disease diagnosis. Their main task is to identify if the detainee or staff member is unwell and determine whether they require hospitalization (refer to Tables 9.8–9.10).

Table 9.8. Tropical Diseases that Present with Fever

Disease	Countries	Incubation	Transmission	Management
Dengue	Most hot climates	3–14 Days	Mosquito No person to person in UK	Symptomatic
Hantavirus	Eastern Europe	2 Days to 8 weeks	No person to person in UK	Symptomatic
Lassa Fever	West Africa			Hospital
Malaria	Sub-Saharan Africa SE. Asia S. America	7 Days to 1 year	Mosquito No person to person in UK	Requires urgent treatment Hospital
Typhoid	Hot climates	Up to 72 h	Oral-fecal	Requires antibiotics
Yellow fever	Sub-Saharan Africa	3–6 Days	Mosquito No person to person in UK	Hospital Parts of South America

Source: Nicholson F. (2011). Infectious diseases: The role of the forensic physician. Clinical Forensic Medicine, 295–340.

The most effective way to accomplish this is by possessing knowledge of the appropriate inquiries to pose and conducting a suitable examination. Tables 9.8–9.10 serve as a helpful reminder to avoid overlooking less common diseases.

Table 9.9. Suspicion of Exotica? History and Examination Aide Memoir

Has the detainee travelled to Africa, South East Asia, the Indian Sub-continent, Central/South America or the Far East in the last 6–12 months
Ascertain whether they received any vaccinations prior to travel and what
Ask if they took malaria prophylaxis, what type and whether they completed the course
Ask if they swam in any stagnant lakes during the trip
If yes to any of the above, ask if they have experienced any of the following symptoms:
A fever/hot or cold flushes/shivering
Diarrhea ±abdominal cramps ±blood or slime in the stool
A rash
Persistent headaches ±light sensitivity
Nausea or vomiting
Aching muscles/joints
A persistent cough (dry or productive) lasting at least 3 weeks
Take temperature
Check the skin for signs of a rash and note its nature and distribution
Check throat
Listen carefully to the lungs for signs of infection/consolidation

Source: Nicholson F. (2011). Infectious diseases: The role of the forensic physician. Clinical Forensic Medicine, 295–340.

Table 9.10. Tropical Diseases that Present with Diarrhea

Disease	Incubation	Infectivity	Transmission	Management
Amoebic Dysentery	Days to months	Years	Oral-fecal	Requires antibiotics
Cholera	Hours to 5 days	3–5 Days after recovery	Oral-fecal Vomit	Requires antibiotics
Giardia	3–25 Days	Months	Oral-fecal	Treat with tinidazole
Malaria	7 Days to 1 year	None	No person-to-person	Urgent treatment Hospital
Typhoid	Up to 72 h	Days to weeks	Oral-fecal	Requires antibiotics

Source: Nicholson F. (2011). Infectious diseases: The role of the forensic physician. Clinical Forensic Medicine, 295–340.

A Closer Look

Postmortem Detection of Hepatitis B, C, and Human Immunodeficiency Virus Genomes

Hepatitis B virus, a major cause of chronic liver disease, is detected by targeting its viral DNA. Postmortem samples often include liver tissue, blood, or other bodily fluids. Given that HBV can be present in low quantities, especially in chronic cases where the virus might be integrated into the host's genome, PCR assays are employed to ensure sensitivity and specificity. The detection process involves extracting DNA from the samples and using primers specific to HBV sequences to amplify and then quantify the viral load.

Similarly, hepatitis C virus detection focuses on RNA, given that HCV is an RNA virus. In postmortem cases, HCV RNA is often identified in blood samples or liver tissues. The process starts with RNA extraction, followed by reverse transcription to convert RNA into complementary DNA (cDNA). This cDNA is then amplified using PCR. The detection of HCV RNA is critical not only for understanding the viral load at the time of death but also for determining the stage of liver disease caused by the infection.

Human immunodeficiency virus detection in postmortem samples can be more complex due to the potential degradation of viral RNA and DNA. HIV, being a retrovirus, integrates its RNA into the host DNA, making the detection of proviral DNA a viable method. The process typically involves the extraction of DNA from tissues such as lymph nodes or blood, followed by PCR amplification of HIV-specific sequences. Additionally, detecting viral RNA in bodily fluids can provide insights into the infection status and progression.

The choice of sample and detection method often depends on the postmortem interval, as the integrity of the samples can affect the sensitivity of the assays. In cases where tissues are decomposed, specialized techniques and rigorous controls are necessary to avoid false negatives. Additionally, contamination and the quality of the samples play significant roles in ensuring accurate detection.

Therefore, the postmortem detection of HBV, HCV, and HIV genomes is a sophisticated process that requires a thorough understanding of molecular biology techniques and careful handling of forensic samples. The ability to accurately detect these viruses postmortem provides invaluable information for forensic analysis, public health monitoring, and epidemiological research, contributing significantly to our understanding of viral infections and their impact on individuals and populations.

Summary

This chapter explores the critical involvement of forensic physicians in managing infectious diseases within legal and medical frameworks. This comprehensive chapter addresses the forensic analysis of infectious disease cases, emphasizing the physician's role in determining cause of death, investigating outbreaks, and contributing to public health responses. It discusses the forensic examination techniques, including autopsy procedures and specimen analysis, crucial for identifying pathogens and understanding disease transmission patterns. The chapter also deals with the legal aspects, highlighting how forensic findings inform legal proceedings and public health policies. With a focus on emerging infectious threats and historical case studies, it underscores the evolving challenges faced by forensic physicians in combating infectious diseases and protecting public health. This information is essential for medical professionals, legal experts, and policymakers seeking a deeper understanding of the intersection between forensic medicine and infectious disease management.

References

1. Bolyard, E. A., Tablan, O. C., Williams, W. W., Pearson, M. L., Shapiro, C. N., & Deitchman, S. D.; & the Hospital Infection Control Practices Advisory Committee. (1998). Guideline for infection control in health care personnel. *American Journal of Infection Control, 26*(3), 289–354. https://doi.org/10.1016/S0196-6553(98)80015-1.
2. Centers for Disease Control (CDC). (1988). Universal precautions for prevention of transmission of human immuno-deficiency virus, hepatitis B virus and other bloodborne pathogens in health-care settings. *MMWR Morbidity and Mortality Weekly Report, 37*(24), 377–388.
3. Centers for Disease Control and Prevention. (1981). Community-acquired methicillin-resistant *Staphylococcus aureus* infections–Michigan. *MMWR Morbidity and Mortality Weekly Report, 30*(13), 185–187.
4. Desmond, R. A., Weiss, H. L., Arani, R. B., et al. (2002). Clinical applications for change-point analysis of herpes zoster pain. *Journal of Pain and Symptom Management, 23*(6), 510–516. https://doi.org/10.1016/S0885-3924(02)00393-7.
5. Gilden, D. H., Vafai, A., Shtram, Y., et al. (1983). Varicella-zoster virus DNA in human sensory ganglia. *Nature, 306*(5939), 478–480. https://doi.org/10.1038/306478a0.
6. Gnann, J. W., Jr, & Whitley, R. J. (2002). Herpes zoster. *New England Journal of Medicine, 347*(5), 340–346. https://doi.org/10.1056/NEJMcp013211.
7. Haustein, U. F., & Hlawa, B. (1989). Treatment of scabies with permethrin versus lindane and benzoyl benzoate. *Acta Dermato-Venereologica, 69*(4), 348–351. https://doi.org/10.2340/00015555-0056.
8. Klutymans, J., Van Belkum, A., & Verbrugh, H. (1989). Nasal carriage of *Staphylococcus aureus*: Epidemiology and control measures. *Infectious Disease Clinics of North America, 3*(4), 901–913. https://doi.org/10.1016/S0891-5520(18)30219-3.
9. Limb, S., Kawar, M., & Forster, G. E. (2002). HIV post-exposure prophylaxis after sexual assault: The experience of a sexual assault service in London. *International Journal of STD & AIDS, 13*(9), 602–605. https://doi.org/10.1258/09564620260216290.
10. Lowry, F. D. (1998). *Staphylococcus aureus* infections. *New England Journal of Medicine, 339*(8), 520–532. https://doi.org/10.1056/NEJM199808203390806.

11. Martinson, F. E., Weigle, K. A., Royce, R. A., Weber, D. J., Suchindran, C. M., & Lemon, S. M. (1998). Risk factors for horizontal transmission of hepatitis B in a rural district in Ghana. *American Journal of Epidemiology*, *147*(5), 478–487. https://doi.org/10.1093/oxfordjournals.aje.a009456.

12. National Occupational Health and Safety Committee. (1994). *National Model Regulations for The Control of Workplace Hazardous Substances*. Commonwealth of Australia [NOHSC:1005].

13. Stark, M. M. (2011). *Clinical Forensic Medicine*. Springer Science & Business Media. http://books.google.ie/books?id=bAAhI7jUZ1IC&pg=PA336&dq=Nicholson,+F.+(2009).+Infectious+diseases+and+an+at-risk+exposure+(Chapter+4).&hl=&cd=1&source=gbs_api.

14. Report from the Unlinked Anonymous Surveys Steering Group. (2001). *Prevalence of HIV and hepatitis infections in the United Kingdom 2000*. Annual report of the Unlinked Anonymous Prevalence Monitoring Programme. Department of Health, London, UK.

INDEX

Printed and bound by CPI Group (UK) Ltd, Croydon, CR0 4YY
18/09/2026
14965061-0001